MANAGING LOW BACK PAIN

Second Edition

MANAGING LOW BACK PAIN

Second Edition

EDITED BY

William H. Kirkaldy-Willis
M.A., M.D., F.R.C.S.(Edin)(C), F.A.C.S.

Emeritus Professor
Department of Orthopaedic Surgery
University Hospital
University of Saskatchewan
College of Medicine
Saskatoon, Saskatchewan, Canada

CHURCHILL LIVINGSTONE
New York, Edinburgh, London, Melbourne   1988

Library of Congress Cataloging-in-Publication Data

Managing low back pain/edited by William H. Kirkaldy-Willis.—2nd ed.
    p.   cm.
    Includes bibliographies and index.
    ISBN 0–443–08535–8
    1. Backache.   2. Backache—Prevention.   I. Kirkaldy-Willis, W. H.
    [DNLM: 1. Backache—diagnosis.   2. Backache—therapy.   WE 755 M2665]
RD768.M37   1988
617′.56—dc 19
DNLM/DLC
for Library of Congress   87–29967
                                                                            C.I.P.

Second Edition © Churchill Livingstone Inc. 1988
First Edition © Churchill Livingstone Inc. 1983

Distributed in the United Kingdom by Churchill Livingstone,
Robert Stevenson House, 1–3 Baxter's Place, Leith Walk, Edinburgh
EH1 3AF, and by associated companies, branches, and representatives
throughout the world.

Accurate indications, adverse reactions, and dosage schedules for
drugs are provided in this book, but it is possible that they
may change. The reader is urged to review the package information
data of the manufacturers of the medications mentioned.

Acquisitions Editor: *Toni M. Tracy*
Copy Editor: *Ann Ruzycka*
Production Designer: *Gloria Brown*
Production Supervisor: *Sharon Tuder*

Printed in the United States of America

First published in 1988

CONTRIBUTORS

Thomas N. Bernard, Jr., M.D.
Orthopaedic Surgeon, Hughston Orthopaedic Clinic, Columbus, Georgia

Charles V. Burton, M.D., F.A.C.S.
Medical Director, Institute for Low Back Care, Minneapolis, Minnesota

A. J. Roy Cameron, Ph.D.
Associate Professor and Chairman, Department of Health Studies, University of Waterloo, Waterloo, Ontario, Canada

J. David Cassidy, D.C., M.Sc., F.C.C.S.(C)
Research Associate, Department of Orthopaedic Surgery, University Hospital, University of Saskatchewan College of Medicine, Saskatoon, Saskatchewan, Canada

Pierre R. Dupuis, M.D., F.R.C.S.(C)
Associate Professor, Department of Orthopaedic Surgery, and Consultant, Pain Management Service, University Hospital, University of Saskatchewan College of Medicine, Saskatoon, Saskatchewan, Canada

Harry F. Farfan, M.Sc., M.D., C.M., F.R.C.S.(C)
Orthopaedic Department, St. Mary's Hospital, Montreal, Quebec, Canada

Kenneth B. Heithoff, M.D.
Medical Director, Center for Diagnostic Imaging; Staff Radiologist, Abbott-Northwestern Hospital, Minneapolis, Minnesota

Elizabeth S. H. Kirkaldy-Willis
The Back School, Department of Rehabilitation Medicine, University of Saskatchewan College of Medicine, Saskatoon, Saskatchewan, Canada

William H. Kirkaldy-Willis, M.A., M.D., F.R.C.S.(Edin)(C), F.A.C.S.
Emeritus Professor, Department of Orthopaedic Surgery, University Hospital, University of Saskatchewan College of Medicine, Saskatoon, Saskatchewan, Canada

Holly Mayer, R.N., M.P.H.
Director, Productive Rehabilitation Institute of Dallas for Ergonomics, Dallas, Texas

Tom G. Mayer, M.D., F.A.C.S.
Associate Clinical Professor, Department of Orthopaedic Surgery, University of Texas Health Science Center, Dallas, Texas

Arlis McQuarrie, B.P.T., M.C.P.A.
Assistant Clinical Professor, School of Physical Therapy, University of Saskatchewan College of Medicine; Senior Physiotherapist, Outpatient Physical Therapy, University Hospital, Saskatoon, Saskatchewan, Canada

Larry F. Shepel, Ph.D.
Head, Department of Psychology, University Hospital, University of Saskatchewan College of Medicine, Saskatoon, Saskatchewan, Canada

Stanley Tchang, M.D., F.R.C.P.(C)
Professor, Department of Medical Imaging, University Hospital, University of Saskatchewan College of Medicine, Saskatoon, Saskatchewan, Canada

Eldon Tunks, M.D., F.R.C.P.(C)
Professor, Department of Psychiatry, McMaster University School of Medicine; Director of Pain

Clinics, Chedoke-McMaster Hospitals, Hamilton, Ontario, Canada

John H. Wedge, M.D., F.R.C.S.(C)
Professor and Head, Department of Surgery, University Hospital, University of Saskatchewan College of Medicine, Saskatoon, Saskatchewan, Canada

James N. Weinstein, D.O.
Associate Professor, Department of Orthopaedics, University of Iowa Hospitals, Iowa City, Iowa

Gordon M. Wyant, C.D., M.D., F.F.A.R.C.S., F.R.C.P.(C)
Emeritus Professor, Department of Anaesthesia, University of Saskatchewan College of Medicine; Director, Pain Management Service, University Hospital, Saskatoon, Saskatchewan, Canada

Ken Yong-Hing, M.B., Ch.B., F.R.C.S. (Glasgow)(C)
Associate Professor and Head, Department of Orthopaedic Surgery, University Hospital, University of Saskatchewan College of Medicine, Saskatoon, Saskatchewan, Canada

FOREWORD

Few physicians in the world have spent more time thinking about the management of low back pain than the editor of this book. This second edition of *Managing Low Back Pain* is not simply a "rehash" of knowledge that can be found elsewhere in the literature. It presents ideas and concepts that are of great importance to the physician or therapist, as he or she considers how to improve the prevention and treatment of low back pain.

Dr. Kirkaldy-Willis has done much to stimulate our thinking. He often presents his answers to problems in such an extremely clear fashion that we are able to verify and expand on these answers to deal with problems with which we are confronted. He has compiled a book which, although initially intended for orthopaedic surgeons, has a message equally cogent for many other health care professionals involved in the management of patients with low back pain and sciatica.

By far the greater part of this work is devoted to the nonsurgical aspects of the management of low back pain. We are not aware of any similar work that deals so thoroughly with the fundamentals of degenerative spine pathology and the pathogenesis of low back pain. New chapters in the second edition discuss anatomy, epidemiology, magnetic resonance imaging, diagnosis, physical therapy, functional rehabilitation, and the pain clinic.

The first section deals with essential principles. These help us to understand the nature of the process that leads to one lesion or another. The second section sets out the knowledge necessary to make a full, accurate, and concise diagnosis for the majority of patients. The third is concerned with treatment, the major emphasis being on nonoperative treatment. This is a reasonable emphasis because we believe there is a real need for more instruction in conservative care, and there has been no paucity of publications devoted to surgery of the lumbar spine.

This book deserves careful study by all concerned with the prevention and treatment of low back pain. It is most appropriate that such a book should become available at the present time to aid a new generation of health care workers. These therapists are well aware of the need for better care for patients suffering from degenerative lesions of the lumbar spine. This book fulfills their need admirably.

L. L. Wiltse, M.D., Long Beach, California
A. H. White, M.D., San Francisco, California

PREFACE TO
THE SECOND EDITION

Since the appearance of the first edition of *Managing Low Back Pain* new knowledge has been acquired, new techniques of diagnosis and treatment have been developed, and a new attitude toward the prevention and management of low back pain has seen the light of day.

Albert Einstein once said, "Imagination is more important than knowledge." With this in mind we have tried to present a solid foundation of fact and theory on which the reader can build. However, there should be room in the physician's armamentarium for any type of knowledge and skill that will prove of value to the patient. We should be prepared to acknowledge new ideas from what H. R. H. The Prince of Wales calls "Complementary Medicine."

The Editor believes that the physician of the future has much to learn by standing with feet firmly planted on the rock of orthodoxy in the low-back country, and reaching out to explore ideas that come from the borderland which separates orthodoxy from complementary practice. The interaction that occurs at this point produces the action.

William H. Kirkaldy-Willis

PREFACE TO THE FIRST EDITION

Though written mainly by orthopaedic surgeons, this book was created to help all those involved in the treatment of patients suffering from low back and leg pain. We believe it will also be of help to postgraduate and undergraduate students.

Richard Foster wrote, "Books are best written in Community." For the thoughts that led to the writing of this book the writer is indebted to a number of different communities: to an outstanding teacher and to students in a biology class at high school in England; to surgeons in London and Edinburgh who were stimulating teachers; and to the staff and patients of a mission hospital in a primitive part of East Africa and of the central hospital in Nairobi: the problems presented by bone and joint tuberculosis and by poliomyelitis were new to the writer and no previous surgeon had tackled them. During the past 18 years he has been working in an entirely different environment in North America. The variety and diversity of these situations has again and again compelled the writer to think hard about each series of problems, often with reluctance, starting from essential principles.

The subject addressed is the degenerative lesion of the lumbar spine produced by repeated minor trauma, as this is the most common. Some space is devoted to the role of developmental lesions. Other lesions, congenital, inflammatory, neoplastic, rheumatoid, and metabolic, are mentioned only for purposes of exclusion. These have been dealt with elsewhere in a thoroughly adequate way.

Throughout this book, more attention has been given to the importance of making an accurate assessment of the patient's problem and, on this foundation, to the formulation of a logical regimen of treatment than to any other aspect of the problem. In the writer's opinion, a logical rather than an empirical approach is most important.

The natural history of spinal degeneration is considered first. Understanding this makes it possible for the physician and therapist to estimate the prognosis in each case and therefore to help the patient grasp the nature of his or her problem and the extent to which treatment may be expected to be of help. For the patient it is important to understand the limitations as well as the benefits of treatment.

Considerable space has been allocated to a consideration of biomechanics, pathology, and pathogenesis. Study of these subjects has helped us to comprehend the nature of the problem and we believe that the physician and therapist need the same fundamental knowledge.

Turning our attention to the clinical picture and to diagnosis, emphasis is placed on the fact that there are at least three aspects to be considered: the framework in which the lesion is found—the personality of the patient; the actual syndrome or lesion present in each patient; and the presence or absence of abnormal movement of the affected segment.

Any decision as to the most rational and suitable form of treatment for each individual is based on the three aspects of the problem mentioned immediately above and the stage, (a) dysfunction phase (decreased movement), (b) unstable phase (increased abnormal movement, or (c) stability phase (stabilization), to which the lesion has progressed.

Details of types of treatment, such as the Spine Education Program, physiotherapy, occupational therapy, manipulation, mobilization, immobilization, and the description of operative techniques, are considered in the third section of the book.

A wise man, Ecclesiastes, writing more than 2,500 years ago, said, "Much learning is a weariness of the flesh." Certainly a great deal has already been written about the problem of low back pain. May it be of some comfort to the present reader to know that while knowledge is undoubtedly required, even more important is the ability to discern the needs of the individual patient and how these can be met most effectively.

William H. Kirkaldy-Willis

ACKNOWLEDGMENTS

It is impossible to acknowledge all the help I have received over many years that has led to the writing of this book. I would, however, like to record my thanks to the following: the staff, fellows, and residents of the Departments of Orthopaedic Surgery, Pathology, and Human Diagnostic Imaging at the University Hospital in Saskatoon; the contributing authors; Mrs. Shirley Stacey and Mr. David Geary, for the illustrations; Mr. John Junor, Mr. David Mandeville, and Mr. R. Van den Buecken, for the photography; Dr. C. V. Burton, Camp International, and Datanet, for the conversion technology computer that greatly facilitated the preparation of the manuscript for the second edition; and my wife, for so much help and encouragement.

William H. Kirkaldy-Willis

CONTENTS

ESSENTIAL PRINCIPLES

1

The Epidemiology and Natural History of Low Back Pain and Spinal Degeneration

J. David Cassidy
John H. Wedge

The ubiquitous nature of pain originating in the lower back is accepted by those involved in treating this complaint regardless of their individual disciplines. Beyond this statement, however, there is little agreement on the nature of the problem. The lack of diagnostic precision, the variation in the perspective of those studying the problem, the poor correlation of symptoms, radiological findings, and pathological changes, and the application of uniform treatment programs to a heterogeneous group of disorders all lead to confusion.

An attempt to understand and correlate the epidemiology, natural history, pathology, and biomechanics of the spine with the clinical presentation is essential if we are to develop rational and effective treatment programs. This chapter will attempt to tie together the available information on the epidemiology and natural history of low back pain with the spectrum of pathological changes seen in the vertebral motion segment.

EPIDEMIOLOGY

Epidemiology is the science concerned with the study of the frequency and distribution of disease in different populations and the various factors that influence these variables. Low back pain has recently become a popular topic for epidemiological investigations. This is the result of several factors including the enormous cost of treatment and disability for this condition. Although the condition is usually the result of a benign process and is self-limiting in the majority of cases, the sheer numbers of those affected are of major concern. Moreover, a small but significant number of those affected develop chronic pain resulting in long-term disability and enormous expense. For these reasons, the factors influencing the occurrence of low back pain are of such importance.

Low back pain is a symptom and not a proper diagnosis. In some cases this symptom can be matched to a pathological diagnosis with a high degree of

Table 1-1 The Taxonomy of Low Back Pain

Symptom Duration	Pathological	Clinical Syndromes
Transient	Disc prolapse	Facet joint
Acute	Osteoporosis	Sacroiliac joint
Recurrent	Spondylitis	Myofascial
Chronic	etc.	etc.

certainty (Table 1-1). In most cases, however, the diagnosis is not certain, and the condition is characterized by the length of the process. Thus, transient low back pain is universal and of little concern. Acute low back pain is more severe and may require treatment, even though most cases recover uneventfully. Recurrent low back pain is of greater concern since it often influences lifestyle and may require a change in occupation. Once low back pain has persisted longer than 6 months, it can be considered a chronic problem. In the clinical setting, however, it is more useful to group these patients into syndrome categories based on current theories of pathogenesis and treatment.

Most of the epidemiological studies available on low back pain are based on symptom duration. Acute and chronic low back pain most probably span a group of heterogeneous disorders with varying etiologies. This fact places some limitation on the conclusions generated from these studies. Other confounding factors include geographical location and target population. In some countries, social factors have a direct affect on the length of disability for low back injuries in industry. The results of studies done on industrial or other selected samples cannot always be extrapolated to the general population. Despite these limitations epidemiological studies have contributed significantly to our knowledge on low back pain. This is particularly true for understanding the natural history of this disorder.

Low Back Pain in Society

Low back pain is common in industrialized nations. In fact, it is so common that only a minority of us will live without suffering from it at some time during our lifetime. It is now generally accepted that between 60% and 80% of the general population will suffer from low back pain someday, and that between 20% and 30% are suffering from it at any given time. These figures are the results of studies undertaken on selected and random samples of different populations in different countries.

The first major studies came from Sweden. In two separate reports published in 1954, Hult[1,2] looked at lifetime incidence and incapacity due to low back pain in males. In the Munkfors investigation,[1] he studied 114 forest workers and 163 industrial workers between the ages of 35 and 39 years. Eighty percent reported a history of lower back disturbances. Of the 55% that reported an incapacity to work because of low back pain, 38% were disabled less than 3 weeks and 17% for more than 3 weeks. The other study included 1,193 men between the ages of 25 and 59 years employed in heavy or light labor. Fifty-three percent of the workers in light industry and 64% of the workers in heavy industry had experienced low back pain. Eleven percent had been incapacitated with low back pain for periods ranging from 3 weeks to 6 months, and 4% had been incapacitated for more than 6 months.

In 1969, Horal[3] reported on a randomly selected group of subjects sicklisted with low back pain in the city of Gothenburg, Sweden and compared them to a control group of subjects that had not been sicklisted for back pain. The two groups consisted of 212 age- and sex-matched pairs for a total of 424 subjects studied with a mean age of 48 years. Overall, low back pain commonly began in the mid thirties, increased until the late fifties, and rapidly declined thereafter. There were no great differences between the sexes. Sixty-seven percent of the control group had a history of low back pain even though they had not been sicklisted for it.

In the same year and city, Hirsch et al.[4] reported their findings on a random sample of 692 Swedish females between the ages of 15 and 71 years. Forty-nine percent of the women gave a positive history for low back pain regardless of age. The lowest incidence was seen in the youngest group aged 15 to 24 years at 18% and the highest incidence in the group aged 45 to 54 at 70%. In the younger years, the pain was usually mild, but after age 35 the back pain was more severe and sciatica became more frequent.

The first report from the United States came from a random sample of the population of Columbus, Ohio in 1973. Nagi et al.[5] interviewed 1,135 men and women between the ages of 18 and 64 years.

Eighteen percent (21% of women and 14% of men) reported that they were "often bothered with back pain." Of that 18%, 62% had undergone x-ray examination, 26% had worn a back support, and 4% had undergone operative treatment. Back pain was most common in subjects over the age of 35, and it remained high until the late fifties. Persons with back complaints reported greater use of health services than other persons with other limiting pathologies and impairments.

In another U.S. study, Frymoyer et al.[6] surveyed 1,221 men between the ages of 18 and 55 years who had been seen in a family practice facility between 1975 and 1978. Seventy percent of the respondents gave a history of low back pain, and in 24% the pain was of considerable severity.

More recently Svensson and Andersson[7] reported on the frequency of low back pain in a random sample of 940, 40- to 47-year-old men in Goteborg, Sweden. Seventy-six percent (716) of the men were personally interviewed, and information about the remaining participants was obtained from the National Insurance Office. According to the information from the interviews, the lifetime incidence of low back pain was 61%. However, this figure was changed to 72% after consulting the insurance records and finding that some of the subjects had forgotten that they had been sicklisted for low back pain in the past. This means that the incidence of low back pain based on the interview had been an underestimation. The prevalence of low back pain in this study was 31% and 10% had a history of sciatica. Low back disability prevented work in close to 4%.

The largest cross-sectional survey on low back pain was reported by Valkenburg and Haanen[8] in 1982. They studied 3,091 men and 3,493 women from a rural and urban district in the Netherlands. The life-time incidence and point prevalence of low back pain was 51% and 22%, respectively, for men and 57% and 30%, respectively, for women. For both men and women, the frequency of low back pain increased up to about the age of 60 years and then decreased thereafter (Table 1-2).

Biering-Sorensen[9] studied all of the inhabitants aged 30, 40, 50, and 60 years of age in a Copenhagen suburb in Denmark. Eighty-two percent (449 men and 479 women) of the population participated in the survey, which included an interview and examination. One year later, a follow-up questionnaire was completed by 99% of the subjects. The lifetime prevalence rates for low back pain ranged from 68% to 70% for men and from 62 to 81% for women (Table 1-3). The incidence of first attacks of low back pain over the follow-up year was highest in the 30-year-olds at 11% and decreased in the older age groups. In women there was an overall increase in low back pain late in life, which may have been related to the onset of postmenopausal osteoporosis.

Individual Risk Factors

Individual risk factors for the development of low back pain have been identified in epidemiological studies (Table 1-4). Age has been shown to be a factor. Low back pain tends to begin in the third decade of life and reach its maximal frequency during the middle ages.[8–10] It tends to be less frequent in the elderly. There is no particular predilection for sex, although operations for disc herniations are performed twice as often in men as in women.[11] This finding probably reflects the need for men to return to work quickly. One study has shown that for the same degree of symptoms, men are more likely to undergo surgery than women.[12]

Table 1-2 Age and Sex-Specific Prevalence Rates of Low Back Pain (LBP)

6584 Subjects	Percentages in Each Age Group							Total Percentage
	20	25	35	45	55	65	75	
3091 Men								
LBP ever	52	51	54	53	54	42	33	51
LBP now	20	21	24	23	27	17	15	22
3493 Women								
LBP ever	46	56	61	65	60	53	46	58
LBP now	24	26	31	33	34	33	28	30

(Data from ref. 8.)

Table 1-3 Occurrence of Low Back Pain in 449 Men and 479 Women 30, 40, 50, and 60 Years Old

Low Back Pain	Percentages in Each Age Group (Men:Women)			
	30 Years	40 Years	50 Years	60 Years
Lifetime prevalence	68:62	69:61	70:68	68:81
One year incidence	11:11	0:6	6:3	6:4
One year prevalence	43:42	48:39	45:46	43:54

(Data from ref. 9.)

Table 1-4 Individual Risk Factors Associated with the Development of Low Back Pain

Positive Association	Questionable Association	No Association
Increasing age	Tallness	Sex
Marked scoliosis	Obesity	Body build
Poor health	Trunk strength	Increased lordosis
Lack of fitness	Intelligence	Most scolioses
Smoking	Economics	Leg lengths
Psychosocial problems		Psychiatric illness
Drug abuse		
Headaches		
Neck pain		
Angina pectoris		
Leg discomfort		
Stomach pains		

Individual height, weight, and body build do not seem to be strongly correlated to the occurrence of low back pain.[2,3,9,13] This is also true for minor postural deviations and leg length differences.[1,2,13,14] Although many clinicians believe that an increase in the lumbar lordosis is an important factor in low back problems, several studies have failed to show any correlation between the degree of lordosis and the occurrence of low back pain.[13,15] With the exception of curves of 80° or more, scoliosis has not proven to be associated with more low back pain than normal.[16,17] Tallness and marked obesity have been found in some studies to carry a risk for the development of low back pain and sciatica.[18,19] Other studies have failed to show such a relationship.[1,2,4]

There are conflicting reports on the association between trunk muscle strength and low back pain. Reduced strength in the abdominal and paravertebral extensor muscles has been found in populations of back pain patients in some studies, but not in others.[13,20–23] This issue is further complicated by

the possibility that individuals with low back pain are less motivated during strength testing because of pain or fear of pain.[23] If there is weakness of the postural muscles, it is not known if it is primary or secondary to the low back pain. There is good evidence, however, that overall physical fitness and conditioning have a significant preventive effect on the occurrence of back injuries.[24]

Some reports suggest that low back pain patients use health care services more than persons with other disabilities.[5] Stress, anxiety, tension, fatigue, and depression have been found to be associated with low back pain.[6,25] Other studies suggest that the population likely to experience future low back pain does not enjoy good general health, even prior to the first episode of low back trouble.[26] Lower limb discomfort, frequent headaches, stomach pains, and angina pectoris are more common in back pain patients.[25,26] There is an increased number of sickness absence days in back pain patients.[7]

Psychological problems are more frequently associated with low back pain. Depression, anxiety, hypochondriasis, and hysteria have been identified as factors related to unfavorable outcomes for both chemonucleolysis and operative treatment of lumbar disc disease.[27,28] A high proportion of chronic back pain sufferers abuse alcohol and drugs.[29] Their general social situation is poor with divorce and family problems more frequent than usual.[30] They tend to have a poorer intellectual capacity, a lower level of education, less income, and more difficulty establishing emotional contacts than the general population.[31] It is not certain whether or not these changes are primary or secondary to the chronic back pain experience itself.

Daily smoking of cigarettes has been identified as a risk factor for both the development of low back pain and prolapsed intervertebral discs in the lumbar spine.[6,25,26,32] Various possible mechanisms might account for this. Smoking produces a chronic cough and this, in turn, gives rise to higher intra-abdominal and intradiscal pressures putting increased mechanical stress on the lumbar discs.[6,33] Repeated coughing, therefore, might be a causative factor in disc ruptures. There is also a positive correlation between cigarette smoking and diminished mineral content of bone.[34] This, in turn, might lead to microfractures of the trabeculae in the lumbar vertebral bodies causing low back pain similar to that experienced by patients with vertebral osteoporosis. Finally, smoking causes a reduction in the vertebral body blood flow that can adversely affect the nutrition of the intervertebral discs.[35] This might promote early degenerative disease in the discs and increase the risk for low back pain.

Low Back Pain in Industry

Since the lifetime incidence of low back pain in society is so high, it is not surprising that industrial studies show that more than half of the working population will be affected by low back pain at some time during their working career.[1-3] Moreover, the problem is most prevalent between the ages of 35 and 55 years, just at the time when the worker is most productive.[31] The annual rate of low back pain for all industrial workers in the United States has been estimated at 2%.[36] Furthermore, back and spine impairments were the chronic conditions most frequently cited in the United States in 1969 to 1970

as the cause for limitation of activities in persons under 45 years of age.[37] In Great Britain, 3.6% of all sickness absence days were due to back pain in 1969 to 1970, and the average absence period for men was 33 days.[38] Swedish health statistics show that about 1% of all work days each year are lost because of back pain, and that back problems account for an average of 12.5% of all sickness absence days with an average absence period of 36 days.[31] No other disease accounted for a greater number of days away from the work place.

Material handling holds the greatest risk for low back injury and lifting is implicated as the main cause in over half the injuries.[2,7,10,35,36] In a 10-year prospective study of employees at the Eastman Kodak Company in Rochester, Rowe[39] found that 35% of the sedentary workers and 45% of the heavy handlers were seen in the medical department for low back pain. Furthermore, more than 4 hours per worker per year were lost because of low back pain, and it was second only to upper respiratory infection in terms of time loss because of illness. Other industrial activities associated with the onset of low back pain have been studied by Snook (Table 1-5).[36]

Other industrial risk factors for the development of low back pain include exposure to prolonged static work postures and vibration.[31] Prolonged sitting and driving of motor vehicles has been particularly implicated in this respect. Several studies have shown that truck drivers have a high incidence of low back pain.[6,35,36] In a Connecticut study, it was estimated that men who are truck drivers are almost five times more likely to develop a lumbar disc herniation than men who are not truck drivers.[40] Amplification of the imparted motion or resonance occurs within the dominant frequency range of many vehicles and in-

Table 1-5 Activities Associated with Industrial Low Back Injuries

Activity	Percentage of Injuries
Lifting	37–49%
Bending	12–14%
Twisting	9–18%
Pulling	9–16%
Falling/slipping	7–13%
Pushing	6–9%
Carrying	5–8%
Lowering	4–7%

(Data from ref. 36.)

dustrial devices (around 5 Hz). As a result, there is a high energy transfer to the spine with increased risk for mechanical damage to the resonating structures. The use of jackhammers has also been cited as a risk factor in low back pain.[35] Prolonged and frequent bending, frequent twisting, monotonous or repetitive work, physically heavy work, and diminished work satisfaction have all been found to be correlated to the occurrence of low back pain.[31,41]

Several studies have confirmed that the cost for the treatment and compensation of industrial low back pain is in excess of that spent on all other industrial injuries combined.[42–44] In 1976, it was estimated that approximately $14 billion was spent in the United States on treatment and compensation for low back pain.[43] By 1983, this figure had risen to $20 billion.[45] Moreover, the vast majority of this cost is absorbed by a relatively small number of claimants who receive permanent total or partial disability payments. In a recent study of back injury claims at the Boeing Company in Washington, 10% of the 900 back injury claims over a 15-month period accounted for 79% of the total back injury costs.[44] Claims related to back injuries constituted 19% of the total injury claims but were responsible for 41% of the total injury costs. In one study, medical costs accounted for only 33% of the total workers' compensation costs, with the rest going towards disability payments (Table 1-6).[42]

Prolonged absenteeism has a profound and adverse effect on the low back injured worker. Records from Washington indicate that workers with back complaints who are absent from work more than 6 months have only a 50% chance of returning to productive employment.[46] If they are absent over 1 year this possibility drops to 25%, and if more than 2 years

it is almost nil. Low back pain patients who have been absent from work for more than 3 months suffer from increased emotional disturbances when compared to those disabled for extremity injuries.[47] In fact, psychological testing is more accurate in predicting return to work than the physician's prognosis. Quite often, the degree of pain reported is out of proportion and inconsistent with the objective evidence of disability, and the discrepancy usually represents an unconscious psychogenic elaboration of symptoms. Moreover, these symptoms will not respond to treatment directed toward the lower back unless appropriate psychological measures are included.

NATURAL HISTORY

Low Back Pain

In most cases low back pain is self-limiting. Ninety percent of patients with acute low back pain improve after 2 months.[10] This percentage declines to 2% to 3% after 6 months, and to 1% after 1 year.[48] Those patients that recover face a 60% recurrence rate over the following 2 years.[10,48] Recurrences are less common during the third year, and accident-related attacks take longer to subside regardless of when they occur. For those patients that recover quickly, it seems likely that the injury involves a minor strain to the posterior facet joints, surrounding ligaments, and muscles. Patients exhibiting pain for longer periods of time have probably sustained more tissue damage and may have injured the disc.[48] However, after 3 to 6 months, psychosocial factors will tend to modulate the pain process and play an increasingly important role in the recovery process.

Spinal Degeneration

An understanding of the biomechanics (Ch. 2) and of the pathology (Ch. 4) is essential to the process of following the natural history through the stages of spinal degeneration. The spectrum of degenerative change is an intervertebral joint is divided into three phases: Phase I—Dysfunction—is the earliest. Minor pathology results in abnormal function of the posterior joints and disk. Phase II—Instability (the unstable phase)—is intermediate. Progressive degeneration

Table 1-6 Percentage Medical and Compensation Costs for Low Back Pain: Approximately $20,000,000,000 U.S. / Year[a]

33% Medical Costs	22% Temporary Disability	45% Permanent Disability
33% Hospitalization		
33% Physicians' fees		
12% Diagnostic tests		
9% Physical therapy		
7% Drugs		
5% Appliances		

[a] 10% of cases account for 80% of total cost (Data from refs. 36, 42, 43, 44, and 45.)

due to repeated trauma produces laxity of both the posterior joint capsule and the annulus. Phase III—Stabilization—is the final stage in the process. Fibrosis of the posterior joints and capsule, loss of disc material, and formation of osteophytes render the segment stable because movement is reduced. In Figure 1-1 the natural history is superimposed on the scheme of pathogenesis. The symptoms, clinical course, and treatment are correlated with the stages in the pathogenesis. This correlation makes it possible to predict the degree to which the natural history can be modified by different treatment methods.

PATHOLOGY

Radiological and postmortem studies suggest that the degenerative changes described in Chapter 4 are progressive and almost universal. The morbidity associated with these changes, however, is episodic and many people never experience symptoms at all. Figure 1-2 is a graphic illustration of the pathogenesis. While the degenerative changes are progressive, the rate of progression is not linear and those factors that alter the rate are poorly understood. Sex, body weight, body habitus, posture, and occupation all probably play a role.

SYMPTOMS

Attempts to correlate symptoms with degenerative changes have met with little success. The peak incidence of disabling symptoms occurs between the ages of 35 and 55. This does not parallel the progression of degeneration. The lack of correlation would suggest that the later stages in the degenerative process have a protective effect and are nature's mechanism for compensating for damage. This teleological explanation has led to the concept of the phases of degeneration, the central theme of this book.

In Figure 1-3 the symptoms of low back pain are plotted against age through the phases of spinal degeneration. The repair reaction can result in return to a symptom-free state in all three phases but is less likely to do so as one moves from one phase to another.

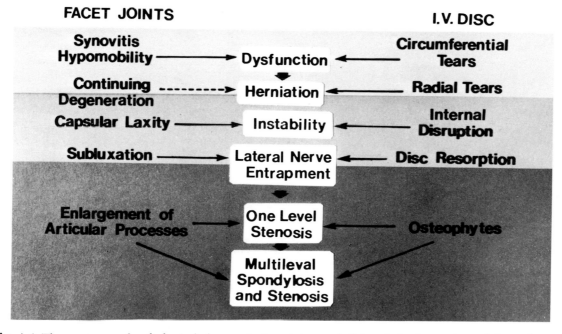

Fig. 1-1 The spectrum of pathological changes in facet joints and disk and the interaction of these changes. The upper light horizontal bar represents dysfunction, the middle darker bar instability, and the lower dark bar stabilization.

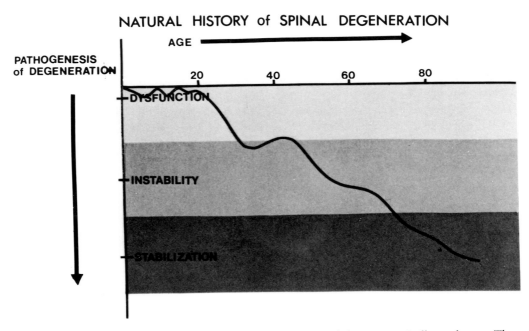

Fig. 1-2 The degenerative process throughout life can be represented diagrammatically as shown. The minor initial lesions may heal, but with time healing is no longer complete.

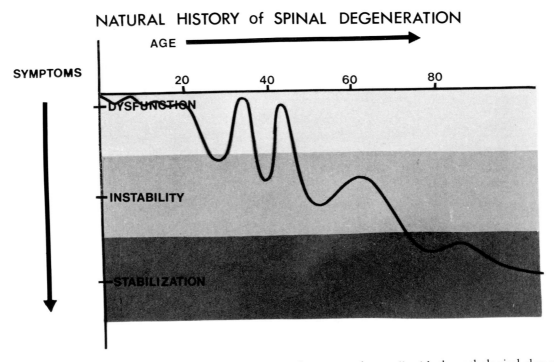

Fig. 1-3 Symptoms through the phases of pathogenesis do not correlate well with the pathological changes. Relief from pain can occur despite the presence of permanent damage. In the later phases, however, symptomatic recovery may not occur.

In the phase of dysfunction, return of the facet joint to the normal position or repair of a capsular tear prevents further damage. A fracture in the lamina may unite without deformity. Each of these examples may represent a single episode of symptoms in a lifetime in the fortunate individual. Injury may occur at more than one level, giving a possible explanation for why several or many acute attacks may not lead to chronicity.

However, if the damage exceeds the capacity of the repair reaction, the condition may pass on to the unstable phase. More severe damage to the three-joint complex can lead to a lengthier period of symptoms and eventually to chronic difficulty. Disk herniation, dynamic lateral entrapment, or other sequelae may occur. Thus, a return to a symptom-free state may not occur, but instead a background state of mild chronic symptoms may exist with superimposed acute attacks from time to time. The picture of the natural history may be complicated by the simultaneous or sequential occurrence of the same process at one or more levels in the lumbar spine.

In the final phase a proliferative repair response may result in stabilizing the segment. This may ex-

plain the decreased incidence of disabling symptoms later in life. However, symptoms may diminish simply because activity is reduced and aggravating factors are avoided.

It is unlikely that the damaged segment can be stabilized in all individuals. This could explain the small group of patients who have continuing severe difficulty late into old age. In addition, the proliferative repair response may lead to compromise of the neural elements, which results in spinal stenosis, the culmination of the degenerative process for an unfortunate few.

TREATMENT

In Figure 1-4 the various forms of treatment are superimposed on the three phases of spinal degeneration. The indications for different treatment will be dealt with in depth in later chapters. An understanding of which forms of treatment are more likely to meet with success throughout the natural history is obviously important if we are to develop a rational plan of management for the individual patient. In general,

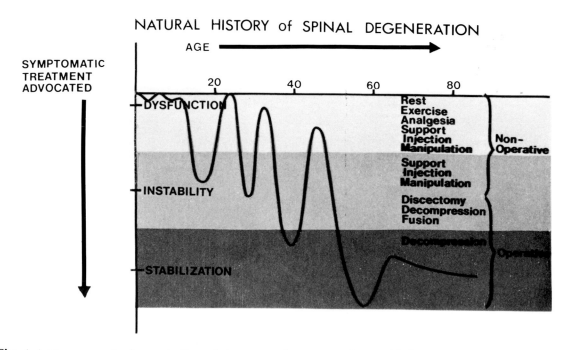

Fig. 1-4 Diagrammatic demonstration of the types of treatment that are likely to meet with success in the different stages of pathogenesis. The curve on the graph represents symptoms.

relatively simple nonsurgical management is likely to meet with success early in the natural history whereas operative procedures may be necessary later. The nature of the surgery obviously depends on the pathology encountered in the later two phases of spinal degeneration.

RESULTS OF TREATMENT

Unfortunately, in the past both nonoperative and operative treatment have been based on the training, discipline, and bias of the individual physician rather than on an understanding of the pathology and the natural history of the disease. Patients have too often been led to believe that a form of treatment is an "all or nothing" phenomenon and that therapeutic methods from different disciplines are mutually exclusive. Counseling the patient should include a realistic explanation of what he or she can expect from a particular form of treatment at that stage in the pathology of spinal degeneration. For example, removing an extruded disc may dramatically relieve suffering

but may not significantly alter the progression of pathological changes or the longterm clinical picture.

Figure 1-5 is a graph superimposed on the three phases. Treatment is more likely to result in a return to a symptom-free state and to have more longterm benefit in the earlier stages of the degenerative process. The expectations for a particular method of treatment are less optimistic as we move along the course of the natural history. Ideally, intervention should take place as soon as it becomes obvious that spontaneous recovery is unlikely or that it will be unacceptably prolonged. In the later stages the patient must understand that expectations are for significant general improvement or relief of a particular part of the problem rather than for a "cure."

CONCLUSION

An attempt has been made to correlate pathological changes, symptoms, diagnosis, and treatment throughout the whole spectrum of degenerative change in the lumbar spine that forms what we call

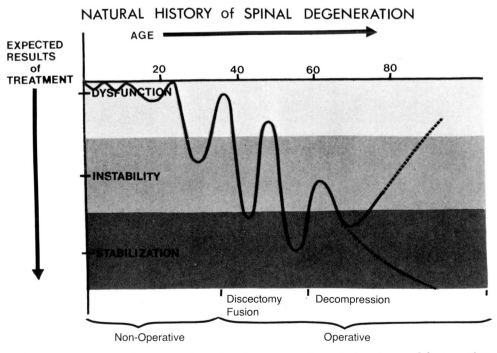

Fig. 1-5 The curve represents the expected results of treatment through the phases of degeneration. Initially nonsurgical measures are almost universally successful in relieving symptoms. In the late stages even surgery is unlikely to result in complete relief of symptoms.

the natural history of the disease. In doing this we find that often there is little correlation between the patient's disability and the degree of damage to the tissues. Factors such as the personality of the patient, secondary gain, and expectations for the future make the picture more complex.

Study of the natural history of this disease enables the physician to gain insight into the disease process, to make a more complete and accurate diagnosis, to formulate a more rational regime of treatment, and to inform the patient in simple terms what may be expected from conservative or operative treatment and even more important what the future holds.

In the final analysis, with cooperation between physician and patient it is possible occasionally to effect a cure, often to arrest the progress for a long time, and nearly always to alleviate the suffering of the patient.

REFERENCES

1. Hult L: The Munkfors investigation. Acta Orthop Scand (Suppl) 16, 1954
2. Hult L: Cervical, dorsal, and lumbar spinal syndromes. Acta Orthop Scand (Suppl) 17, 1954
3. Horal J: The clinical appearance of low back disorders in the city of Gothenberg, Sweden. Acta Orthop Scand (Suppl) 118, 1969
4. Hirsch C, Jonsson B, Lewin T: Low-back symptoms in a Swedish female population. Clin Orthop 63: 171, 1969
5. Nagi SZ, Riley LE, Newby LG: A social epidemiology of back pain in a general population. J Chronic Dis 26: 769, 1973
6. Frymoyer JW, Pope MH, Costanza MC, et al: Epidemiologic studies of low-back pain. Spine 5: 419, 1980
7. Svensson HO, Andersson GBJ: Low back pain in forty to forty-seven year old men. I. Frequency of occurrence and impact on medical services. Scand J Rehabil Med 14: 47, 1982
8. Valkenburg HA, Haanen HCM: The epidemiology of low back pain. In White AA, Gordon SL (eds): Idiopathic Low Back Pain. CV Mosby, St. Louis, 1982
9. Biering-Sorensen F: A prospective study of low back pain in a general population. I. Occurrence, recurrence and aetiology. Scand J Rehabil Med 15: 71, 1983
10. Bergquist-Ullman M, Larsson U: Acute low back pain in industry. Acta Orthop Scand (Suppl) 170, 1977
11. Sprangfort EV: The lumbar disc herniation, a computer-aided analysis of 2504 operations. Acta Orthop Scand (Suppl) 142, 1972
12. Kelsey JL, Ostfeld AM: Demographic characteristics of persons with acute herniated lumbar intervertebral disc. J Chronic Dis 28: 37, 1975
13. Pope MH, Bevins T, Wilder DG, et al: The relationship between anthropometric, postural, muscular, and mobility characteristics of males ages 18–55. Spine 10: 644, 1985
14. Dieck GS, Kelsey JL, Goel VK, et al: An epidemiologic study of the relationship between postural asymmetry in the teen years and subsequent back and neck pain. Spine 10: 872, 1985
15. Hansson T, Bigos S, Beecher P, et al: The lumbar lordosis in acute and chronic low-back pain. Spine 10: 154, 1985
16. Nachemson AL: Adult scoliosis and back pain. Spine 4: 513, 1979
17. Jackson RP, Simmons EH, Stripinis D: Incidence and severity of back pain in adult idiopathic scoliosis. Spine 8: 749, 1983
18. Kelsey JL: An epidemiological study of acute herniated lumbar intervertebral discs. Rheumatol Rehabil 14: 144, 1975
19. Ikata T: Statistical and dynamic studies of lesions due to overloading on the spine. Shikoku Acta Med 40: 262, 1965
20. Addison R, Schultz A: Trunk strengths in patients seeking hospitalization for chronic low back disorders. Spine 5: 539, 1980
21. McNeill T, Warwick D, Andersson G, et al: Trunk strengths in attempted flexion, extension, and lateral bending in healthy subjects and patients with low back disorders. Spine 5, 529, 1980
22. Nicolaisen T, Jorgensen K: Trunk strength, back muscle endurance and low-back trouble. Scand J Rehabil Med 17: 121, 1985
23. Pope MH, Rosen JC, Wilder DG, et al: The relation between biomechanical and psychological factors in patients with low back pain. Spine 5: 173, 1980
24. Cady LD, Bischoff DP, O'Connell ER, et al: Strength and fitness and subsequent back injuries in firefighters. J Occup Med 21: 269, 1979
25. Svensson H-O, Vedin A, Wilhelmsson C, et al: Low back pain in relation to other diseases and cardiovascular risk factors. Spine 8: 277, 1983
26. Biering-Sorensen F, Thomsen C: Medical, social and occupational history as risk indicators for low-back trouble in a general population. Spine 11: 720, 1986
27. Wifling FG, Klonoff H, Kokan P: Psychological, demographic and orthopaedic factors associated with prediction of outcome of spinal fusion. Clin Orthop 90: 153, 1973
28. Wiltse LL, Rocchio PD: Preparative psychological tests as predictors of success of chemonucleolysis in the treatment of the low back syndrome. J Bone Joint Surg 57A: 478, 1975

29. Raskink R, Glover MB: Profile of a low back derelict. J Occup Med 17: 258, 1975

30. Magora A: Investigation of the relation between low back pain and occupation. 5. Psychological aspects. Scand J Rehabil Med 5: 186, 1973

31. Andersson GBJ: Epidemiologic aspects on low-back pain in industry. Spine 6: 53, 1981

32. Kelsey JL, Githens PB, O'Conner T, et al: Acute prolapsed lumbar intervertebral disc. An epidemiologic study with special reference to driving automobiles and cigarette smoking. Spine 9: 608, 1984

33. Nachemson AL, Elfstrom G: Intravital dynamic pressure measurements in lumbar discs. Scand J Rehabil Med (Suppl) 1, 1970

34. Daniell HW: Osteoporosis of the slender smoker. Arch Intern Med 136: 298, 1976

35. Frymoyer JW, Pope MH, Clements FH, et al: Risk factors in low-back pain: an epidemiological survey. J Bone Joint Surg 65A: 213, 1983

36. Snook SH: Low back pain in industry. In White AA, Gordon SL (eds): Idiopathic Low Back Pain. CV Mosby, St. Louis, 1982

37. Kelsey JL: Epidemiology of Musculoskeletal Disorders. Oxford, New York, 1982

38. Benn RT, Wood PHN: Pain in the back: an attempt to estimate the size of the problem. Rheumatol Rehabil 14: 121, 1975

39. Rowe ML: Low back pain in industry: a position paper. J Occup Med 11: 161, 1969

40. Kelsey JL, Hardy RJ: Driving of motor vehicles as a risk factor for acute herniated lumbar intervertebral disc. Am J Epidemiol 102: 63, 1975

41. Svensson H-O, Andersson GBJ: Low-back pain in 40- to 47- year old men: work history and work environment factors. Spine 8: 272, 1983

42. Leavitt SS, Johnson TL, Beyer RD: The process of recovery: patterns in industrial back injury. 1. Costs and other quantitative measures of effort. Indust Med Surg 40: 7, 1971

43. Akeson WH, Murphy RW: Low back pain. Clin Orthop 129: 2, 1977

44. Spengler DM, Bigos SJ, Martin NA, et al: Back injuries in industry: a retrospective study. 1. Overview and cost analysis. Spine 11: 241, 1986

45. Genant HK: Preface. In Genant HK (ed): Spine Update 1984: Perspectives in Radiology, Orthopaedic Surgery, and Neurosurgery. Radiology Research and Education Foundation, San Francisco, 1983

46. McGill CM: Industrial back problems: a control program. J Occup Med 10: 174, 1968

47. Beals RK, Hickman NW: Industrial injuries of the back and extremities. J Bone Joint Surg 54A: 1593, 1972

48. Nachemson AL: The natural course of low back pain. In White AA, Gordon SL (eds): Idiopathic Low Back Pain. CV Mosby, St. Louis, 1982

2

Biomechanics of the Lumbar Spine

Harry F. Farfan

Some understanding of biomechanics, difficult as this is for many clinicians, enables us to define the etiology of the lesion in the lumbar spine. It is of special value in deciding if the cause of injury is compression, with fracture of a cartilage disc plate followed by a slow degenerative process in disc and posterior joints, or torsion, involving more rapid failure of posterior joints and disc.

To date there is no consensus on the normal mechanism of the spine. This lack creates a very real problem. How can we understand the abnormal when the normal is not known? In the absence of a method to measure internal stresses directly, a possible approach to understanding the normal mechanism is by mathematical simulation. The more closely the simulation approximates in vivo observations, the more confidence we have that the simulation is a true representation. In scientific endeavor the descriptive hypothesis remains just that until it can be formulated in terms that can be treated rigidly in mathematical terms and subject to a rigid experimental proof. In this presentation a mathematical formulation of the normal lumbar spinal mechanism is presented in descriptive terms.

In the body all motion is initiated through the agency of active muscle contraction, which in turn is controlled and coordinated by the central nervous system (CNS). While ligament and capsule may be called on to support a load, these tissues remain passive and unable to initiate a motion. Almost without exception, it is these passive elements that are injured. It therefore falls to the muscular system and its control mechanism to protect the organism from injury.

Mechanical structures fail because they are unable to support the stresses induced by the loads applied to them. Two systems are involved: the passive structural members that provide local support and the appropriate muscle groups that act to minimize the risk of failure.

Because the lumbar tissues are undoubtedly injured more often than those of the extremities in performing an upper extremity task, the spinal mechanism becomes a pertinent example of the interaction between muscle on the one hand and ligament, bone, and joint on the other.

THE SPINAL MECHANISM

Among special adaptations in humans are the modifications that permit them to maintain an upright posture—a capability shared with other anthropoids, notably the chimpanzee and the gibbon. Humans, however, are unique in their ability to lift and carry heavy objects and to perform, in bipedal stance, the

15

accelerated trunk movement necessary for throwing objects.

Hip Extensor Muscle

The main muscle power for maintaining the trunk upright resides in the hip and thighs. The muscles of the hips and lower extremities have been studied extensively in relation to bipedal motion, but surprisingly little attention has been paid to their function in supporting the trunk, upper extremities, and head.[1]

In humans, the relatively long anteverted femoral neck puts the gluteal attachments well behind the center of rotation of the hip, giving them extension power regardless of the degree of hip flexion. The extensive attachment of the gluteus maximus to the iliotibial band further increase the leverage of this muscle. By far the most significant modification is the greatly increased anterior-posterior (A-P) diameter of the pelvis, which permits the posterior migration of the glutei, increasing both their leverage and their bulk.

The effectiveness of the hip extensors is somewhat diminished when the hip is fully flexed, as in the squatting position. Thus, flexion at the knees to below the 90° position is not a good method of lifting.

We may estimate, using a conservative force density of muscle contraction (50 lb/in²), that the glutei and hamstrings together can generate a moment greater than 15,000 in-lb, which is enough for men in the 50th percentile by weight to manage their own weight above the pelvis (one-half body weight) plus an external load of three times body weight. This estimation is supported by results of weight-lifting championships, where the 150-lb athlete lifts 450 lb, developing a maximum external moment of the order of 10,000 in-lb. No other sport imposes such high moments on the spinal mechanism. In rowing for example, the maximum moment is only equivalent to a 200-lb lift.

If we examine the weight lift in greater detail, we see that maximum moment occurs early in the lift when the barbell clears the knees. The attitude of the trunk as measured by a line drawn through hip and shoulder is approximately 70° to the vertical. As the upright position is obtained, the moment decreases to zero. To raise the weight above the head does not require the balancing of large moments but

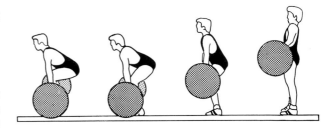

Fig. 2-1 Dead lift. The maximum moment occurs when the barbell clears the knees. Raising the weight above the head does not involve large moments.

rather an enormous coordination to maintain the moments near zero (Fig. 2–1).

Trunk Musculature

Surprisingly, the trunk musculature is much weaker than the hip extensor system. The spinal musculature has a cross-sectional area of approximately 10 in², firing at a density of 50 to 100 lb/in² at approximately 2–2.5 in. behind the center of the disc. It can generate a moment of only 2000 to 3000 in-lb, which is only 20% of that required for a 450-lb lift. Though the extensor muscle system in humans is proportionally more developed than that in other anthropoids, it is still grossly inadequate to handle the large moments that are required.

The paraspinal muscles, such as the sacrospinalis, run at a slight angle to the long axis and therefore in contracting generate a small component to shear in the plane of the disk. This component is too small to balance the shear of 525 lb induced by the combination of body weight and barbell.

The Ligamentous Systems

The missing moment is supplied by the ligamentous system, which may conveniently be considered as two separate but interdependent systems. The first consists of the midline ligaments, the supra- and interspinous ligaments, the facet joint capsules, the ligamentum flavum, and the posterior longitudinal ligament, and the second consists of the lumbodorsal fascia (LDF).

No tension is present in these ligaments unless they are stretched. Stretching occurs through forward rotation of the intervertebral joints. With the hands gripping the barbells, the hip extensors rotate the pelvis backward while the spine rotates forward. As previously pointed out, ample hip extensor power is present to rotate the pelvis and stretch the ligaments to the required tension.

It is essential that the hip be free to extend. Should hip extension be limited by arthritis or flexion contracture, the important posterior ligament tension is no longer available. In these instances, the individual must resort to using the spine extensors, with the reduced capacity to lift, thus further increasing the stress on the intervertebral joints. Hence the common problem of a back disorder complicating the diseased hip (Fig. 2–2).

The supraspinous-interspinous ligament system has an angulated attachment to the spinous process. Below the level of L3, the continuation of these ligaments is placed behind the spinous process of L4, L5, and first-to-third sacral segments. This arrangement also is unique to humans among the primates. It ensures that when these ligaments are stretched, they exert a component of shear force backward on each vertebra, more than sufficient to counteract the shear caused by body weight and barbell.

The Posterior Lamella of the Lumbodorsal Fascia

At the posterior midline the LDF blends with the midline longitudinal ligaments. Below the level of the posterior iliac spine, the lateral margin of the

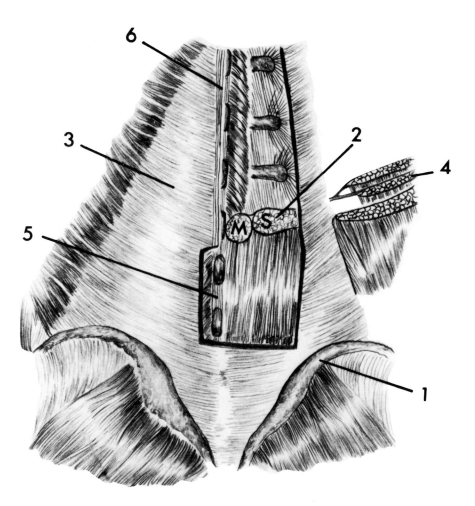

Fig. 2-2 The ligamentous system. 1. Iliac Crest. 2. Sacrospinalis and multifidus. 3. Lumbo-dorsal fascia. 4. Internal oblique and transversus abdominis attached to lumbo-dorsal fascia. 5. Interspinous ligament. 6. Supraspinous ligament.

sheet is firmly attached to the ilium. Above L2, it is attached to both the tips of the transverse processes and the ribs. However, between the levels of L2 and iliac crest, its lateral edge forms the posterior attachment of the internal oblique and transversus abdominis muscles.

With flexion, this ligamentous sheet is stretched and—precisely because it is stretched—should also become narrowed. However, bony restraints at the upper and lower ends prevent narrowing while contraction of internal oblique and transversus abdominis muscles contribute the restraint for the mid-portion.[3]

Preventing the lumbodorsal fascia from narrowing as it is stretched causes its longitudinal tension to increase. Thus with the powerful internal oblique muscle attached to its margin, the probability exists that tension can be generated in the lumbodorsal fascia by abdominal muscle contraction, even without flexion of the spine. This means that in the first arc of rotation, when the midline ligament is still slack, useful tension may be present in the fascia. The efficiency of this system is low in normal upright lordosis and high when the spine is flexed. The efficiency of the internal oblique muscle in this regard will be greatest if its pull is in the tangential plane of the lumbodorsal fascia. This obtains when the abdominal cavity is rounded by a small internal pressure.

This ligamentous sheet, because it follows the contour of the spine, does not create shearing forces; the internal oblique and transversus abdominis muscles, because they lie almost transversely to the spine, do not produce compression. Thus these muscles produce extensor moment without adding appreciably to the compression or shear felt by the intervertebral joint.

The Balance between Muscle and Ligament

Both the ligamentous systems described above are placed behind the musculature. The muscle acting at the center of cross-sectional area had a much shorter lever arm. Therefore, muscle contraction produces a greater compressive force on the disc than an equivalent tension in the ligament. It is important to realise that the penalty of using the paraspinal muscle instead of the ligament is increased stress at the intervertebral joint.

Consider a simple diagram of the spinal mechanism

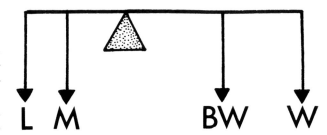

Fig. 2-3 Moments due to external loads are balanced by moments generated internally. External loads: BW, body weight above disc acting through center of gravity of upper body; W, weight held in hands. Internal loads: L, tension developed in ligamentous system; M, tension developed in trunk musculature.

(Fig. 2–3). Both muscle (M) and ligament (L) forces are used to balance the body weight (BW) and the barbell (W). It is clearly more efficient to manage the load with ligament tension alone, because compression stress is less than when muscle is used.

Mathematically there may be an infinite number of ways to combine ligament and muscle tensions or strategies to balance a given weight. However, physiologically there are constraints. To lift a very heavy load, a technique that depends almost entirely on using the ligament is preferred because stress levels are lowest. For maximal external loads, we *must* rely on a ligament strategy. Therefore, there is a unique method of lifting the maximal weight, and no variation can be tolerated. Evidence that the proper use of ligament strategy is an acquired skill exists.

Relying solely on the ligament has its drawbacks. The first is that in many body positions the ligament is largely inoperative because it is slack for the first 45° of forward flexion. For smaller external loads (BW + 50 lb) a ligament strategy can be used, but the spine must be in a flexed position. Secondly, the ligament is a passive structure, whereas muscle contraction implies some measure of active control and hence a mechanism that may act to prevent injury. Even with heavier lifts the trunk muscles remain active, remaining available to provide fine control in case of accident. Using a muscle strategy permits greater variation in trunk attitude. However, for this increased freedom the body tends to pay the price of increased spinal stress because the muscle is used.

Does this mean that the stresses in the spine vary with the choice of strategy? Not necessarily, if a system exists whereby stresses caused by intermediate strategies can be minimized. We believe that this is the role of the abdominal muscle mechanism. As mentioned above, the abdominal musculature produces longitudinal posterior tensions with reduced compression and shear. Calculations show that when the abdominal mechanism functions properly, it tends to reduce stress when the midline ligaments are unavailable.

STABILITY OF THE LUMBAR SPINE

It has been determined that the unsupported upright spinal column can support only 5 lb before it buckles or collapses. With the body in an upright relaxed stance, the center of gravity of the upper half of the body is some 14 inches above the lumbosacral joint. This is equivalent to balancing a weight of approximately 75 lb at the end of a 14-inch flexible rod. Clearly this feat cannot be accomplished without some mechanism of stabilization. There is no problem with the thoracic segments that are stabilized at the back, front, and sides by the ribs. The only available support system for neck or lumbar regions is the musculature. No means of maintaining the trunk and upper extremities in a given position could exist without the stabilizing effects of the peripheral trunk musculature, especially if the ligamentous system is slack.

In the absence of muscle and ligament support, we can expect the spine to buckle under body weight. Buckling in the saggital plane would be motion in the normal mode and therefore not dangerous (Fig. 2–4).

Buckling in the lateral or vertical modes, however, could endanger the intervertebral joints. In both instances, the tendency to buckling is increased as the imposed load is increased, and the intervertebral joint is rotated laterally (sidebend). With lateral rotation, the facet joints induce a dangerous torsion at the joint.

The paravertebral muscles are poorly placed to counteract the dangerous types of buckling. The abdominal muscles, particularly the lower digitations of the external oblique, seem well placed to control buckling by lateral bend and the psoas to protect against vertical collapse. The obliques are ideally placed to counteract torque. The amount of torque contributed by the abdominals is very small (approximately 300–400 in-lb). This small contribution is sufficient to afford some valuable protection for the intervertebral joint.

The generation of torque, by pitching a ball, for example, is produced from motion imparted to the

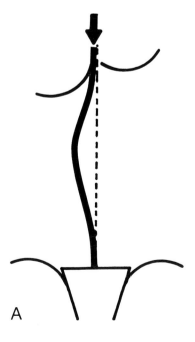 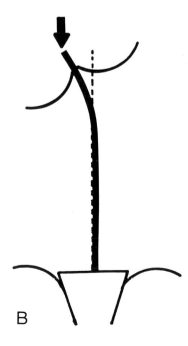

Fig. 2-4 Two forms of buckling under increased axial load (↓) **(A)** Axial buckling prevented by the psoas muscles. **(B)** Lateral bend controlled by laterally placed musculature. Both forms of buckling induce a torsion at the intervertebral joints because lateral bend is accompanied by axial rotation.

A

B

pelvis by the lower extremities and transmitted to the upper extremities through the trunk, which must become rigid at the crucial moment. The torque at the upper extremities, therefore, derives principally from the angular momentum imparted to the trunk by the lower extremities. However, this torque must be transmitted to the upper extremities via a rigid torso.

The stability of the spine depends greatly on the conditions obtaining at the joint itself (the point "P" in Fig. 2–5). Redraw Figure 2–5 so that P is free to move between stops S and S1, representing an increased abnormal motion at the joint, as caused by injury, for example. Any tendency to lateral bend would immediately cause P to move towards the appropriate stop, and this motion cannot be controlled satisfactorily by muscle acting at a distance to P. The point "P" is mechanically unstable. This instability results not so much because the joint permits movement—slight degrees of motion (called deformation) are normal—but because when 1 mm of deformation is called for, the joint yields more than this (Fig. 2–5).

We see, therefore, that the integrity of the spinal mechanism depends on the controlled interaction between the musculature: on the hip extensors for the power for heavy exertion, on the paraspinal musculature for lighter tasks, and on the abdominal musculature for the balance between ligament and spinal motion and for adjusting the whole system to the task to be performed. A loss of efficiency in any of these components leads to a loss of control that may precipitate an injury at the intervertebral joint.

HUMAN LOCOMOTION

In normal human locomotion, the movement of the mass of shoulder girdle and lower extremities alternates in direction with the movement of the mass of the pelvis and lower extremities. The movement of these two counter-rotating masses constitutes a vertically oscillating pendulum, which, in common with other similar systems, minimizes the energy consumption.

The rotating masses of the shoulders are joined by a flexible vertebral column to the counter-rotating mass of the pelvis. This column must transmit torque,

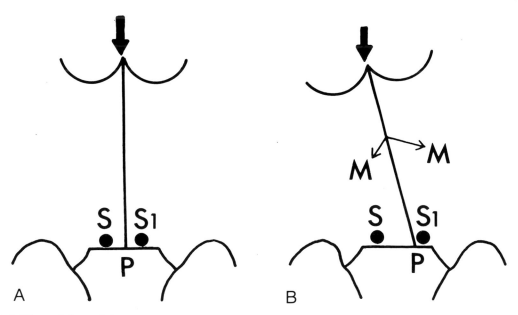

Fig. 2–5 The stability of the spine depends on two factors **(A)** Conditions obtaining at the joint (P). P can move between the stops S and S1. **(B)** Any tendency to lateral bend causes P to move toward the appropriate stop, and this motion cannot be controlled by muscle acting at a distance to P. The point P is mechanically unstable.

first in one direction, then in the other. As the speed of forward motion increases, the rate of oscillation must increase to keep pace with the legs. Thence, the requirement for torque must also increase.

The torque transmittable by an IV joint is increased when it is compressed. When the compression force on the IV joint is increased, it becomes flexed. Thus, to increase torque transmission, the lumbar lordosis must be reduced and the spine placed under compression by active muscular contration of the abdominals and erector spinae.

The power for initiating and maintaining this spine oscillation is primarily from the erector spinae. These muscles induce a lateral bend of the spine. In the lumbar region, by virtue of the special orientation of the facet joints, contraction of erector spinae on one side causes a rotation of the spine to the opposite side; the hips go one way and the shoulders go the other way. At each step, the spine moves from extension and lateral bend, on one side, to neutral bend and diminished lordosis or flexion, to lateral bend and extension on the other side. As speed is increased, the amplitude of the movement is reduced as the discs become stiffer.

Thus, in walking, the spine moves in its normal coordinated manner, which keeps its energy consumption at a minimum. If the spine is kept in a fixed position, the energy consumption is no longer minimal, and accordingly the stresses increase. Thus, carrying a heavy load requiring full spinal flexion, the individual can not walk except by shuffling. Carrying a large weight in one hand prevents the alternating movements necessary for walking. A large light load, carried in front with the arms, prevents forward bending.

Thus, by upsetting the normal spinal movements, we increase the potential for injury, particularly in the torsion mode.

THE INTERVERTEBRAL JOINT

The disc, facet joints, and their complementary ligament and muscle systems all appear to respond to stress at the intervertebral joint. The stress at that joint can be represented in general terms as:

$$\text{Stress} = \sqrt{C^2 + S^2}$$

where

C is compression force and
S is shear force.

The amount of stress at the joint can be manipulated by changing the spinal geometry through muscle action. Calculations show that in life normal spinal function can be achieved by choosing the combination of ligament tension and muscle force that produces the minimum stress at the intervertebral joint. This simulated system is not very sensitive to compression. This is to be expected because the column must withstand very high compressive loads, often more than 1 ton. On the other hand, the system is very sensitive to shear. Correspondingly, in the laboratory, we find that the intervertebral joint is relatively much weaker in shear. Basically, then, the organism seems to respond to imposed loads by attempting to reduce shear to a minimum and to equalize stress at all joints.

AXIAL COMPRESSION LOADING: THE DISC

The *main support* for a compression load is the vertebral body annulus column. The upper lumbar facet joints are unable to support a compression force in the axial direction. At the two lower intervertebral joints, the facets may support up to 20% of the axial compression.

The *compression strength* of the vertebral body resides virtually in its thin cortical shell, which per unit cross-sectional area is as strong as the femur. The cancellous core of the vertebral body may increase the strength of the unit by a hydraulic mechanism. Under a slowly increasing compression load, the fluid content of the vertebral body may be squeezed out into extracellular space through the veins or through small canals through the cortex. When the rate of deformation is increased, these channels are not large enough to permit the greater rate of outflow. Therefore, the internal pressure in the vertebral body rises, making the whole structure more rigid. This hydraulic system depends on the rate of loading and makes the vertebral body the shock-absorbing system for the disc, which is stiffer and stronger than that body. Shock absorption is a role sometimes erroneously ascribed to the disc.

The *endplate* of the vertebral body is the weak point of the disc. It is the site of failure when compression loads become excessive. The endplate may be over-stressed by two different mechanisms. First, when compression is applied peripherally to an oval-shaped plate, stresses develop in the plate in the line of its long axis. Fissure fractures in the endplate can be created experimentally by this method of compressing the annulus in the absence of the nucleus. Second, in the presence of a hydrostatic nucleus or when the disc cavity contains sufficient firm material to act as a punch as the endplates are forced closer together. The result is a depressed fracture. The endplate itself is reinforced around its periphery at the point where the annulus is attached.

Compression Loading

After a compression load is applied, the nucleus of the disc takes approximately 1 sec to attain its highest pressure. The annulus therefore takes on the initial load, and as it deforms under the load, the nucleus pressure develops to redistribute the load to the best advantage. This mechanism explains why the disc may function quite successfully without a nucleus.

The concentric arrangement of the collagenous layers of the annulus ensures that when the disc is placed in tension, shear, or rotation, the individual fibers are always in tension. When compressed in the presence of a functioning nucleus, the annular fibers are again stressed in tension. This arrangement ensures that should the annulus fail, the failure would be at the annulus-endplate interface where, as with other ligamentous attachments, healing is most likely to occur.

Motion at the Disc

Motion is a function of the properties of the annulus and does not depend on the nucleus. The functioning annulus can be depicted diagrammatically as in Figure 2–6. There is a point in the disc at which, when compression is applied, the disc is compressed but no forward, backward, or sideways rotation occurs. We may call this the neutral point. When the load is applied eccentrically away from this point, the joint rotates (flexes) in the direction of the eccentric load. In the symmetric disc, applying the load in the sagittal plane results in forward or backward rotation, with no tendency for lateral bending. In this situation,

all the applied force goes to provide the desired motion, and we may call this the preferred line of the axis of motion. In the symmetric vertebra, this preferred line lies in the sagittal plane. In either scoliotic or asymmetric joints, the preferred line apparently does not coincide with the sagittal plane.

The eccentricity of the applied load in the normal disc cannot be further forward than the mid-point of the annulus. A load applied in front of the annulus will put the posterior annulus in tension. This can occur accidentally as in a sudden fall on the backside. The combination of rising nucleus pressure and tension in the posterior annulus may cause the disc to rupture and its contents to explode into the neural canal.

The fact that the point of load application remains within the confines of the annulus implies that the disc itself has no need to support a moment. Indeed in the laboratory, the maximum moment supportable by the annulus is of the order of 200 to 300 in-lb.

Compression Failure

It can be seen from the above discussion that with axial loading the disc is always compressed with a force approximately equal to the weight of the body supported by the joint and that additional compression due to ligament or muscle tension results whenever the spine moves from the neutral upright position. Thus, at L5-S1 the average force in men is BW/2, or 75 lb, and the disc area approximately 2.5 to 3.0 in^2. This is equivalent to a pressure of 25 to 30 lb/in^2. Pressure is increased with forward flexion because of the tension in muscle and ligament needed to support the body in this position. When failure occurs, it is not the annulus but the endplate that fails. It is extremely difficult to cause annular failure by compression.

The spinal mechanism seems well equipped to support and to react to compression load. An accidental axial overload can be imposed by an uncoordinated lift when the spinal musculature takes on too much load. Asymmetries in the disc and/or the facet joints may act to concentrate the stresses, thereby increasing the risk. Less frequently, increased axial load may occur accidentally as in a fall onto the backside. Details of traumatic injuries depend on an analysis of forces obtaining at the time of trauma and are outside the scope of this discussion.

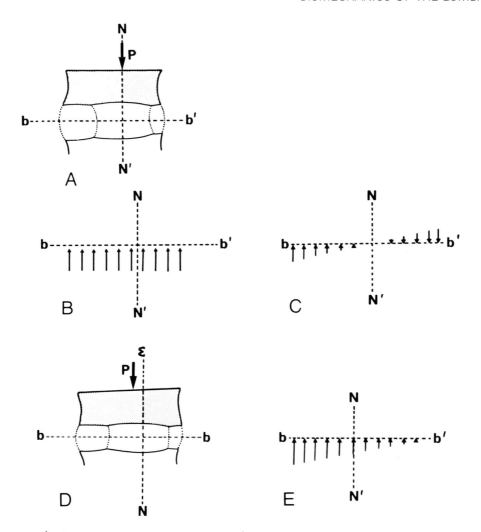

Fig. 2-6 (A) NN[1], the neutral axis of the IV joint; bb[1], the bisector of the disc. When force P is applied in the neutral axis, the joint has no tendency to rotate, flex, or extend. **(B)** The load P is supported over the cross-sectional are of the disc, as shown diagrammatically. **(C)** If a pure rotation (or a moment)—flexion, for example—could be applied to the disc, the distribution of stress would appear as shown here. **(D)** When the disc is flexed, stress is distributed by applying the force P at some eccentricity (ϵ) from the neutral axis. Thus both compression and moment act on the disc, and the posterior annulus does not go into tension. **(E)** As shown in (E), this is obtained by adding algebraically the arrows in (B) and (C).

SHEARING FORCES AND TORSION: THE FACET JOINTS

As stated above, the midline posterior ligamentous system develops posterior shearing forces at the disc to counteract the forward shearing forces due to body weight that arise when the body bends forward. Muscles such as the sacrospinalis, multifidus, and psoas may also create shear forces that combine to produce a smaller posterior shear force.

The neural arch and its appendates are so arranged as to add considerable resistance to forward shear. The disc, with its large central cavity, does not appear to be an ideal structure for supporting shear force. In fact, its shear strength is probably less than 200 lb. Under normal circumstances it is doubtful that any shear is felt by the disc, because of the protection afforded by ligament, muscle, and facet joints.

Axial torsion is a normal motion of the human spine. The fact that much of its design is evidently antitorsional is because this capacity to resist torque allows its transmission through the spine between pelvis and shoulder. This capacity for torque transmission can be greatly increased by flexion, or by its equivalent, an increasing compression load.

The Facet Joints

The facet joints are carried on articular processes that themselves arise from the neural arch. The *superior articular process* is squat and strong. Because of this, it shows little deflection when loaded at 90° to its articular surface. Its facet joint projects above the endplate just far enough to allow the joint's center to lie in the transverse plane of the disc.

The *inferior articular process* is much longer and extends over the back of the vertebral body in such a way that the center of its articular surface lies in the transverse plane of the disc. Because of its length, this process is more easily deflected by load and may deflect as much as 8 to 9° before fracture occurs. The articular process, pedicle, and neural arch all exhibit proportionally the same strength as femoral bone. However, it is always difficult to visualize the fact that some deflection of bone normally occurs.

The *synovial joint* has a very low coefficient of friction. Its design is such that it can support a load at 90° to the plane or curved surface in which motion takes place. The facets may therefore support a load in the plane of the disc. They are clearly capable of supporting shear forces when the spinal column is in the flexed position. They are also oriented 90° to the direction of motion imposed by axial torsion because the center of this motion is within the disc. Thus, like all synovial joints, the facet joints are weight-bearing. By virtue of this function, these joints are capable of absorbing some 700 to 800 lb of shear force whereas the disc probably supports less than 200 lb. The maximum shear that the intervertebral joints may be called on to support is probably less than 500 lb. The facet resistance to torsion nearly doubles the torque strength of the whole intervertebral joint. Thus loss of function by the facet joints may have a serious impact on the strength of the whole joint, and it is not difficult to understand why

the intervertebral joint deteriorates when a facet joint is damaged.

Stable and Unstable Injuries to the Intervertebral Joint

In the case of injury resulting in endplate failure, a "back-up" system—namely, the posterior midline ligaments, the facets, and the disc annulus—is present to protect against a repetition of damaging forces. Should injury occur, this system survives and is available at the site of injury to maintain a certain degree of spine stability (Fig. 2–5A).

In the case of accidental torsional injury, simultaneous damage to the disc annulus and facet joints removes the local back-up mechanism of stabilization. Except for the antitorsional activity by abdominal muscles, the joint has no protection against torsion. The muscles, however, are too far removed from the site of injury to control the local effects at the intervertebral joint (see Fig. 2–5A).

The proper function of the facet joints depends on the integrity of their articular processes, which in turn rely on the integrity of the neural arches that support them. Therefore, it is important to understand the forces that affect the neural arch as a whole.

The normal force impinging on the neural arch is shown in Figure 2–7. The shear force pushing back

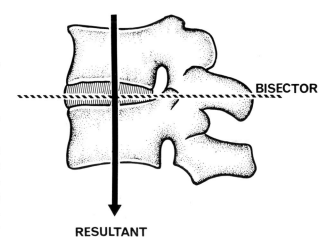

Fig. 2-7 The muscles and ligaments apply tension to the spine while the facet joints support the shear force in the plane of the disc. The forces combine to apply a twisting force to the neural arch so that stress is concentrated at the pars inter articularis.

on the inferior articular process and the downward pull of the midline structures create a stress concentration at the pars interarticularis. The stress is magnified when torsional forces are added to the facet joints in the direction of axial rotation of the intervertebral joint. It is predictable, therefore, that a torsional injury is the most likely cause of spondylolysis. The second most likely cause is overload with the spine in the flexed or almost fully flexed position, particularly if the erector spinae muscles contract strongly at the same time.

THE THREE-JOINT COMPLEX

Because the facet joints form two of the three articulations of an intervertebral joint, motion at one site must reflect motion at the other two. The instantaneous center of motion for the whole intervertebral joint—for flexion, extension, and torsion—has been found to be near the center of the disc. This must also be the center of motion for the facet joints. The facet joints do not interfere with flexion or extension but are squarely opposed to axial rotation, allowing only approximately 2° to 3° of rotation. When rotation is forced, the facets impose a flexion or forward rotation at the disc and a lateral bend towards the side of the impacted facet joint (coupled motion).

TORSIONAL FAILURE

The force required to induce 3° of axial rotation is generally large enough to deform the neural arch appreciably or even to produce crush injuries to the facet joint.

The forward rotation imposed by the facet joints is not normal in the sense that the annulus is forced into tension or, rather, into reduced compression. The tensile stress added to the torsional stress imposed by the axial rotation together render the annulus more vulnerable. This vulnerability is reduced if the compression load is simultaneously increased to compensate. The difference can make a 20% difference to the torque strength. Hence the inadvisability of doing torsional exercises without either muscle control or some external load.

Forced rotation of 2° to 3° may also damage the annulus. In torsion only half of the annulus is loaded in tension because of the alternating arrangement of its fibers. The highest stresses are attained first in the outermost fibers and predictably, they fail at the ligament-bone interface. As predictably, they fail at the posterolateral angles, which act as "stress risers." The distortion and tearing of the outer annular fibers are greatest at these points and are sufficiently large to interfere with the neural canal content.

AGING AND DEGENERATION

A very high percentage of in vitro experimentation has been on intervertebral joints obtained at autopsy. The average age of the specimens is 60 to 65 yr. It thus happens that, theoretically at least, we should know more about the damaged intervertebral joint than the normal one. However, it is precisely because we are not sure of the normal that we have problems interpreting the laboratory results and separating "aging changes" from "degeneration."

In my opinion, considerable evidence exists to support the point of view that aging and degenerative changes are not synonymous and that degenerative changes do not appear unless the joint has been damaged by trauma. Many elderly joints prove to be just as strong in torsion or compression as the younger ones. Furthermore, degenerated joints appear to be stiffer than normal but fail before the healthier ones. This is a typical mechanical characteristic of scar tissue and scar implies injury.

THE RESULT OF COMPRESSION AND TORSIONAL INJURY

Compression Overload

As shown above, the failure in compression overload is a fractured endplate. Little or no damage to the annulus or the facet joints occurs. Should the fracture seal off and no damage to the nucleus ensue, we may conclude that joint function is restored to normal. However, this is usually not the case, because the scar in the endplate remains a weakness and the character of the nucleus undergoes a change that renders it less efficient. The net result is loss of stiffness of the annulus and therefore of the whole joint. In mechanical terms, greater deformation results for any given load. Under such conditions the facet joints become abnormal because of the abnormal call for weight bearing on their surfaces, which are not optimized for this function. This would be especially true of spines submitted to repeated axial loadings, such as is the case with truck drivers and farmers.

The joint with a fractured endplate also shows a reduced resistance to torsion and in the appropriate circumstances tends to be prone to torsional strains.

Creep

Because the intervertebral joint loses stiffness following injury, the "creep" characteristics of the joint are changed. "Creep" is the gradual deformation of the intervertebral joint under a constant load. Creep deformation is greater and occurs more rapidly in the injured joint, which tends to creep in the direction of the injury. Thus, with a fractured endplate, the disc creeps to a reduced thickness. With torsional failure, the joint tends to creep into the rotated position of injury. This phenomenon accounts for the appearance of symptoms as the day passes by.

Loss of Stiffness

The loss of joint stiffness affects the entire function of the joint. For instance, the center of motion may be markedly shifted from its normal position. This affects the system of forces acting in the joint, upsetting the normal muscle-ligament balance and the resultant joint motion.

Loss of Annular Substance

The gradual loss of annular substance and of facet articular cartilage leads to a permanent loss of vertical height of the disc. The vascular portions of disc and facet joint act to proliferate scar and at the capsule or peripheral annulus—where ligament is inserted into bone—osteophyte formation is induced. The mechanical importance of these changes is that mechanical deformation at the joint is reduced and joint strength is improved.

Torsion

The second and major mode of injury is torsion. Abnormal motions may occur because asymmetries are present in the intervertebral joint, disc or facet joint; minor torque forces may develop when the intervertebral joint is compressed; or else, in the presence of a minor asymmetry a torque may be induced at the intervertebral joint in the performance of a task. In torsional injury, damage occurs simultaneously to the peripheral annulus and the facets. The neural arch may be deformed. Torque resistance at the joint is reduced by this injury. The surviving structures of the intervertebral joint are not able to compensate for the injury and abnormal deformations may occur at the joint.

Severe Injury

When the intervertebral joint is badly damaged, the degree of axial rotational deformation is uncontrollable and therefore the joint is mechanically unstable. Because all local torque-resistant structures are damaged simultaneously, the organism has no replacement mechanism to tide it over until healing is complete. The only surviving antitorque mechanism is that provided by the abdominal muscles, which cannot react fast enough to protect from the unexpected overload.

At first the remaining intact deeper layers of annulus offer a resistance to further torsion as do the deformed facet joints. However, the reduced diameter of the remaining undamaged annulus and the acquired deformation of neural arch do not offer the original resistance to torque. Also, a greater degree of rotation can occur before the undamaged annular fibers and deformed neural arch offer any resistance. The damaged annular layers heal with scar formation, but the deformed neural arch does not correct. The intervertebral joint is left with a reduced resistance to torque at the annulus and an abnormal amount of motion permitted by the neural arch.

The deformed neural arch permits the intervertebral joint to settle in a new position, and should the annulus heal, we have a stabilized deformity that at best is weak, in which the neural arch has returned to its relatively normal appearance but with the vertebral bodies displaced relative to each other.

CONCLUSIONS

Mechanical failures are predictable when the functions of the individual structural members are understood within the confines of the whole system. A knowledge of the mechanical behavior of each member allows the site of failure to be predicted.

When the precise location of failure has been determined, a knowledge of pathology makes it possible to predict local reactions to the injury and therefore the pathogenesis of the symptomatology.

At this stage of our understanding we can say that injury occurs in one of two modes: first by direct force or axial overload with initial damage to the disk alone, either through compression that causes the endplate to fracture or tension, tensile rupture of posterior annulus with explosive rupture of the disk; or, second, by indirect force or torsional overload with the initial damage occurring simultaneously to facet and annulus.

We may also add that bending overload equals torsional overload because of coupled motion; that the direct and indirect force overload may be combined but the features of torsional overload predominate; and that because the site of failure depends on stress distribution and on local geometric features, we must distinguish injuries at the L4–5 from those at the L5–S1 joints.

These diagnoses are precise *etiological* diagnoses and not to be confused with syndromes such as low back pain, combined low back pain and sciatica, or sciatica. The clinical syndrome can never be a scientific basis for a disease classification. For this we must have the etiological diagnosis.

The clinician must relate the symptomatology to the etiologic diagnosis. Various modes of treatment can then be related to etiology in a rational way rather than to symptomatology, as is all too common at present.

REFERENCES

1. Farfan HF: Biomechanical advantage of lordosis and hip extension for upright activity in man compared with other anthropoids. Spine 3: 336, 1978
2. Farfan HF, Gracovetsky S, Lamy C: Mechanism of the lumbar spine. Spine 6: 249, 1981
3. Gracovetsky S, Farfan HF, Hellerer C: The abdominal mechanism. Spine 11(4): 317, 1985

3

The Anatomy of the Lumbosacral Spine

Pierre R. Dupuis

The lumbosacral spine is made of the five lumbar vertebrae, the sacrum, and coccyx. It is a complex structure made of bony elements linked by joint capsules and ligaments and governed by multiple layers of muscles.[1-3]

THE BONY ELEMENTS

Body of the Lumbar Vertebrae

The body of the lumbar vertebrae (Fig. 3-1) is a large and heavy kidney-shaped structure. It is wider from side to side and its posterior aspect is from moderately concave at the first segment to flat or mildly convex at the fifth. The size of the vertebral bodies increases from L1 to L5 because of the increasing loads each body has to carry. It is made of dense cancellous bone enclosed in a rather thin cortical shell. On the front and the sides, multiple small foramina for arterial supply and venous drainage pierce the cortex. Dorsally, a number of larger arterial foramina and one or more large orifices accommodate the basivertebral veins. The upper and lower surfaces or endplates are flat and rough except for a smooth peripheral ring originating from the fusion of the ring apophysis at maturity. On the posterior aspect of the upper smooth ring, on either side of the midline, are two small lips projecting upward towards two corresponding indentations on the posterior aspect of the lower smooth ring of the vertebra above. They most probably represent remnants of the uncovertebral joints found in the cervical spine.

Vertebral Arch

The vertebral arch is a horseshoe-shaped structure made of the lamina and pedicles. Projecting from it are seven processes: paired superior and inferior articular processes, a spinous process and paired transverse processes. The pedicles are short and stocky and are attached to the cranial half of the body. At the first lumbar, they point directly backwards but will point progressively more laterally from thereon down. The lamina are broad flat structures blending in medially with the spinous processes. The latter are flat, broad, and rectangular and project directly backwards from the lamina. The transverse processes project laterally and slightly posteriorly from the junction of the pedicles and lamina and, together with the spinous process, serve as levers for the muscles and ligaments that attach to them. The articular processes project from the lamina. The superior processes bear a mildly concave articular surface and face medially and

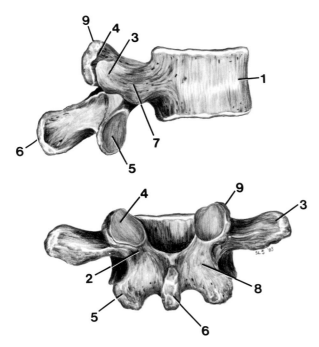

Fig. 3-1 Typical lumbar vertebra viewed from the side (top) and the back (bottom). 1. body; 2. pars interarticularis; 3. transverse process; 4. superior facet; 5. inferior facet; 6. spinous process; 7. pedicle; 8. lamina; 9. mamillary process. (Dupuis PR, Kirkaldy-Willis WH: The spine: integrated function and pathophysiology. In Cruess RL, Rennie WRJ (eds): Adult Orthopaedics. Churchill Livingstone, New York, 1984.)

slightly posteriorly. The inferior processes point laterally and slightly anteriorly and their articular surface is mildly convex.

Facet Joints

The facet joints (Fig. 3-2) are typical synovial joints. The articulating surfaces are made of hyaline cartilage. In the lumbar spine, their capsules are thick and fibrous and cover the dorsal aspect of the joint. The ventral capsule is made of an extension of ligamentum flavum. The deltoid space determined by the capsule or flavum on one side and the junction of the rounded edges of the superior and inferior articular cartilagenous surfaces on the other, is filled by a similarly shaped fibrous rim. On this rim, mostly at the proximal and distal poles, fibroadipose or adipose enlargements or miniscoids may be found.[4,5]

Sacrum

The sacrum (Fig. 3-3), a narrow wedge-shaped structure, is made of five fused vertebrae. Proximally it articulates with the fifth lumbar vertebra, laterally with the ilium, and distally with the coccyx. On the midline of its dorsal convex surface, are four more-or-less united spinous processes called the median sacral crest. On each side of this crest and slightly medial to the posterior sacral foramina, a series of fused zygapophyseal joints form the intermediate crest. Laterally to the posterior sacral foramina, the fused transverse and costal processes of the sacral vertebrae form, proximally the ala of the sacrum and distally, the lateral sacral crest. The endopelvic surface is concave. It displays four pairs of pelvic sacral foramina opposite the dorsal sacral foramina. This surface is also scored by horizontal crests that represent the sites of intervertebral fusion of the sacral vertebrae. On the outer aspect of the fused transverse processes sits a broad, ear-shaped articular surface called the auricular surface. This surface, which points laterally and slightly posteriorly, articulates with the ilium. The very tip of the sacrum is formed by the undersurface of the body of the fifth sacral vertebra, which articulates with the coccyx. This fifth sacral vertebral is devoid of lamina and spinous process, determining a hiatus called the sacral cornua.

Coccyx

The coccyx (Fig. 3-4) consists of three to five variably fused vertebral bodies. The first and largest segment articulates through a rudimentary disc with the lower surface of the fifth sacral vertebra. Posteriorly its roof is also deficient, determining a coccygeal cornua.

THE INNER ARCHITECTURE OF THE VERTEBRA

The trabecular arrangement of the vertebral spongiosa[6,7] is determined by the stresses to which it is exposed. There are three trabecular systems (Fig. 3-5)—one vertical and two oblique. The vertical trabecular system runs from one endplate to the other. The superior oblique system spreads out to the spinous and superior articular processes from the supe-

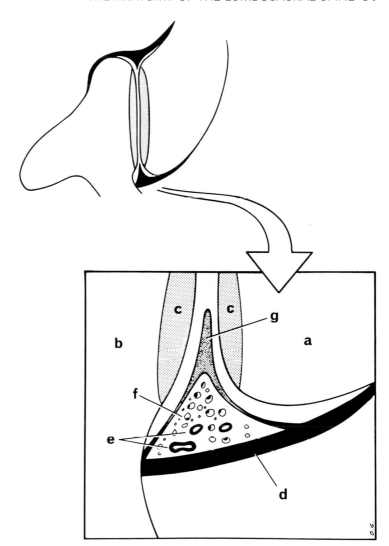

Fig. 3-2 Diagrammatic representation of the fibro-adipose meniscoid of a facet joint according to Engel and Bogduk.[4,5] a. inferior articular process of the vertebra above; b. superior articular process of the vertebra below; c. articular cartilage; d. joint capsule; e. blood vessels; f. adipose tissue cells of the base of the meniscoid; g. fibrous cap of the meniscoid.

rior endplate by way of the pedicles. The inferior oblique system spreads out to the spinous and inferior articular processes from the inferior endplate also by way of the pedicles. The crisscrossing of the three systems creates a very light but also very resistant structure.

THE SPINAL CANAL

The configuration of the spinal canal is primarily determined by the shape of the posterior aspect of the vertebral body and the direction to which the pedicles point. Because the posterior aspect of the

vertebral body is moderately concave at the first lumbar segment and flat or even slightly convex at the fifth segment and the pedicles project directly back at the first segment but slightly more laterally at each of the next four segments, the shape of the canal will evolve from an oval on its side at L1 to a frank triangular shape at L5 (Fig. 3-6).

THE NERVE ROOT CANAL

The nerve root canal[8,9] is a funnel-shaped structure that contains the lumbar spinal nerve. It begins at the exit of the nerve from the dura. In the upper

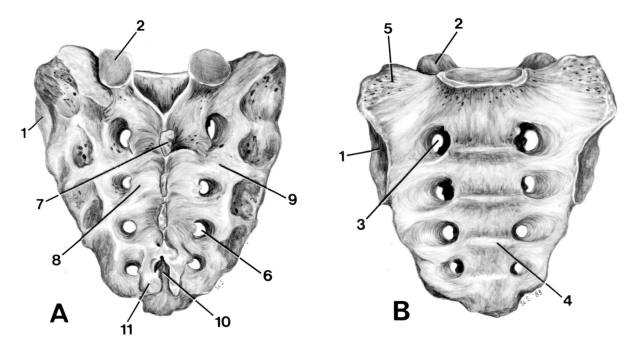

Fig. 3-3 The sacrum viewed **(A)** from the back and **(B)** from the front. 1. auricular surface; 2. articular process; 3. anterior sacral foramen; 4. bony crest where anterior body fusion has occurred; 5. ala; 6. posterior sacral foramen; 7. median sacral crest; 8. intermediate sacral crest; 9. lateral sacral crest; 10. sacral hiatus; 11. cornua. (Dupuis PR, Kirkaldy-Willis WH: The spine: integrated function and pathophysiology. In Cruess RL, Rennie WRJ (eds): Adult Orthopaedics. Churchill Livingstone, New York, 1984.)

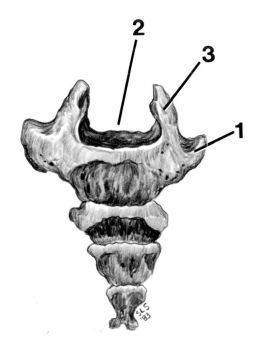

Fig. 3-4 The coccyx. 1. transverse process; 2. hiatus; 3. cornua. (Dupuis PR, Kirkaldy-Willis WH: The spine: integrated function and pathophysiology. In Cruess RL, Rennie WRJ (eds): Adult Orthopaedics. Churchill Livingstone, New York, 1984.)

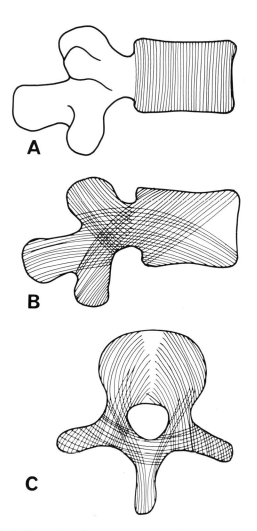

Fig. 3-5 The trabecular arrangement of the typical lumbar vertebra according to Gallois and Japoit,[6] and Kapanji.[7] **(A)** The vertical trabecular system. **(B)** Superior and inferior oblique systems. **(C)** Oblique systems viewed from above. (Dupuis PR, Kirkaldy-Willis WH: The spine: integrated function and pathophysiology. In Cruess RL, Rennie WRJ (eds): Adult Orthopaedics. Churchill Livingstone, New York, 1984.)

lumbar segments it runs frankly laterally but from thereon distally, progressively more downward. It ends at the outer aspect of the intervertebral foramen. The inner half is delimited posteriorly by ligamentum flavum and anteriorly by annulus fibrosus and the posterior aspect of the body of the vertebra below

it. The outer half is determined dorsally by the pars interarticularis and articular joint covered with flavum, cranially and caudally by the pedicles and ventrally by the posterior aspect of the vertebra and disc of the level below.

THE INTERVERTEBRAL DISC AND ENDPLATES

The intervertebral disc links two adjacent vertebral bodies. It contributes one third of the length of the lumbar spine (20% in the thoracic spine and cervical spine) and is made of three distinct components. The first component, the nucleus pulposus, is a gellike substance made of a meshwork of collagen fibrils suspended in a mucoprotein base made of water and various mucopolysaccharides (approximately 88% of water in the young and 70% in the elderly). It forms approximately 40% of the total cross-sectional area of the disc. This central nucleus will differentiate from its periphery outwards into the concentric fibrocartilagenous lamellae of the annulus fibrosus, which forms the second component and the outer boundaries of the disc (Figs. 3-7A and 3-8A). From the nucleoannular interface outward, the thickness of lamellae increases gradually. In each lamella, the collagen fibers run an oblique and helicoidal course with a 30° orientation to the plane of the joint. The fibers of the adjacent lamellae have a similar arrangement but run a course in the opposite direction so that they determine an interception angle of roughly 120° to each other (Fig. 3-7B). The fibers of the outermost annular lamella attach to the vertebral body by mingling with the periosteal fibrils. The outer two thirds of the annulus fibrosus anchors firmly to the vertebral body above and below with penetrating Sharpey's fibers while the inner one third attaches loosely to the cartilagenous endplate, the third component of the disc (Fig. 3-8C). Both endplates are made of hyaline cartilage resting on a flat subchondral bone plate supported by the spongiosa of the vertebral body. On this bony endplate are multiple small perforations that permit direct contact between the vascular buds of the marrow and the cartilagenous plate (Fig. 3-8B). This is one of the main nutritional pathways for the disc.

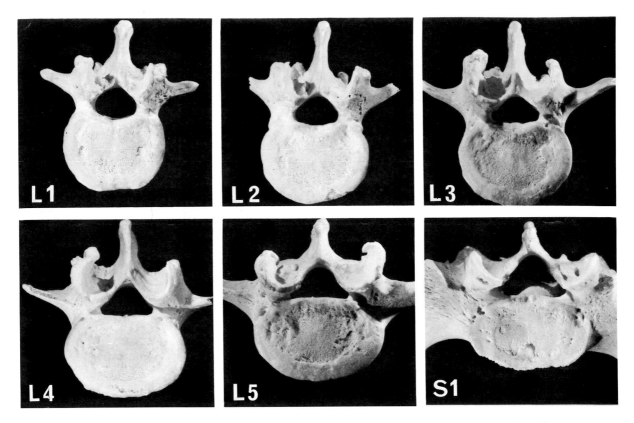

Fig. 3-6 The changing shape of the spinal canal from L1 to S1. The vertebrae are viewed from above. From L1 to S1 the spinal canal changes from an oval on its side to a more trefoil shape as the posterior wall of the vertebrae changes from concave to convex, and the pedicles grow shorter and broader, migrate more laterally, and project more posterolaterally.

THE LIGAMENTS OF THE SPINE

Anterior Longitudinal Ligament

The anterior longitudinal ligament (Fig. 3-9) is a long fibrous structure originating from the anterior and basilar aspect of the occipital bone and ending at the upper and anterior part of the sacrum. Its fibers run a longitudinal course and attach to the anterior surface of all vertebral bodies. Its long fibers extend over four or five vertebral bodies. Some medium fibers extend over two or three bodies; short fibers attach firmly to and mingle with the fibers of the outermost annular fibers and the adjacent periosteal fibrils of two adjacent vertebrae.

Posterior Longitudinal Ligament

Situated on the posterior surface of the vertebral body, the posterior longitudinal ligament (Fig. 3-10) is the extension of the tectorial membrane, which arises from the basilar aspect of the occipital bone at the foramen magnum. From the second vertebra to the coccyx, it attaches to the superior margin of the vertebral bodies and discs, its fibers spanning two to four vertebral bodies. It is broad, flat, and

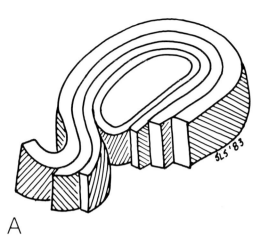

A

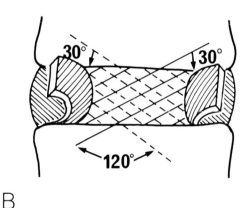

B

Fig. 3-7 (A) Lamellar arrangement of annulus fibrosus. Note the increasing thickness of each lamella from nucleus pulposus outward. **(B)** Orientation of the collagen fibers in each lamella. The fibers run a 30° oblique course to the horizontal plane. This arrangement runs in the opposite direction in adjacent lamellae. (Dupuis PR, Kirkaldy-Willis WH: The spine: integrated function and pathophysiology. In Cruess RL, Rennie WRJ (eds): Adult Orthopaedics. Churchill Livingstone, New York, 1984.)

smooth in the cervical area but quickly narrows down considerably in the thoracic and lumbar spines, where it gives thin lateral expansions to the annulus fibrosus at each level, giving it a denticulated aspect.

Capsular Ligaments

The capsular ligaments attach to the margins of adjacent articular processes. They are particularly well developed in the lumbar spine where they are thick and their taut fibers run a course perpendicular to the axis of the joint.

Ligamentum Flavum

The ligamentum flavum (Fig. 3-11) takes its name from the light yellow color it gets from its 80% elastin content. Its upper attachment is to the anterior surface of the lamina above, and its lower attachment is to the upper posterior edge of the lamina below. At each level its lateral extension forms the anterior capsule of the zygapophyseal joint and attaches proximally and distally to the inferior border of the pedicle above and the superior border of the pedicle below, forming a portion of the foramenal roof.

Interspinous Ligament

The interspinous ligament (Fig. 3-9) is a collection of fibers extending from the base of one spinous process to the tip of the next. It is rudimentary in the cervical spine where it blends with ligamentum nuchae, membranous in the thoracic spine and broad and thick in the lumbar spine.

Supraspinous Ligament

The supraspinous ligament (Fig. 3-9) extends as a well-defined, cordlike structure from the tip of the seventh cervical vertebra to the median sacral crest, attaching to every spinous process. In the lumbar spine it is broad and thick but much thinner in the thoracic spine.

Intertransverse Ligaments

The intertransverse ligaments (Fig. 3-11) run from transverse process to transverse process. While relatively ill defined in the cervical spine, they present as round and thick cords from tip to tip of transverse processes in the thoracic spine and as thin membranous structures from border to border of transverse

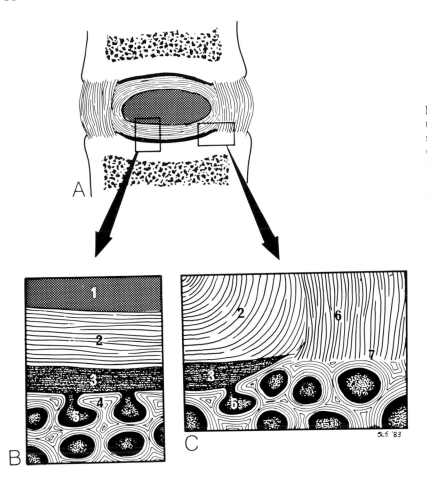

Fig. 3-8 Arrangement of the fibrocartilagenous fibers of the annulus fibrosus. **(A)** Fibers are arranged in a concentric lamellar fashion. **(B)** Magnified view of the central part of the disc. 1. nucleus pulposus; 2. annulus fibrosus; 3. horizontal disposition of the collagen fibers of the cartilagenous endplate; 4. bony endplate; 5. vascular channel in direct contact with cartilagenous endplate. **(C)** Fiber arrangement of the peripheral part of the disc. 6. outer fibers of annulus fibrosus; 7. anchoring of the fibers to the bony endplate (Sharpey-type fibers). Dupuis PR, Kirkaldy-Willis WH: The spine: integrated function and pathophysiology. In Cruess RL, Rennie WRJ (eds): Adult Orthopaedics. Churchill Livingstone, New York, 1984.)

processes in the lumbar spine. They are intimately connected to the deep musculature of the back.

Iliolumbar Ligament

The iliolumbar ligament (Fig. 3-12) is thick, broad, and deltoid. Its proximal attachment is to the tip and anterior part of the fifth transverse process. It usually divides into two bands, the upper one attaching to the iliac crest in front of the sacroiliac joint, the lower one running and blending in with the ventral sacroiliac ligaments. The iliolumbar ligament is a major stabilizer of L5 on the sacrum. On occasion, a weak attachment from the tip of the fourth lumbar transverse process also blends in.

Sacroiliac Ligaments

The sacroiliac ligaments (Fig. 3-12) are made of the short and long sacroiliac ligaments posteriorly and the anterior sacroiliac ligament. The short sacroiliac ligament (interosseous ligament) is the joint's major stabilizer. This thick and massive structure fills the space immediately behind and above the joint. It is made up of deep and more superficial bands, which blend and form a fibrous sheet covering the entire posterior part of the joint. It is covered by the dorsal or long sacroiliac ligament that consists of numerous fiber fascicles running in a vertical and oblique fashion from the intermediate and lateral sacral crests to the posterior iliac spine and adjacent

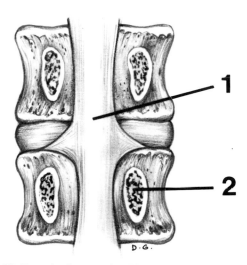

Fig. 3-10 Posterior longitudinal ligament. The motion segment is viewed from the back with posterior elements removed: 1. posterior longitudinal ligament with lateral expansions; 2. pedicle.

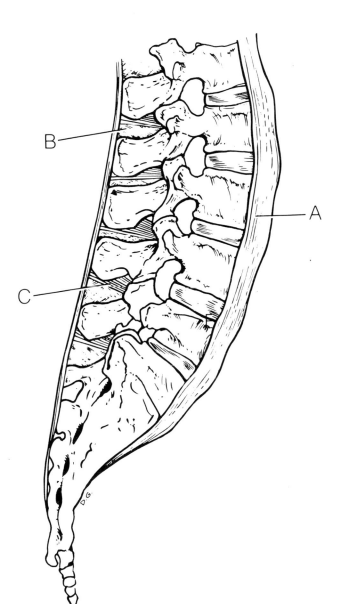

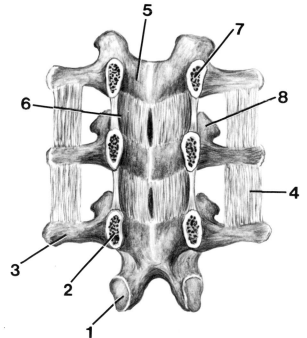

Fig. 3-9 Lumbosacral spine viewed from the side: a. anterior longitudinal ligament; b. supraspinous ligament; c. interspinous ligament.

Fig. 3-11 View of the posterior elements from the front, vertebral body excised. 1. inferior articular facet; 2. pedicle; 3. transverse process; 4. intertransverse ligament; 5. lamina; 6. ligamentum flavum; 7. pedicle; 8. superior articular facet. (Dupuis PR, Kirkaldy-Willis WH: The spine: integrated function and pathophysiology. In Cruess RL, Rennie WRJ (eds): Adult Orthopaedics. Churchill Livingstone, New York, 1984.)

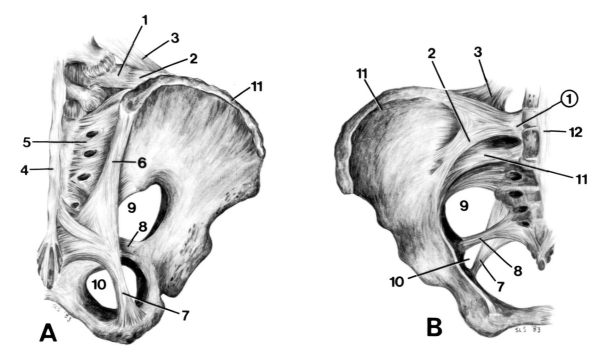

Fig. 3-12 The pelvis viewed **(A)** from the back and **(B)** from the front with ligaments: 1. transverse process of L5; 2. iliolumbar ligament; 3. participating attachment to the iliolumbar ligament from the transverse process of L4; 4. supraspinous ligament; 5. short posterior sacroiliac ligament; 6. long posterior sacroiliac ligament; 7. sacrotuberous ligament; 8. sacrospinous ligament; 9. greater sciatic foramen; 10. lesser sciatic foramen; 11. anterior sacroiliac ligament; 12. anterior longitudinal ligament. (Dupuis PR, Kirkaldy-Willis WH: The spine: integrated function and pathophysiology. In Cruess RL, Rennie WRJ (eds): Adult Orthopaedics. Churchill Livingstone, New York, 1984.)

ilium. Anteriorly, the anterior sacroiliac ligament is a weak thickening of the capsular ligaments. This thin ligament runs from the anterior surface of the lateral portion of the sacrum to the margins of the auricular surface of the ilium.

Vertebropelvic Ligaments

The vertebropelvic ligaments (Fig. 3-12) further stabilize the sacrum on the pelvis. The sacrotuberous ligament runs from the fourth and fifth transverse tubercles and adjacent lateral margins of the sacrum downward and laterally to the inner margin of the ischial tuberosity. The sacrospinous ligament runs from the lateral margins of the sacrum and coccyx to the ischial spine. These ligaments and attachments determine the greater sciatic foramen above and lesser sciatic foramen below.

THE VASCULAR SUPPLY TO THE LUMBAR SPINE

The Arterial Supply

The arterial supply[10,11] to the first four lumbar vertebrae comes from pairs of segmental arteries arising from the posterior and lateral aspect of the aortic wall at every level. The small segmental arteries subserving the fifth lumbar vertebra, the sacrum, and coccyx arise from the median sacral artery. This is a branch of variable caliber originating from the back of the aorta just above its bifurcation and ending in the coccygeal body. On the way down it anastomoses with the iliolumbar artery and lateral sacral arteries and sends branches to the pelvic sacral foramina. In the lumbar spine, each segmental or lumbar artery gives off two sets of branches before entering the sacral foramen (Fig. 3-13A). First, very short branches penetrate directly the waist of the body. Second, longer descending and ascending branches form a dense network on the front and sides of the body.

Some of these penetrate the vertebra near the endplate, and others form a very fine vascular mesh over the longitudinal ligament and annulus. Just proximal to the foramen the lumbar arteries divide into three ter-

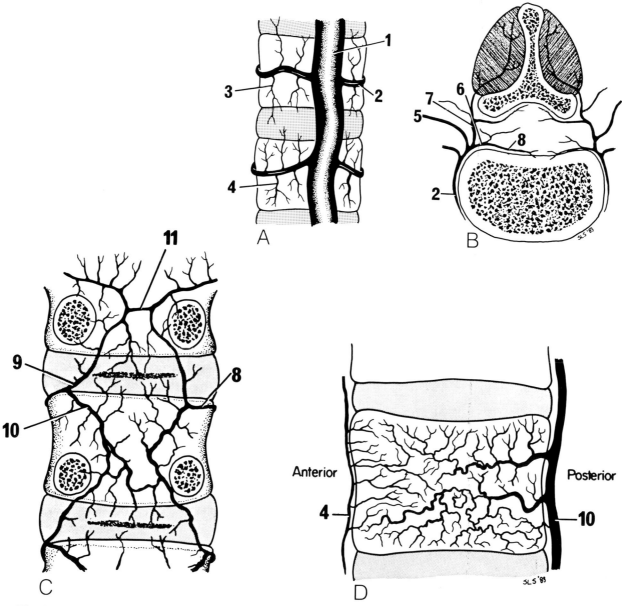

Fig. 3-13 Vascular supply to the spine. Spine viewed **(A)** from the front and **(B)** from above (axial cut): 1. aorta; 2. segmental artery; 3. long ascending and descending branches; 4. short ascending and descending branches; 5. anterior branch of segmental artery; 6. spinal branch of segmental artery; 7. posterior branch of segmental artery; 8. anterior division of spinal branch. Spine viewed **(C)** from the back with posterior elements removed and **(D)** from the side (midbody sagittal cut): 9. ascending limb of anterior spinal branch; 10. descending limb of anterior spinal branch; 11. transverse anastomosis between left and right systems. (Figs. A-D from Dupuis PR, Kirkaldy-Willis WH: The spine: integrated function and pathophysiology. In Cruess RL, Rennie WRJ (eds): Adult Orthopaedics. Churchill Livingstone, New York, 1984.)

minal branches (Fig. 3-13B). An anterior branch supplies both the nerve, which exits the foramen, and the trunk muscles. A spinal branch enters the foramen and further divides into anterior, posterior, and radicular branches. Finally, the posterior branch courses backward crossing over the pars interarticularis to end into the spinal musculature but not before giving branches to the apophyseal joints and corresponding posterior aspect of the lamina. In the canal, the posterior spinal branch forms a finely woven mesh on the anterior surface of the lamina and flavum, and the anterior spinal branch immediately divides into ascending and descending limbs, which anastomose with levels above and below forming a regular arcuate system (Fig. 3-13C). The left and right systems are linked at every level by transverse anastomoses running underneath the posterior longitudinal ligament. From the transverse anastomoses, both arcuate systems, and the external vessels running on the front sides of the vertebra, arteries penetrate the body and join into an arterial grid in its centrum (Fig. 3-13D). From this grid, branches ascend and descend toward the endplates ending in fine networks of vascular buds, which pass vertically into the vertebral endplate where they form a capillary bed (Fig. 3-14).

The Venous Drainage

The vascular pattern for venous drainage closely resembles its arterial supply.[11-14] At the endplate, venous drainage comes from a postcapillary venous network that empties into a subarticular horizontal collecting system through vertical channels perforating the endplates (Fig. 3-14). From that system, venules drain into a large central venous grid (Fig. 3-15) from which one or two large basivertebral veins arise. These in turn drain into the internal vertebral venous plexus. This plexus lies within the spinal canal between the dura mater and the vertebra. The basic framework is made up of two pairs of longitudinally oriented valveless venous strips, one anterior to the dural sac and one posterior, which anastomose with one another and with the external venous plexus (Fig. 3-16). The posterior pair is smaller, plexiform, and

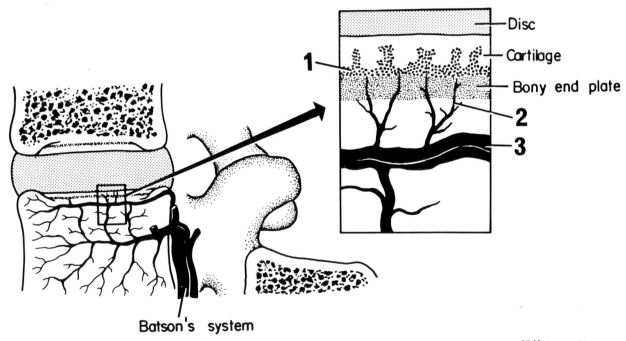

Batson's system

Fig. 3-14 Vascular arrangement at the vertebral endplate according to Crock and Yoshizawa.[10,11] 1. capillary bed in direct contact with the endplate cartilage; 2. postcapillary venous network; 3. subarticular horizontal collecting system. (Dupuis PR, Kirkaldy-Willis WH: The spine: integrated function and pathophysiology. In Cruess RL, Rennie WRJ (eds): Adult Orthopaedics. Churchill Livingstone, New York, 1984.)

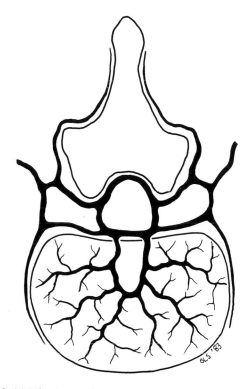

Fig. 3-15 The internal and external systems for venous drainage of a vertebra. It closely follows the pattern for arterial supply. (Dupuis PR, Kirkaldy-Willis WH: The spine: integrated function and pathophysiology. In Cruess RL, Rennie WRJ (eds): Adult Orthopaedics. Churchill Livingstone, New York, 1984.)

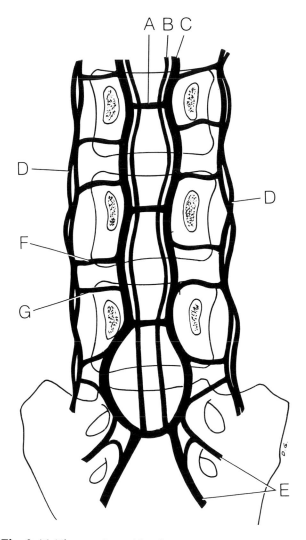

Fig. 3-16 The anterior epidural venous system of the spinal canal: a. transverse venous anastomosis. It joins the left and right systems and runs under the posterior longitudinal ligament where it collects from the basivertebral veins; b. medial epidural vein; c. lateral epidural vein; d. left and right ascending lumbar veins; e. lateral sacral veins; f. superior vein of the foramen; g. inferior vein of the foramen.

lies on the anterior aspect of the vertebral arches. The anterior pair of venous strips has a surprisingly constant arrangement. On each side of the midline two veins, the lateral and medial epidural veins, run longitudinally. At each vertebral level the left and right systems are joined by a midbody transverse anastomosis. At the level of each disc the pair of veins on both sides arc out toward the foramen. On each side, just cranial and just caudal to the disc, a superior and inferior foramenal vein join the epidural system to the ascending lumbar vein of the external vertebral plexus. In front of the lumbosacral disc, the arrangement of the veins is different and quite characteristic. The lateral epidural veins arc out more laterally than at the other levels and the medial veins assume an almost straight trajectory on the midline. At the sacral level the epidural veins are connected to the two main lateral sacral veins of the external plexus. The anterior external plexus lies in front of the vertebral body, disc, and anterior longitudinal ligament and communicates with the segmental veins, the left ascending lumbar vein, and when present, the right ascending lumbar vein. The posterior external venous plexuses are on the posterior surface of the lamina and around the spinous process, articular and transverse processes, and anastomose with the internal plexus and end in the segmental or lumbar veins (Fig. 3-15).

THE NERVE SUPPLY TO THE LUMBOSACRAL SPINE

The External Vertebral Nerve Supply

The periosteum and bone of the vertebrae are supplied by a multitude of small branches originating from the autonomic nervous system, paravertebral plexuses, and overlying muscles (Fig. 3-17B).[15–17]

One can find complex encapsulated endings and free nerve endings. They mediate pain and proprioception. Neither the nucleus pulposus nor the annulus fibrosus has a nerve supply except for the outermost layers of the annulus, which contain free nerve endings that probably mediate pain. The anterior longitudinal ligament is richly innervated by nerve fibers from the sympathetic system. The fibers overlap from side to side and from level to level.

The posterior elements are supplied by the medial branch of the posterior primary ramus (Fig. 3-17A). Anatomically, the anterior and posterior rami arise from the spinal nerve just as it exits the foramen where it gives a small direct branch to the facet joint.

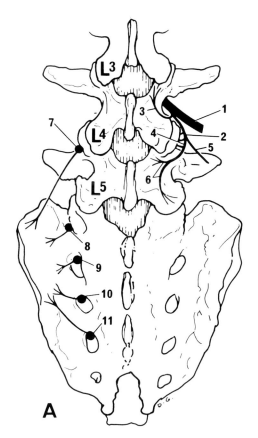

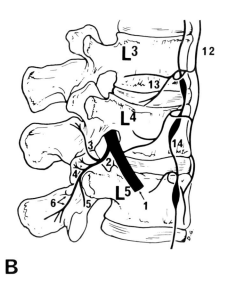

Fig. 3-17 Nerve supply to the lumbosacral spine viewed **(A)** from the back and **(B)** from the side: 1. anterior primary ramus; 2. posterior primary ramus with direct branches to facet; 3. ascending facet branch; 4. medial division of posterior primary ramus; 5. lateral division of posterior primary ramus; 6. descending facet branch; 7–11. direct branches from posterior primary rami (L4–S3) to posterior sacroiliac joint; 12. recurrent branches of gray ramus to anterior longitudinal ligament; 13. branches from gray ramus to disc; 14. sympathetic chain.

The anterior primary ramus will participate in the formation of the lumbar and sacral plexuses but also will give off a few nerve twigs to the adjacent annular fibers. The posterior primary ramus divides into medial and lateral branches just after it gives off an ascending facet branch to the posterior aspect of the joint immediately above. The lateral branch courses laterally on the transverse process and supplies the superficial spinal musculature. The medial branch courses medially and, as it exits through the intertransverse ligament, immediately crosses the superior aspect of the transverse process at its most medial edge and courses in a trough made of the superior process overhang and transverse process where it is firmly fixed by the mamillo-accessory ligament stretching across from the accessory process to the mamillary process.[18] It then hooks sharply medially then gently caudomedially where it ends in the deep musculature of the spine. In its course, as it emerges from under the ligament, it supplies the caudal aspect of the joint above and the rostral aspect of the one below. Therefore, each medial branch of the posterior primary ramus participates in the innervation of three joints.

The Sacroiliac Joint

The sacroiliac joint (Fig. 3–17A) gets its innervation from branches originating from the posterior primary ramus of L4, the posterior primary ramus of L5, and the posterior primary ramus of S1. Also some fine branches from S2 and sometimes S3 may contribute.

The Internal Vertebral Nerve Supply

The structures inside the spinal canal are subserved by the recurrent meningeal nerve (sinuvertebralis). Rarely a single nerve, it is usually composed of two to four nerve filaments originating from the anterior primary ramus just distal to its division. Each nerve filament receives one or more twigs from the neighboring gray ramus communicans or directly from the sympathetic ganglion. They return to the spinal canal through the intervertebral foramen, ventral to the dorsal root ganglion and cranial to the disc. Some

fine branches pass dorsal to the ganglion and are distributed to the dorsal dura, ligamentum flavum, and periosteum. The majority of the fibers remain anterior and divide into transverse, ascending, and descending branches spanning more than one level cranially and caudally. They anastomose freely from side to side and level to level. Some branches supply the periosteum of the vertebra and penetrate the body with the vascular supply. Other branches supply the anterior dura and root sleeves, posterior longitudinal ligament, outermost fibers of the annulus fibrosus, and surrounding soft tissues.

THE LUMBOSACRAL SPINE MUSCULATURE

The musculature governing the lumbosacral spine can be divided in four functional groups: the extensors, the flexors, the lateral flexors, and the rotators. Flexion and extension demand synergystic muscle action from both the left and right muscle groups.

The Extensors

The extensors are arranged in three layers. The most superficial layer (Fig. 3–18A) is made of the large fleshy sacrospinalis (erector spinae). It ascends from its attachments on the dorsal part of the iliac crest, the median and lateral sacral crests, and the spinous processes of the sacrum and lumbar spine. A single muscle in the lower lumbar spine, it progressively divides into three distinct columns as it reaches the upper lumbar spine, which from lateral to medial are iliocostalis, longissimus, and spinalis.

Just deep to the sacrospinalis lies the intermediate layer (Fig. 3–18B) made of multifidus. This three-layered fasciculated muscle originates on the sacrum from the laminar area just medial to the posterior sacral foramina, from the tendinous origins of sacrospinalis and the medial surface of the posterior and superior iliac spine. In the lumbar spine it originates from the mamillary processes. From its origin, each fasciculus is directed cranially and medially toward the inferior and medial margin of the lamina and adjacent spinous process. The superficial layer attaches from three to four levels above, the intermedi-

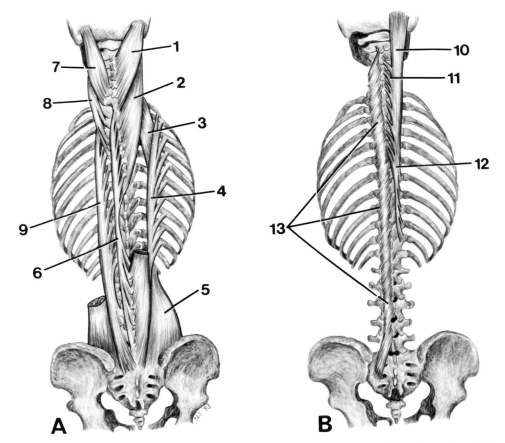

Fig. 3-18 Muscles of the spinal column. **(A)** Superficial layer and **(B)** intermediate layer: 1. splenius capitis; 2. splenius cervicis; 3. iliocostalis cervicis; 4. iliocostalis thoracis; 5. iliocostalis lumborum; 6. spinalis thoracis; 7. longissimus capitis; 8. longissimus cervicis; 9. longissimus thoracis; 10. semispinalis capitis (spinalis capitis is blended in this muscle); 11. semispinalis cervicis; 12. semispinalis thoracis; 13. multifidus. (Dupuis PR, Kirkaldy-Willis WH: The spine: integrated function and pathophysiology. In Cruess RL, Rennie WRJ (eds): Adult Orthopaedics. Churchill Livingstone, New York, 1984.)

ate layer two levels above and the deep layer, one level above. Multifidus acts both as an extensor and a rotator.

The deep layer of the extensors (Fig. 3-19) is made of a multitude of small muscles arranged from level to level. Interspinalis consists of short fasciculi attached between the spinous processes of contiguous vertebrae. Intertransversarius consists of two to three slips of muscles, a ventrolateral one that bridges adjacent transverse processes, a dorsolateral slip that bridges the accessory process of one vertebra to the transverse process of the other, and a medial slip that bridges the accessory process of one vertebra

with the mamillary process of the other. Rotatores lumborum are small irregular and variable muscles connecting the upper and posterior part of the transverse process of the vertebra below to the inferior and lateral border of the lamina of the vertebra above.

The Forward Flexors of the Lumbar Spine

Flexors of the lumbar spine can be divided into an iliothoracic (extrinsic) group and a femorospinal (intrinsic) group. The iliothoracic group is made of the abdominal wall muscles, rectus abdominus, obli-

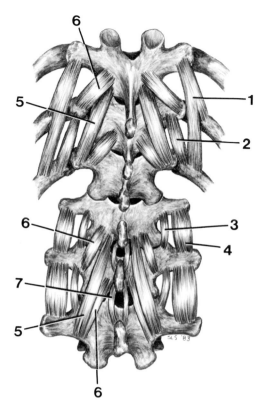

Fig. 3-19 Muscles of the spinal column at the thoracolumbar junction. The deep layer: 1. levator costarum longus; 2. levator costarum brevis; 3. intertransversarius medialis; 4. intertransversarius lateralis; 5. rotator longus; 6. rotator brevis; interspinalis. (Dupuis PR, Kirkaldy-Willis WH: The spine: integrated function and pathophysiology. In Cruess RL, Rennie WRJ (eds): Adult Orthopaedics. Churchill Livingstone, New York, 1984.)

quus externus, obliquus internus, and intertransversarius. The femorospinal group (Fig. 3-20) is made up of psoas major and iliacus muscles.

The Lateral Flexors of the Lumbar Spine

Pure lateral flexion, although possible, is not natural to the lumbar spine. It is normally a combination of side bending and rotation. Pure lateral bending can theoretically be achieved if the rotatory component of this coupled motion is neutralized by an antagonist group of muscles. Normally side bending is brought about by ipsilateral contraction of both obliquus abdominis, intertransversarius and quadratus

lumborum (Fig. 3-20). Of these only unilateral contraction of quadratus lumborum can bring about pure lateral flexion. Simultaneous contraction of both quadratus lumborum muscles will produce some extension of the lumbar spine.

The Lumbar Spine Rotators

Rotation of the lumbar spine is brought about by unilateral contraction of muscles that follow an oblique direction of pull; the more oblique the course the more important the rotational effect. Most of the extensors and lateral flexors follow an oblique course and produce rotation when their primary component has been neutralized by antagonist muscle groups.

THE CONTENTS OF THE LUMBAR SPINAL CANAL

The lumbar spinal canal contains, supports, and protects the distal part of the lumbar enlargement of the spinal cord proximally (the conus medullaris) and the cauda equina and spinal nerves distally. This part of the conus medullaris, which is within the boundaries of the lumbar spine, tapers out at the lower first or upper second lumbar vertebral level into a fine connective tissue filament, the filum terminale, which descends and attaches to the first coccygeal segment. This very lower part of the central nervous system is ensheathed in three meninges. The pia mater closely invests the conus medullaris and rootlets. The dura mater and pia arachnoid are separated from the pia mater by the subarachnoid space filled with cerebrospinal fluid. Pia arachnoid and dura mater are separated by a potential space called the subdural space. From the proximal lumbar spine, dura mater and pia arachnoid continue down and join with the filum terminale at the level of the distal border of the first or proximal border of the second sacral segment. Dura mater and pia arachnoid also ensheath the spinal nerves to their point of exit. At L1 the spinal nerves exit the dural sac almost at right angle. Their course within the nerve root canal is almost horizontal, and each spinal nerve is rather short. However, from there downward, the nerve roots exit the dura slightly more proximal than their foramenal exit point at each level, causing their course

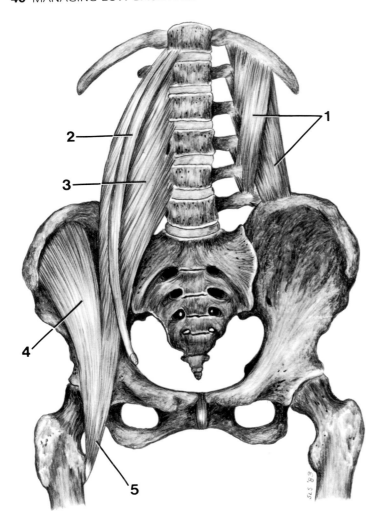

Fig. 3-20 Muscles of the spinal column. The intrinsic flexors of the lumbar spine: 1. two layers of quadratus lumborum; 2. psoas minor; 3. psoas major; 4. iliacus; 5. conjoined attachment of psoas and iliacus on and around the lesser femoral trochanter. (Dupuis PR, Kirkaldy-Willis WH: The spine: integrated function and pathophysiology. In Cruess RL, Rennie WRJ (eds): Adult Orthopaedics. Churchill Livingstone, New York, 1984.)

to be more and more oblique and their length to increase. This is more apparent with the fifth lumbar and first sacral nerve roots.

The dural sac, its contents, and the spinal nerves are not freely mobile structures. The dural sac within the spinal canal and nerve roots within the spinal and foramenal canals are stabilized by a series of ligamentous attachments that also define a specific range of motion for each. Spencer et al.[19] recently reviewed the literature and Hofmann's original description[20] on the fixation systems of the lumbosacral nerve roots and reported on the results of their spinal dissections. They describe three distinct arrangements of ligamentous fixation for the thecal sac and spinal nerves.

Dural Attachment Complex

The dural attachment complex (Figs. 3-21 and 3-22) is made of connective tissue bands or ligaments segmentally distributed along the lumbar spine with varied levels of development, at times absent. Three groups of ligaments are recognized. The first group extends from the anterior dura to the posterior longitudinal ligament (midline Hofmann ligament). The second group extends from the anterolateral dura to the lateral extension of the posterior longitudinal ligament (lateral Hofmann ligament). Finally, the third group extends from the dural extension of the proximal root sleeve to the posterior longitudinal ligament

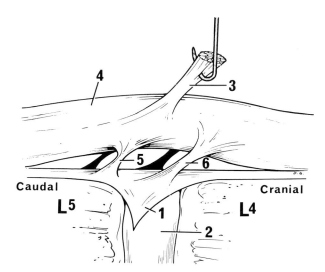

Fig. 3-21 Diagrammatic representation of the dural ligamentous complex (Hofmann): 1. posterior longitudinal ligament and lateral expansion; 2. annulus fibrosus; 3. transected lumbar nerve root retracted posteriorly and cranially; 4. lumbar dural sac; 5. midline dural ligament; 6. lateral dural ligament.

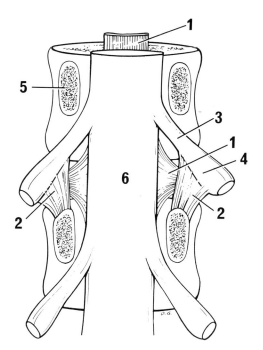

Fig. 3-22 Diagrammatic representation of the lateral root ligament: 1. posterior longitudinal ligament and lateral expansion; 2. lateral root ligament; 3. spinal nerve; 4. spinal ganglion; 5. pedicle; 6. lumbar dural sac.

and periosteum of the inferior pedicle (lateral root ligament).

Intraneural Complex

The intraneural complex is found within the dural sheath of the nerve roots.[21] The anterior and posterior rootlets are quite free within the dural sac and the short proximal dural root pouch at the point of exit from the thecal sac. At the bottom of this short pouch the nerve sleeve proper is formed and the rootlets enter independently a bitubular conduit lined by pia arachnoid, itself firmly attached to the dural sleeve. There, between the pia arachnoid and pia mater investing the rootlets in the vicinity of the dural rootlet ostea, strands of fibers are found to form a most solid dura-arachnoid-rootlet bond. At the level of the ganglion, the dural sleeve ends to form the fibrous sheath of the anterior primary ramus. Both the ganglion and primary ramus are firmly adherent to this sheath, which continues distally as the epineurium.

Foramenal Complex

The foramenal complex extends from lateral aspect of the ganglion as multiple filaments or bands of fibrous tissue originating from the sheath to the circumference of the foramen, sometimes in a spokelike fashion. Distinct extensions to the joint capsule and periosteum of the pedicles can often be identified.[19,21]

REFERENCES

1. Brash JC (ed): Cunningham's Textbook of Anatomy, 9th Ed. Oxford University Press, London, 1951
2. Warwick R, Williams PL (eds): Gray's Anatomy, 35th Ed. Longman, Edinburgh, 1973
3. Hollinshead EWH: Anatomy for Surgeons, 2nd Ed. Vol. 3. Harper & Row, New York, 1969
4. Bogduk N, Engel R: The menisci of the lumbar zygapophyseal joints: a review of their anatomy and clinical significance. Spine 9: 454, 1984
5. Engel R, Bogduk N: The menisci of the lumbar zygapophyseal joints. J Anat 135: 795, 1982
6. Gallois J, Japoit T: Architecture intérieure des vertèbres du point de vue statique et physiologique. Rev Chir (Paris) 63: 688, 1925
7. Kapanji IA: Physiologie articulaire. Tronc et rachis. Vol. 3. Maloîne, Paris, 1972

8. Bose K, Balasubramaniam P: Nerve root canals of the lumbar spine. Spine 9: 16, 1984

9. Crock HV: Normal and pathological anatomy of the lumbar spinal nerve root canals. J Bone Joint Surg 63B: 487, 1981

10. Crock HV, Yoshizawa H: The blood supply of the lumbar vertebral column. Clin Orthop 115: 6, 1976

11. Crock HV, Yoshizawa H: The Blood Supply of the Vertebral Column and Spinal Cord in Man. Springer-Verlag, New York, 1977

12. Théron J, Moret J: Anatomic radiology. p. 27. In Théron J, Moret J (eds): Spinal Phlebography. Springer-Verlag, Berlin, 1978

13. Théron J, Moret J: Technique, pitfalls, complications. p. 33. In Théron J, Moret J (eds): Spinal Phlebography. Springer-Verlag, Berlin, 1978

14. Wilkie R, Beetham R: Trans-femoral lumbar epidural venography. Spine 5: 424, 1980

15. Bogduk N: The innervation of the lumbar spine. Spine 8: 286, 1983

16. Edgar MA, Ghadially JA: Innervation of the lumbar spine. Clin Orthop 115: 35, 1976

17. Paris SV: Symposium on evaluation and care of lumbar spine problems: anatomy as related to function and pain. Orthop Clin N Am 14: 475, 1983

18. Bogduk N: The lumbar mamillo-accessory ligament. Spine 6: 162, 1981

19. Spencer DL, Irwin GL, Miller JAA: Anatomy and significance of fixation of the lumbosacral nerve roots in sciatica. Spine 8: 672, 1983

20. Hofmann M: Die Befestigung der Dura mater im Wirbelcanal. Arch F Anat Physio (Anat Abt): 403, 1899

21. Sunderland S: Meningeal-neural relations in the intervertebral foramen. J Neurosurg 40: 756, 1974

4

The Pathology and Pathogenesis of Low Back Pain

William H. Kirkaldy-Willis

Study of the etiology, pathogenesis, and pathology of low back pain helps physician and therapist to understand the nature of the process and to correlate it with the clinical picture. The knowledge thus gained makes an accurate and complete diagnosis possible and facilitates the formulation of a logical plan for treatment.

The necessary knowledge is acquired (1) by study of work done on myofascial syndromes by Travell and Simons[1] and (2) by study of autopsy specimens, correlating these findings with the clinical picture, stress radiographs, myelograms, CT images, and other laboratory tests.

This chapter will describe the role of muscle in low back pain and the changes seen sequentially in bone, joint, and adjacent soft tissues as the process of degeneration advances.

The initial cause of lumbar spine dysfunction must be found in pathophysiology. Function is altered, but structure is normal. We know much less about this than about the pathological and anatomical changes that are seen as the process of degeneration unfolds and progresses. The ways in which pathophysiology can be studied are clearly described in the book *Myofascial Pain and Dysfunction* by Travell and Simons.[1]

PATHOPHYSIOLOGY

Some understanding of lumbar spine dysfunction is almost certainly the most important step in elucidating the ways in which the process of degeneration starts. It is also the most difficult step. In this chapter less will be written about pathophysiology than about pathoanatomy simply because we know less about the former. Three aspects of the problem must be considered: (1) emotional factors, (2) changes in muscle, and (3) changes in the facet joints and intervertebral disc. Figure 4–1 presents an overall view of these factors.

Emotional Factors

The most common aspect pertains to tension, stress, anxiety, fear, resentment, and depression—emotions experienced by all of us at one time or another. Undoubtedly other factors such as repeated minor trauma come into play to localize the site of vascular change to be discussed later.

Review of case histories shows that patients who later develop low back pain have often been under stress before experiencing pain and that the episode of trauma resulting in pain is minor. Often an interval

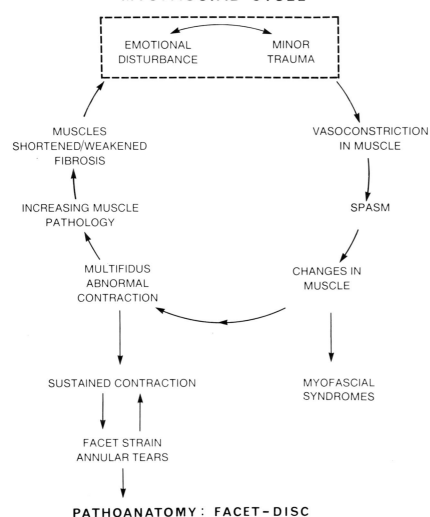

PATHOPHYSIOLOGY: OVERVIEW
MYOFASCIAL CYCLE

EMOTIONAL DISTURBANCE ⟷ MINOR TRAUMA

MUSCLES SHORTENED/WEAKENED FIBROSIS

VASOCONSTRICTION IN MUSCLE

INCREASING MUSCLE PATHOLOGY

SPASM

MULTIFIDUS ABNORMAL CONTRACTION

CHANGES IN MUSCLE

SUSTAINED CONTRACTION

MYOFASCIAL SYNDROMES

FACET STRAIN ANNULAR TEARS

PATHOANATOMY : FACET–DISC INTERACTION

Fig. 4-1 The pathophysiology of low back pain includes emotional factors, changes in muscle, and changes in the facet joints and intervertebral disc.

of several hours or days intevenes between the preceived episode of trauma and the onset of the pain. The writer has had three attacks of moderately severe low back pain over a period of 25 years. On no occasion was he aware of more than minimal trauma. On two occasions he had been under tension and stress. This parallels the experience of many people with low back pain.

We need also to consider injury to muscle and/or posterior facet joint as a possible initiating cause. The muscles activating an intervertebral joint or the joint itself may be responsible for the patient's symptoms.

Often both are involved. We do not know whether a strain to the joint comes first, followed by a contraction of muscle to protect the joint or whether the initiating factor is abnormal muscle function, which leads to a joint strain (Table 4-1, Fig. 4-2).

Table 4-1 Emotional Disturbances

Tension	Stress
Anxiety	Fear
Uncertainty	Resentment
Depression	

EMOTIONS AND TRAUMA

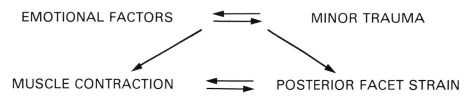

Fig. 4-2 The relationship between emotions and trauma in low back pain.

Vasoconstriction in Muscle

It is postulated that emotional disturbance acts through the autonomic nervous system to produce local areas of vasoconstriction in muscle. In one experiment where the thermocouple needle was inserted into a trigger point zone in muscle, the temperature was higher than that of the surrounding tissue.[1] After 15 to 60 sec the temperature fell to that of the adjacent tissue. This suggests that the trigger point zone is a region of increased metabolism and/or decreased circulation. In another experiment the rate at which radioactive sodium iodide was eliminated from a trigger point zone was measured and was found to be slower than that from normal tissue.[1] It was thought that this was a result of impaired local circulation, thus supporting the theory that vasoconstriction occurs in trigger point zones in muscle.

Changes in Muscle

Changes in trigger point zones in muscle have been recorded by several different investigators. Mielhke et al.* observed mild dystrophic changes in histological sections of these zones, variation in the width of muscle fibers, an increase in the number of nuclei, and an arrangement of nuclei in chains.[1] In a similar study Brendstrup et al.* noted a metachromatic staining of mucopolysaccharides. In ultramicroscopic studies Awad* observed the presence of giant sarcomeres, lipid droplets, and mast cells in trigger point zones. Fassbender* noted swelling of mitochondria and degeneration of the I and A bands in his electromicroscopy studies of these zones. Later, the contrac-

tile elements were replaced by a fine granular residue within the sarcolemma sheath. He considered these changes similar to those seen in ischemic muscle in the dog (Fig. 4-3).

Abnormal Contraction of Muscle

Vasoconstriction and sustained muscle contraction with accumulation of metabolites leads to muscle fatigue. This in turn leads to changes in the recruitment of motor units in an individual muscle and in muscle groups used for a particular movement. One result of these changes is an altered pattern of muscle contraction with sudden violent uncontrolled contractions of involuntary and other muscles (Fig. 4-4).

MULTIFIDUS

This rotator muscle of the lumbar spine is largely a postoral muscle, which is controlled in an involuntarily. It is commonly affected. Uncontrolled contractions produce torsional injury to facet joints and disc. Injury to these structures leads to reflex sustained contraction of the muscle. In other words, the multifidus myofascial syndrome is an integral part of the posterior joint or facet syndrome.

OTHER MYOFASCIAL SYNDROMES IN BACK AND LEG

These syndromes are commonly associated with low back and leg pain. Each of these may be a primary lesion or secondary to another type of lesion (e.g., disc herniation). They will be considered in detail in Chapter 10 (Table 4-2, Figs. 4-3 and 4-4).

---

*As cited in Ref. 1.

VASO CONSTRICTION IN MUSCLE

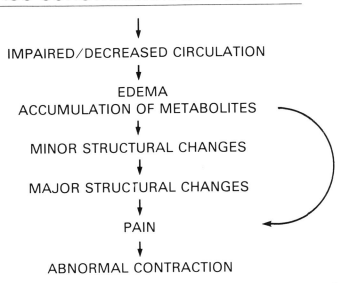

IMPAIRED/DECREASED CIRCULATION

EDEMA
ACCUMULATION OF METABOLITES

MINOR STRUCTURAL CHANGES

MAJOR STRUCTURAL CHANGES

PAIN

ABNORMAL CONTRACTION

Fig. 4-3 Flow chart demonstrating role of vasoconstriction in muscle in producing back pain.

ABNORMAL MUSCLE CONTRACTION

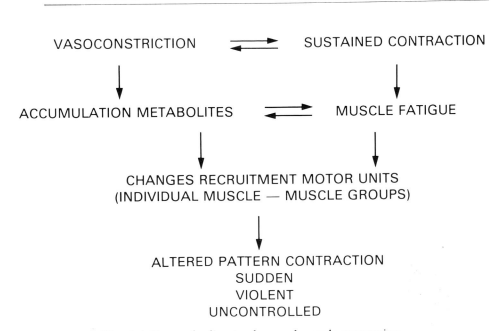

VASOCONSTRICTION ⇄ SUSTAINED CONTRACTION

ACCUMULATION METABOLITES ⇄ MUSCLE FATIGUE

CHANGES RECRUITMENT MOTOR UNITS
(INDIVIDUAL MUSCLE — MUSCLE GROUPS)

ALTERED PATTERN CONTRACTION
SUDDEN
VIOLENT
UNCONTROLLED

Fig. 4-4 Factors leading to abnormal muscle contraction.

Table 4-2 Myofascial Syndromes in the Back and Leg

Multifidus	Quadratus lumborum
Gluteus medius	Piriformis
Gluteus maximus	Tensor fasc. lat.
Hamstring	

MUSCLE SYNDROMES IN NECK AND SHOULDER GIRDLE

These syndromes also are important because they are involved in posture. Correct posture, so important for the function of the lumbar spine, is dependent on neck and shoulder girdle muscles as well as on the flexors and extensors of the spine and hip.

PROGRESSION OF THE LESION

Torsional injury, produced as previously described by contraction of multifidus, initiates lesions in the posterior facet joints and disc. Each recurrent strong contraction tends to cause further injury. In this way the process of degenerative change is initiated and continued to produce the pathological entities to be described in the remainder of this chapter. We need to remember that compression injury and a combination of rotation and compression are also factors in pathogenesis (Fig. 4-5).

Increasing Muscle Pathology

Janda[2] has described with great clarity the way in which certain muscles shorten as a result of the process just described and how other muscles become weakened. The flexors of the hip, external rotators of the hip, hamstring muscles, and spine extensors shorten.

Antagonistic muscles become weakened due to reciprocal inhibition. These include hip extensors, hip internal rotators, quadriceps, and spinal flexors—the abdominal muscles. The result of these long-term changes in muscle is that spinal movement becomes grossly restricted and painful, a restriction that is learned as well as structural from fibrosis (Fig. 4-6).

Further Emotional Disturbance

The combination of restriction of movement of the lumbar spine and pain on movement results in further emotional changes, depression becoming dominant in many patients. This is often called the chronic pain syndrome.

Summary

Much of pathophysiology is speculative at present. But it is a great help to have a theory on which to work. As our knowledge increases, it is often necessary to revise the theory. When, in a later chapter, we come to consider the role of the Spine Education Program we shall see that dealing with abnormalities of function is most important both in treating and preventing lumbar spine degeneration.

PATHOANATOMY

The Mechanism of Injury

Two different mechanisms are involved: rotational strains and compressive forces. Rotational strains affect mainly the L4–5 joint because of the alignment of the posterior facets and because the L5-S1 joint is often protected by the bony architecture and strong

POSTERIOR JOINT SYNDROME

Fig. 4-5 Contraction of the multifidus initiates posterior joint syndrome.

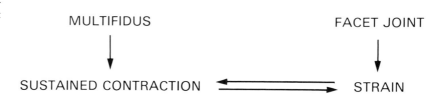

CONTINUING PATHOLOGY
IN MUSCLE

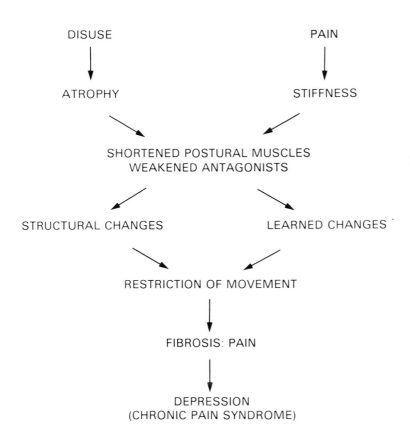

Fig. 4-6 Continuing pathology in muscle. Long-term changes in muscle results in painful, restricted movement as well as depression.

ligaments, thus causing rotational stresses to fall on the L4–5 joint. Compressive forces such as falls onto the buttocks most commonly affect the L5-S1 joint because it is often protected and because the disc is wedgeshaped. Rotational stresses lead to changes in both posterior joints and disc. Compressive forces affect the disc first and changes are not seen in the posterior joints until a later stage.

The Level at Risk

The earliest changes are seen in the L4–5 joint in approximately two thirds of patients and in the L5-S1 joint in the remaining third. The L5-S1 joint is often protected because it is seated deep in the pelvis and because the L5 transverse processes are large,

with short, strong ligaments connecting them to the ilium.

The Three-Joint Complex

At any one level the intervertebral joint is made up of three parts, formed by two posterior facet joints and a disc. Changes affecting the posterior joints also affect the disc and vice versa. The rotational stresses mentioned above most often result in injury to all three parts. They will be described below. Compressive forces usually result in fractures of the cartilage plates of the disc; these are followed by slow degeneration of the disc and resultant stress on the posterior joints at a later date. They may also cause the annulus to rupture explosively at its insertion into the vertebral body bone.

Three Phases in the Degenerative Process

The spectrum of degenerative change in an intervertebral joint can be divided into three phases: dysfunction, instability (the unstable phase), and stabilization (Fig. 4-7). In phase I, normal function of the three-part complex is interrupted as the result of injury. Examination of the patient reveals that on one or other side of the spine at either L4–5 or L5-S1 the segmental posterior muscles are in a state of hypertonic contraction. Normal movement is restricted in one or other direction. In Phase II, examination of the patient demonstrates the presence of abnormal increased movement. Laxity of the posterior joint capsule and of the annulus fibrosus is seen in autopsy specimens. As degenerative changes become advanced (Phase III) the unstable segment regains its stability because fibrosis is present and osteophytes form around the posterior joints and within and around the disc.

Changes in the Posterior Facet Joints

The changes that occur in the posterior facet joints (Figs. 4-8 and 4-9) are the same as those seen in any diarthrodial joint. The earliest change is *synovitis,* which may persist with the formation of a *synovial fold* that projects into the joint between the cartilage

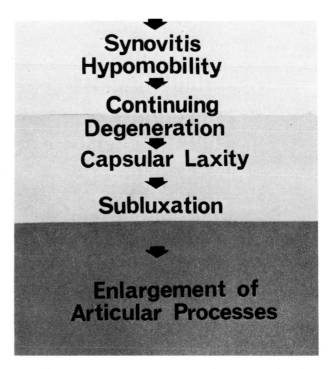

Fig. 4-8 Progressive degenerative changes in the facet joints. The three phases are colored as in Figure 4-7.

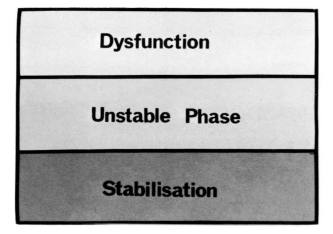

Fig. 4-7 The three phases of the degenerative process. Dysfunction, pale gray; unstable phase, darker shade; stabilization, darkest shade.

surfaces. Later on minimal *degeneration of articular cartilages* occurs and this gradually but increasingly becomes more marked. Sometimes an *intra-articular adhesion* is seen passing from one articular surface to the other. Still later *the capsule becomes lax.* Increasing laxity allows *subluxation* of the joint surfaces to occur. Continuing degeneration (due to repeated rotational strains) results in the formation of subperiosteal osteophytes. These produce *enlargement of both the inferior and the superior facets.* The end result is that the joints become grossly degenerated with almost complete loss of articular cartilage, the formation of bulbous facets (due to subperiosteal new bone formation), and marked periarticular fibrosis. This, together with similar changes in the disc, produces a stable segment with much reduced movement.

The progressive changes are shown in Figure 4-8. It will be appreciated that the early changes occur during Phase I, intermediate changes during Phase II and late changes during Phase III. For simplicity the three phases are shown in horizontal blocks of different shades of gray. In fact there is a gradual

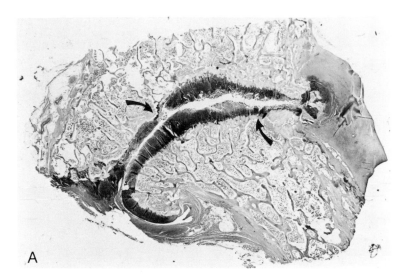

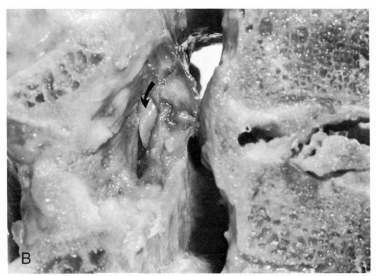

Fig. 4-9 Pathological changes in the facet joints. **(A)** Histological section. The inferior facet (below) shows thinning of cartilage and crevice formation (arrow); the superior facet (above) shows thinning of cartilage at each end of the section and erosion in the center (arrow). **(B)** Macroscopic parasagittal section. A large synovial tag is present in the upper part of the posterior facet (arrow). **(C)** Histological section. Marked subluxation of the dark staining cartilage surfaces and a large intra-articular synovial fold (arrow) are present. (*Figure continues.*)

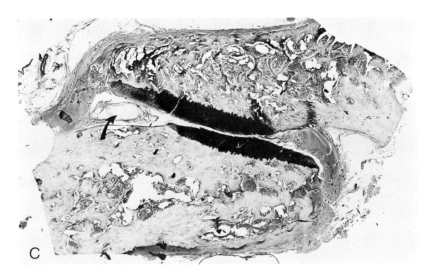

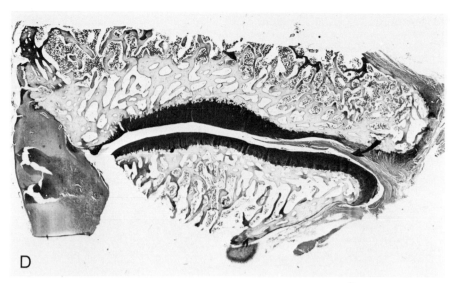

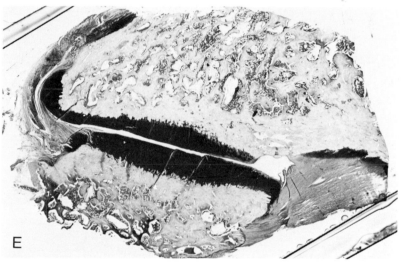

Fig. 4-9 (*Continued*). **(D)** Histological section. Note the long fibrous fold between the cartilage surfaces (arrow). **(E)** Histological section. The dark staining cartilage surfaces are markedly subluxated. **(F)** Histological section demonstrating capsular laxity and instability. A large space that extends deep to the lax capsule is present on the left (arrow). (*Figure continues.*)

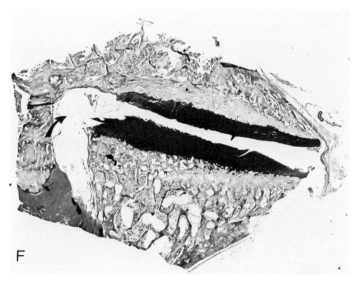

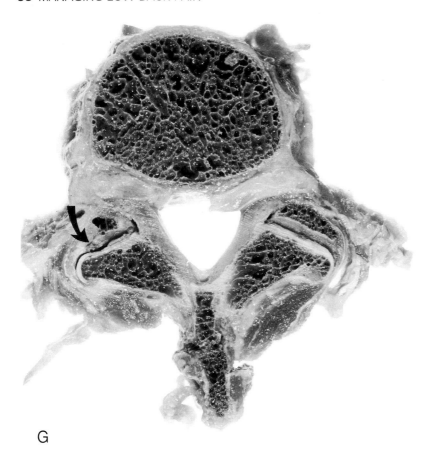

G

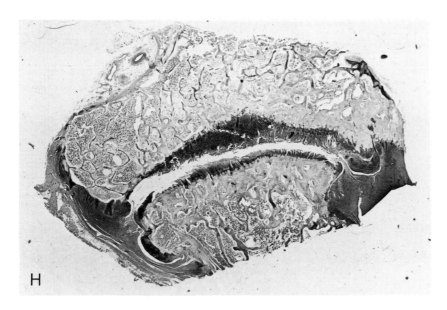

H

Fig. 4-9 (*Continued*). **(G)** Macroscopic transverse section at L5-S1. Marked degeneration of the facet joint is present on the left; the articular cartilage is thin and irregular (arrow); the facet joint on the right is normal. **(H)** Histological section. The superior articular facet (upper picture) is enlarged; marked degeneration is present on both cartilage surfaces. (Fig. F from Cassidy JD, Potter GE: Motion examination of the lumbar spine. Manipulative Physiol Therapeut 2:151, 1979.)

transition from Phase I to II and from II to III. These changes are illustrated in Figure 4-9A–H.

Changes in the Intervertebral Disc

Figure 4-10 schematizes the sequence of changes seen in the disc and demonstrates the phases during which they occur. Here again there is no hard and fast delineation between Phases I and II or Phases II and III.

Recurrent rotational strains produce first a number of small *circumferential tears* in the annulus fibrosus. Later on these become larger and coalesce to form *radial tears* that pass from the annulus into the nucleus pulposus. At a still later stage these tears increase further in size until the disc is completely disrupted internally. The large tear now passes from front to back and side to side of the disc. The normal disc height is greatly reduced because of loss of proteoglycans and water from the nucleus. The annulus becomes lax and bulges right around the circumference of the disc. This generalized bulge must be distinguished from a disc herniation, which is a local protrusion. With further degeneration and loss of disc con-

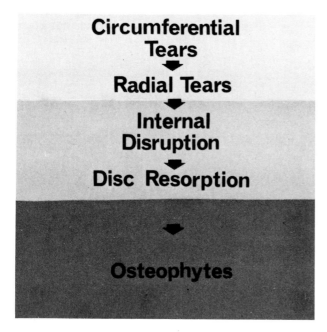

Fig. 4-10 Progressive degenerative changes in the disc. The three phases are colored as above.

tents the disc space is represented by a thin slit between the vertebral bodies filled with fibrous tissue. Vertebral body bone on either side of the disc is dense and sclerotic. This condition is called *disc resorption*. Finally, the disc is anchored by peripheral osteophytes that pass around its circumference. Occasionally the end result is bony ankylosis. The changes described above are shown in Figure 4-11A–F.

The Interaction of Changes in Facet Joints and Disc

In some patients the changes seen during the course of the progressive degenerative process affect mainly the facet joints. In others they affect mainly the disc. More commonly the whole three-joint complex at L4–5 or at L5-S1 is affected; posterior joint changes produce a reaction on the disc and vice versa.

The process of change is illustrated in Figure 4-12. The light gray upper horizontal bar represents dysfunction, the darker middle bar the unstable phase, and the darkest lower bar stabilization. The vertical column on the left shows changes in the facet joints, the right column changes in the disc, and the center column the interaction of changes in the component parts of the complex.

The earliest changes—synovitis and minor strains in the facet joints (with hypomobility) together with minor rotational strains of the annulus leading to the formation of circumferential tears—produce a state of dysfunction. As this dysfunction becomes more severe, leading to the formation of radial tears in the annulus, a localized bulging or protrusion of the annulus that is called a disc herniation may occur, often caused by relatively minor further trauma. The disc contents protrude into the spinal canal. The tear in the annulus may be complete, with the disc contents extruded into the canal. As seen in Figure 4-13, disc herniation occurs most commonly at the end of Phase I or at the beginning of Phase II, but it may occur during Phase III as well. Continuing degeneration that produces capsular laxity of the posterior joints and causes internal disruption of the disc results in segmental instability (Phase II). This phase is characterized by *abnormal increased movement* of the spinal segment, as opposed to *the abnormal decreased movement* found during dysfunction (Phase I).

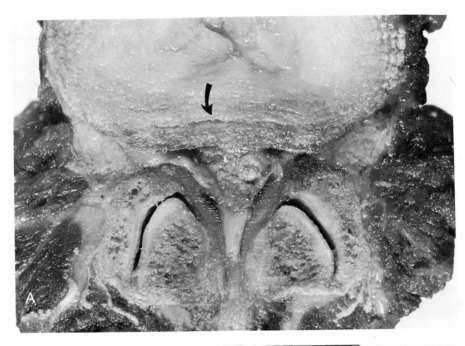

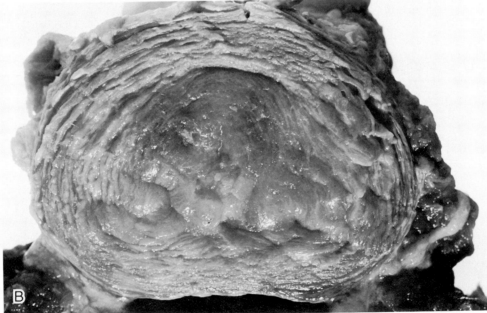

Fig. 4-11 Pathological changes in the disc. **(A)** Macroscopic transverse section at L4–5. Part of the disc is shown above and the facet joints are shown below. A transverse circumferential tear is seen in the annulus fibrosus (arrow). **(B)** Macroscopic transverse section at L4–5 to show the whole disc. Numerous circumferential tears are visible, especially in the upper part of the picture. (*Figure continues.*)

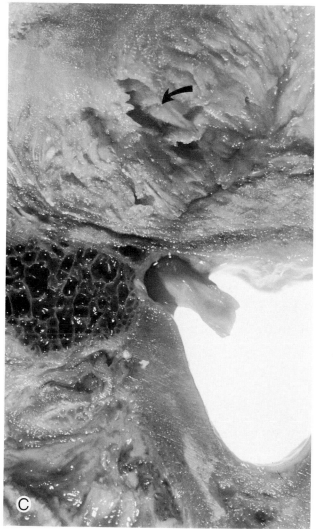

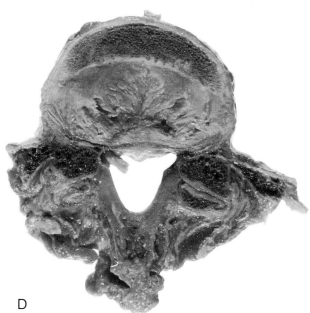

Fig. 4-11 (*Continued*). **(C)** Macroscopic transverse section at L4–5 showing part of the disc (above). The arrow points to one large radial tear. **(D)** Macroscopic transverse section at L4–5. Several radial tears are coalescing; early signs of internal disruption are present. (*Figure continues.*)

LATERAL SPINE NERVE ENTRAPMENT

Lateral spinal nerve entrapment, a relatively common lesion, is seen either late in Phase II or early in Phase III; that is, sometimes we encounter this type of nerve entrapment when the spine is unstable and on other occasions when it is again stabilized (see Fig. 4-12).

The nerve canal is shown in diagrammatic form in Figure 4-13D. It extends from the dura to the foramen. The lateral part of this canal, in which lateral nerve entrapment takes place, runs from the medial edge of the superior facet to the foramen.

Lateral Entrapment with Instability

As previously described and shown in Figure 4-14, the capsule of the posterior facets is lax and permits subluxation of these joints to occur. In the disc internal disruption results in loss both of height and stability,

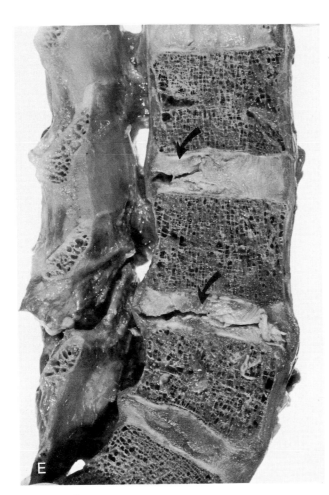
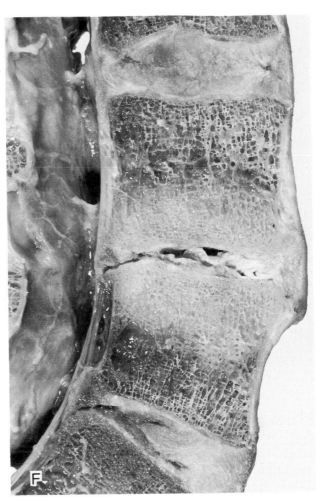

Fig. 4-11 (*Continued*). **(E)** Macroscopic sagittal section of the lumbar spine. The upper arrow points to a disc showing early internal disruption; the lower arrow points to a disc characterized by severe internal disruption. **(F)** Macroscopic sagittal section of the lumbar spine. The central disc demonstrates marked resorption; the disc itself is a narrow slit; vertebral body bone on either side is sclerotic. (Fig. F from Kirkaldy-Willis WH, Wedge JH, Yong-Hing K, Reilly J: Pathology and pathogenesis of lumbar spondylosis and stenosis. Spine 3:323, 1978.)

with annular bulging. The sequelae of loss of disc height are fourfold: subluxation of the facet joints; upward and forward displacement of the superior on the inferior facets; diminution in size of the intervertebral foramen; and, even more important, narrowing of the lateral canal medial to the foramen.

The way in which the foramen is diminished in size is shown in Figure 4-13E. The two vertebrae in the upper picture are positioned to demonstrate normal alignment of the facet, a normal disc height, and a normal foramen. In the lower picture the verte-

brae have been approximated to simulate loss of disc height, subluxation of facets, and narrowing of the intervertebral foramen. In the presence of instability the lax facet capsule allows the superior facet to move backward and forward with rotation. This is illustrated in Figures 4-14A and B. In Figure 4-14A, a sagittal section of an autopsy specimen, the posterior joint at L4–5 is markedly eroded and the capsule appears to be very lax. Note the distance between the anterior aspect of the superior facet and the posterior surface of the annulus. This is the lateral canal. In

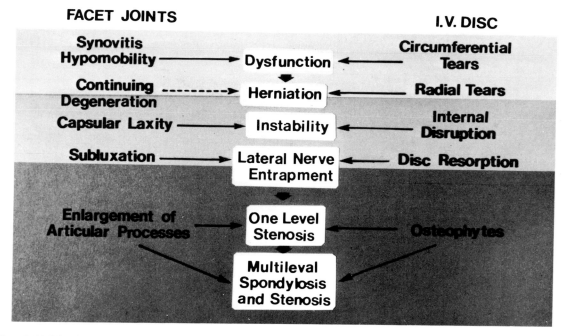

FACET JOINTS **I.V. DISC**

Synovitis Hypomobility → Dysfunction ← Circumferential Tears

Continuing Degeneration ⟶ Herniation ← Radial Tears

Capsular Laxity → Instability ← Internal Disruption

Subluxation → Lateral Nerve Entrapment ← Disc Resorption

Enlargement of Articular Processes → One Level Stenosis ← Osteophytes

Multileval Spondylosis and Stenosis

Fig. 4-12 The interaction of facet joint and disc changes. Changes in the facet joints appear on the left and changes in the disc on the right. Lesions that occur as a result of the interaction of these changes are seen in the center.

Figure 4-14B, from the same specimen, the spinous process of L5 has been rotated; the superior facet has moved anteriorly; the joint space has opened; the anterior aspect of the superior facet is now almost touching the annulus; and the lateral canal is markedly narrowed. The same phenomena are shown in cross section in Figure 4-14C and D. In this kind of entrapment, each time that rotation occurs between L4 and L5 the superior facet impinges on the spinal nerve in the lateral canal. We can thus call this lesion a recurrent dynamic entrapment. Abnormal flexion-extension movement can produce the same effect. As will be seen in Chapter 10 this type of lesion can be demonstrated by the CT scan.

Lateral Entrapment with a Fixed Deformity

Fixed-deformity lateral entrapment occurs in a similar way to that described above. It is encountered during Phase III at a point when the degenerative changes are sufficiently advanced to stabilize the affected segment (Fig. 4-15A). Little or no movement takes place at the affected level. Thus the narrowing

of the lateral canal is fixed because of a permanent deformity. Two factors are involved in producing the entrapment: subluxation of posterior facets, which allows the superior facet to move upward and forward (Fig. 4-15E), and enlargement of this facet by osteophytes, which further narrows the lateral canal (Figs 4-15A and B). The importance of lateral entrapment will be seen when we consider diagnosis and treatment.

CENTRAL STENOSIS

At One Level

Stenosis is encountered mainly at the L4–5 level but also occurs at the L3–4, L5–S1, and other levels. The pathogenesis of this lesion is similar to that of lateral entrapment (lateral stenosis). Narrowing of the central spinal canal is produced mainly by osteophytic enlargement of the two inferior facets, but the superior facets may also contribute. Central stenosis and lateral stenosis may occur as separate entities. They may also be combined. Central stenosis may

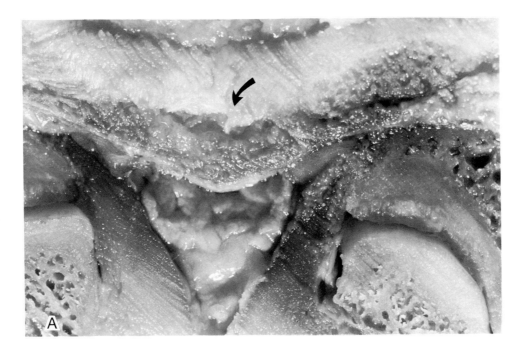

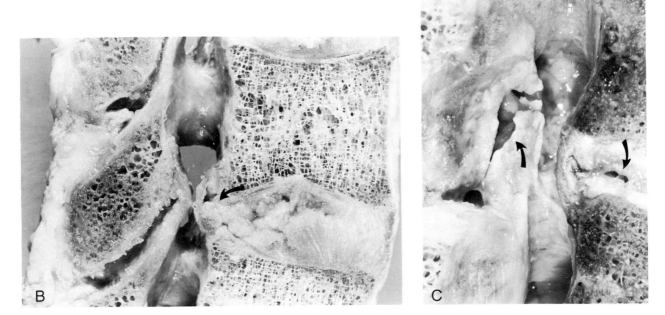

Fig. 4-13 Lesions occurring as a result of the interaction of changes in facets and disc. **(A)** Macroscopic transverse section at L5-S1. The arrow points to a large central disc herniation. **(B)** Macroscopic sagittal section at the L4–5 level demonstrates the presence of a large disc herniation (the arrow), which has ruptured into the spinal canal. **(C)** Macroscopic sagittal section of facet joint and posterior disc at L4–5 demonstrates the presence of instability, the result of marked degeneration of the facet joint (left arrow) and of internal disruption of the disc (right arrow).

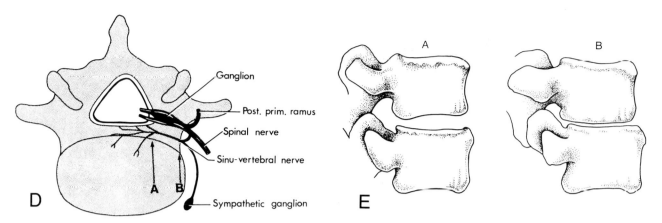

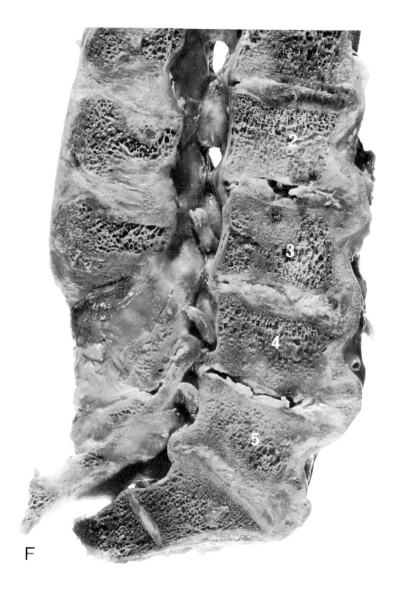

Fig. 4-13 (*Continued*). **(D)** Diagram of transverse section of the lumbar spine. The lateral part of the nerve canal—the site of lateral nerve entrapment—is between the two arrows. **(E)** Drawings of two vertebrae. A shows a normal disc. Note the size of the foramen. B shows marked reduction of disc height, retrospondylolisthesis of the upper on the lower vertebra, subluxation of posterior facets and reduction in size of the foramen. **(F)** Macroscopic sagittal section of the lumbar spine showing degenerative changes at several levels. The L1–2 disc is normal. The L2–3 disc shows marked internal disruption. The L3–4 disc shows early disruption. The L4–5 joint demonstrates very marked disruption. The L5–S1 disc shows resorption. There is marked encroachment on the central canal at the lowest three levels. (Fig. C from Kirkaldy-Willis, Wedge JH, Yong-Hing K, Reilly J: Pathology and pathogenesis of lumbar spondylosis and stenosis. Spine 3:319, 1978.)

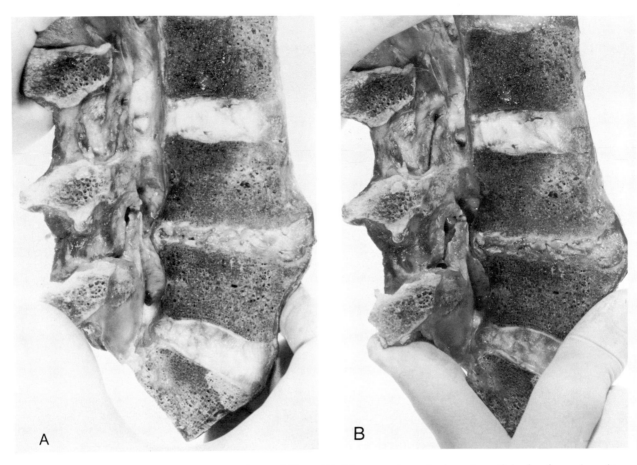

Fig. 4-14 Dynamic lateral stenosis with instability. **(A)** Macroscopic sagittal section of the lumbar spine. At the L4–5 level there is erosion of the facet joint and internal disruption of the disc. This joint complex is unstable. Note the size of the lateral canal between the anterior surface of the superior facet and the posterior aspect of the disc. **(B)** The same specimen. The spinous process of L5 has been rotated toward the observer. The facet joint has opened, the superior facet has rotated toward the back of the disc, and the lateral canal has become narrow.

be seen during Phase II in an unstable spine. It occurs more commonly during Phase III, when the spine is again stabilized as shown in Figure 4-12. The cauda equina and its blood vessels are often compromised to a greater extent than individual spinal nerves.

Spread of Changes to Affect Several Levels

In the early stages the lesion is confined to one level, as stated previously, but later on the degenerative process spreads to involve several levels. The way in which this takes place is not well understood. It is thought that either increased or decreased movement at one level predisposes to strains at levels above and below this. Some experimental work supports this view. In Figure 4-15F, a longitudinal sagittal section of an autopsy specimen obtained many years after a successful posterior fusion from L3 to the sacrum, the discs below the site of fusion are normal. At L2–3, just above the top of the fusion, the posterior joints are markedly degenerate and the disc is disrupted internally. The stiffness produced by the fusion from L3 to the sacrum protects this area and subsequent strains affect the L2–3 level, with resultant spondylosis and stenosis at this level. Involvment of a second and then of subsequent levels first produces the changes seen in Phase I, progresses to Phase II,

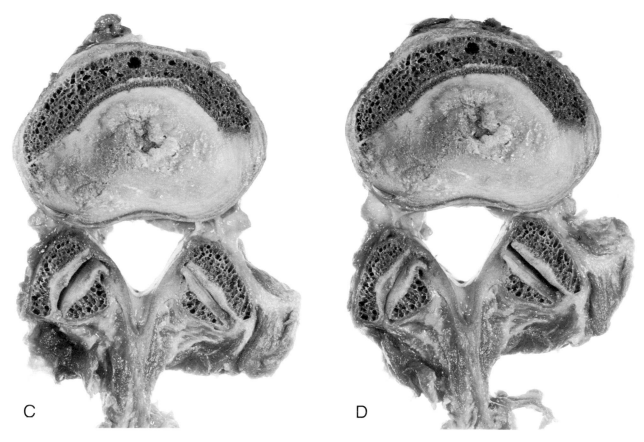

C   D

Fig. 4-14 (*Continued*). **(C)** Macroscopic transverse section at L4–5 demonstrates the effect of instability on the lateral canals. Rotation has opened the left facet joint; the left superior facet has shifted toward the back of the disc, the left lateral canal is narrow. **(D)** The same specimen. Rotation in the opposite direction has opened the right posterior joint; the right superior facet has moved toward the back of the disc; the right lateral canal is narrow. (Figs. A, B from Reilly J, Yong-Hing K, MacKay RW, Kirkaldy-Willis WH: Pathological anatomy of the lumbar spine. In Helfet AJ, Gruebel-Lee DM (eds): Disorders of the Lumbar Spine. JB Lipincott, Philadelphia, 1978.)

and in the end reaches Phase III. In some cases the whole lumbar spine becomes spondylotic, and stenosis—both central and lateral—may be present at several levels. Frequently some degree of scoliosis with a rotational element is present.

Developmental Stenosis

Abnormal development of the spine during the growth years frequently results in a central canal that is smaller than normal. This may involve one segment, one part, or all of the lumbar spinal canal. The coronal or sagittal diameter or both may be affected. A severe form of this abnormality is seen in achondroplasia. More commonly the cause of the narrowing is unknown. Figures 4-15C and D demonstrate one type of developmental stenosis. Of itself this change does not produce symptoms. Together with a small disc herniation or minor degenerative stenosis severe symptoms may result. Thus developmental stenosis is regarded as an enhancing factor.

Lesions That Act Directly to Produce Stenosis

Certain lesions can produce stenosis in a direct way without degenerative or developmental narrowing of the central or lateral spinal canals. Stenosis may

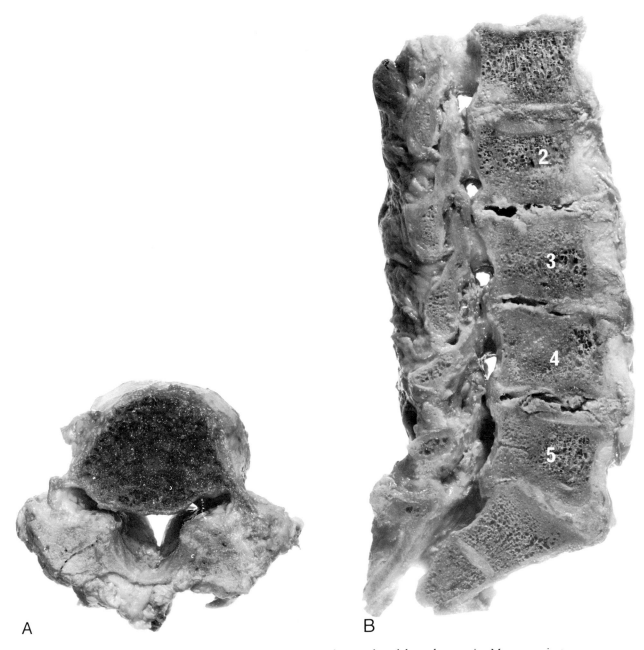

A

B

Fig. 4-15 Other lesions in the lumbar spine. **(A)** Fixed central and lateral stenosis. Macroscopic transverse section at L5-S1 demonstrates fixed central and lateral stenosis seen in phase III (stabilization). The central canal is markedly narrowed by enlarged inferior facets; the right lateral canal is narrow because of facet subluxation; the left lateral canal is very narrow from both subluxation and osteophyte formation. **(B)** Multilevel stenosis. Macroscopic sagittal section of lumbar spine shows internally disrupted discs at the L2–3, L3–4, and L4–5 levels and resorption at the L5-S1 level, with retrospondylolisthesis of L5 on S1. The lateral canals are narrow at every level. (*Figure continues.*)

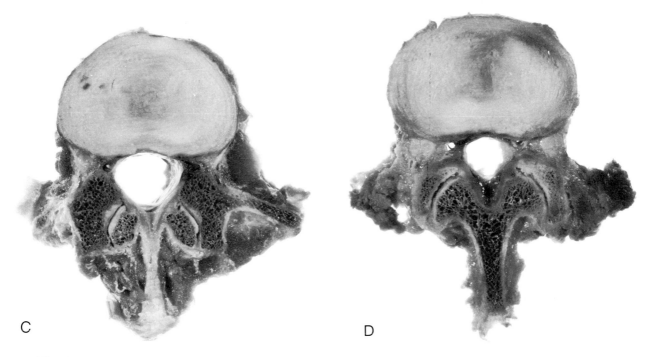

C   D

Fig. 4-15 (*Continued*). **(C)** Development stenosis. In macroscopic transverse section at L3–4, note the size of the normal central canal. **(D)** The same specimen at L4–5. At this level the central canal is small, segmental developmental stenosis has occurred. (*Figure continues.*)

be produced by a *vertebral body fracture*. Late changes following fracture may result in narrowing the canal (Fig. 4-15E). In *degenerative spondylolisthesis,* commonly seen at the L4–5 level, the L5 spinal nerve may be entrapped between the inferior articular facet of L4 (which has slipped forward) and the back of the body of L5. (Fig. 4-16A). In *isthmic spondylolisthesis* at the L5-S1 level the L5 nerve may entrapped by the pars interarticularis just cranial to the fracture (Fig. 4-16B). *Following laminectomy* fibrous tissue scarring may compress the dura and cauda equina or involve spinal nerves. *Fusion operations* may result in stenosis. Most frequently stenosis is caused by continuing degenerative changes at the cranial end of the fusion, but hypertrophic new bone formation underneath the fusion may narrow the spinal canal (Fig. 4-15F). In *Paget's disease* enlargement of a vertebral body may cause stenosis. In *fluorosis,* commonly encountered in some parts of India, new bone formation within the spinal canal may compromise the cauda equina.

A Combination of Factors

Nerve entrapment may be caused by only one of the lesions discussed above, but quite often two or more causes operate together to have a more pronounced effect. Three examples are disc herniation with degenerative stenosis, disc herniation with developmental stenosis, and disc herniation with both degenerative and developmental stenosis.

Venous Hypertension

Throughout this chapter we have been concerned mainly with the way in which one or another kind of lesion causes pain by entrapping spinal nerves and those of the cauda equina. Previous authors have demonstrated experimentally that degenerative changes in the spine are often accompanied by venous hypertension in bone adjacent to a joint. Such hypertension may produce pain by causing pressure on small nerves in bone, annulus fibrosus, or ligaments. It may inter-

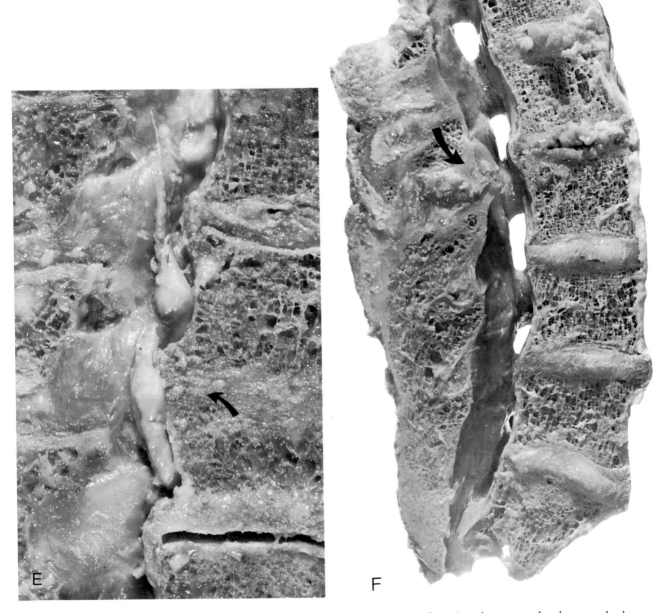

Fig. 4–15 (*Continued*). **(E)** Post–traumatic stenosis. Macroscopic sagittal section shows two lumbar vertebral bodies that are fused as a result of previous trauma with fracture. New bone formation at the site of the fusion has narrowed the central canal (arrow). **(F)** Postfusion stenosis. Microscopic sagittal section of a lumbar spine with a posterior fusion done 20 years previously. A solid posterior mass of bone is present from L3 to the sacrum. The discs in front are well preserved. At the L2–3 level the disc is disrupted and the posterior facet joints are enlarged to produce central stenosis (arrow). (Figs. C and D from Kirkaldy-Willis WH, Heithoff KB, Bowen CVA, Shannon R: Pathological anatomy of lumbar spondylosis and stenosis correlated with the CT scan. In Post MJD (ed): Radiographic Evaluation of the Spine. © 1980 Masson Publishing USA Inc., New York. Fig. F from Kirkaldy-Willis WH, Wedge JH, Yong-Hing K, Reilly J: Pathology and pathogenesis of lumbar spondylosis and stenosis. Spine 3:319, 1978.)

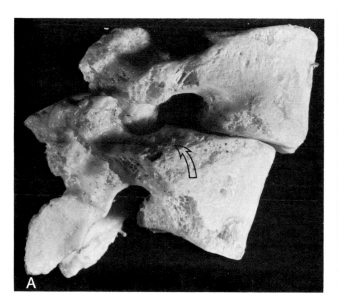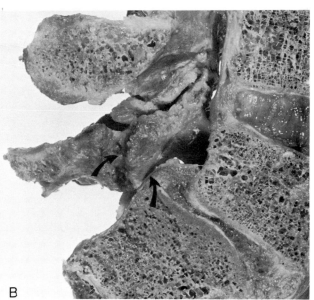

Fig. 4-16 Spondylolisthesis and other lesions. **(A)** Degenerative spondylolisthesis. The upper vertebra (L4) has slipped forward on the lower (L5). The inferior facet of L4 is almost touching the back of the body of L5 (arrow) and the L5 nerve is entrapped at this level. (Specimen courtesy H. F. Farfan, M.D.) **(B)** Isthmic spondylolisthesis. In macroscopic sagittal section of lumbosacral spine, the defect in the pars interarticularis is clearly seen (left arrow). The L5 nerve is entrapped between the back of the sacrum and the bone of the pars just above the defect (left arrow). (*Figure continues.*)

fere with the circulation of the spinal nerves or those of the cauda equina. The bizarre sensations in the legs of a patient with spinal stenosis may be due in part to venous hypertension.

An Overall View

The whole picture of degenerative changes, the effect of developmental stenosis, and the effects of direct factors is shown in Figure 4-17. This demonstrates the way in which an enhancing factor—developmental stenosis—may accentuate the degenerative process and the way in which spondylolisthesis, trauma, Paget's disease, fluorosis and fusion may produce one-level or multilevel spinal stenosis.

Summary

The pathology and pathogenesis of degenerative and other lesions in the lumbar spine are viewed in an overall perspective. This has two components: (1) three horizontal bars demonstrating the three phases—dysfunction, the unstable phase, and stabilization (Fig. 4-1)—and (2) three vertical columns setting out changes in the facets and in the disc, and the interaction of these two (Fig. 4-12). A composite picture is obtained by superimposing (1) on (2). This way of looking at changes in the lumbar spine will be employed again in later chapters as we consider diagnosis, prognosis, and treatment.

THE SACROILIAC JOINT: A GREAT ENIGMA

The Joint

The sacroiliac joint is a synovial joint. The articular cartilage on the sacrum is more than twice as thick as that on the ilium. The former is hyaline and the latter is fibrocartilage. The joint has a thick capsule with strong ligaments anteriorly and posteriorly, reinforced by the sacrotuberous and sacrospinous ligaments and by a massive ligament that passes from

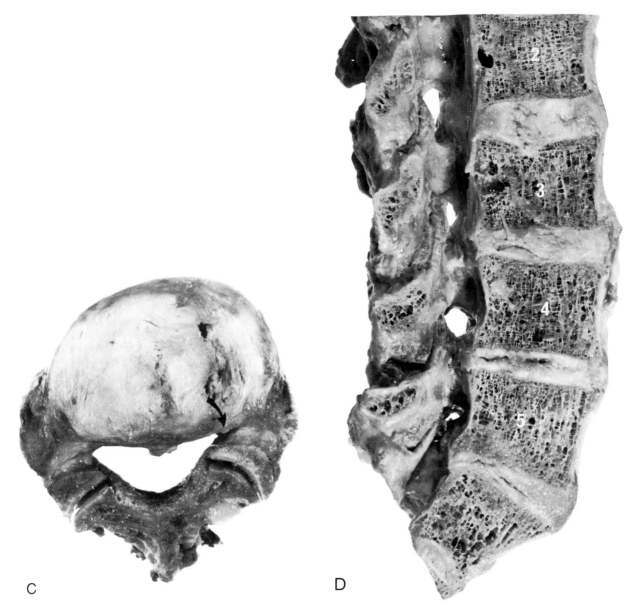

C   D

Fig. 4-16 *(Continued).* **(C)** Lesion of unknown origin. In macroscopic transverse section at the level of the L5-S1 disc, the vertebral body is asymmetrical in shape. The pedicle on the right (arrow) is shorter than that on the left. The left lamina is shorter than the right lamina. The changes may be developmental or may result from rotational trauma to the neural arch. **(D)** Sequential changes in the lumbar spine. Macroscopic sagittal section demonstrates an old fracture of the upper cartilage plate of L3 with herniation of the L2–3 nucleus pulposus into the body of L3 (a Schmorl's node). Early disc disruption is present at L3–4, and marked disruption at L4–5. At L5-S1 the disc has been resorbed. The L2–3, L3–4, and L5-S1 foramina are small. (Fig. A from Farfan HF, Reilly J, Yong-Hing K, et al: Pathological anatomy of the lumbar spine. In Helfet AJ, Gruebel-Lee DM (eds): Disorders of the Lumbar Spine. JB Lippincott, Philadelphia, 1978. Fig. C from Kirkaldy-Willis WH, Heithoff KB, Bowen CVA, Shannon R: Pathological anatomy of lumbar spondylosis and stenosis correlated with the CT Scan. In Post MJD: Radiographic Evaluation of the Spine. © 1980 Masson Publishing USA Inc., New York.)

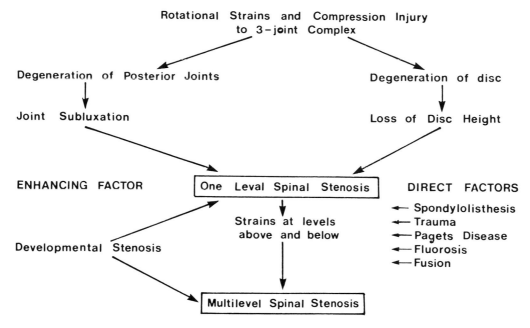

Rotational Strains and Compression Injury
to 3-joint Complex

Degeneration of Posterior Joints   Degeneration of disc

Joint Subluxation   Loss of Disc Height

ENHANCING FACTOR   One Leval Spinal Stenosis   DIRECT FACTORS

◄— Spondylolisthesis
◄— Trauma
Strains at levels   ◄—Pagets Disease
above and below   ◄—Fluorosis

Developmental Stenosis   ◄—Fusion

Multilevel Spinal Stenosis

Fig. 4-17 Diagrammatic demonstration of how the enhancing factor (developmental stenosis) and direct factors (spondylolisthesis, trauma, Paget's disease, fluorosis, and spinal fusion) can cause spinal stenosis or supplement any underlying degenerative change.

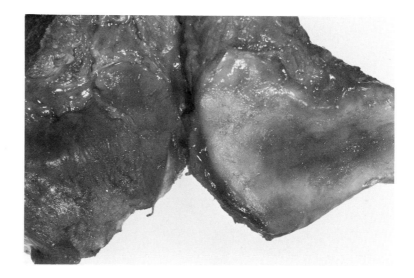

Fig. 4-18 A sacroiliac joint opened like a clam shell. On the right the glistening hyaline carti- lage covering the sacrum. On the left the dull fibrocartilage over the ilium.

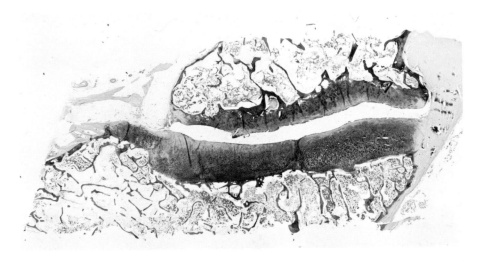

Fig. 4-19 Low power microscopic section of a sacroiliac joint. The sacral cartilage is more than twice as thick as that on the ilium.

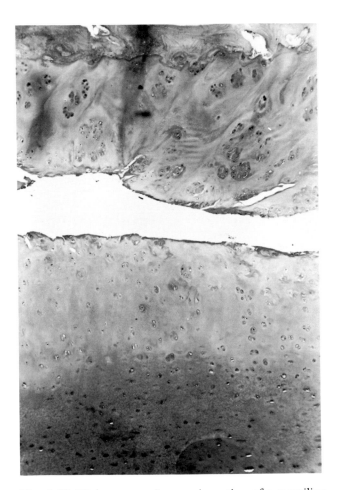

Fig. 4-20 High power microscopic section of a sacroiliac joint. Below, the thick hyaline cartilage over the sacrum, above the thin iliac fibrocartilage. There is marked clumping of chondrocytes in the latter.

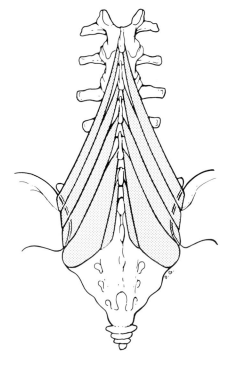

Fig. 4-21 Schematic drawing to demonstrate the insertion of the five slips of the multifidus muscle into ilium, joint, and sacrum. (Redrawn from Mcintosh JE, Valencia F, Bogduk N, Munro RR: The morphology of the human lumbar multifidus. Clin Biomech 1:196, 1986.)

sacrum to ilium at the midpoint of the joint posteriorly. The joint is C-shaped with the wings of the "C" facing posteriorly.

It is difficult to fit the changes that take place into the progressive pathology of the lumbar and lumbosacral spine. Over the decades the iliac cartilage degenerates more than the sacral cartilage. Late in life there is often a fibrous and occasionally a bony ankylosis of the joint (Figs. 4-18, to 4-20).

We shall see in later chapters that this joint is often inculpated in more than one fifth of the cases of low back pain. This pain can be relieved by simple methods of treatment.

The Muscle

The slips of multifidus muscle from L1 to L5 fan out laterally as they reach their insertion and are attached to the ilium (L1), to the sacroiliac joint (L2), and to the back of the sacrum (L3, L4, L5) (Fig. 4-21).

It is not unlikely that the lesion called a sacroiliac syndrome is in fact a myofascial syndrome involving part of the multifidus muscle that inserts into ilium, joint, and sacrum.

REFERENCES

1. Travell JG, Simons DG: Myofascial Pain and Dysfunction. The Trigger Point Manual. Williams & Wilkins, Baltimore, 1984.
2. Janda V: Muscles, central nervous motor regulation and back problems. In Korr IM (ed): The Neurobiologic Mechanisms in Manipulative Therapy. Plenum Press, New York, 1978.

SUGGESTED READINGS

Arnoldi CC: Interosseous hypertension. Clin Orthop Rel Res 115:30, 1970

Kirkaldy-Willis WH, Heithoff KB, Bowen, CVA, Shannon R: Pathological anatomy of lumbar spondylosis and stenosis correlated with CT scan. In Post MJD (ed): Radiologic Evaluation of the Spine. Masson Publishing, New York, 1980.

Kirkaldy-Willis WH, Wedge JH, Young Hing K, Reilly J: Pathology and pathogenesis of lumbar spondylosis and stenosis. Spine 3:319, 1978

Reilly J, Young Hing K, MacKay RW, Kirkaldy-Willis WH: Pathological anatomy of the lumbar spine. In Helfet AJ, Grnebel Lee DM (eds): Disorders of the Lumbar Spine. JB Lippincott, Philadelphia, 1978

5

The Mediation of Pain

William H. Kirkaldy-Willis

THE PROBLEM

The presenting symptom in nearly every patient with a mechanical or degenerative lesion in the lumbar spine is pain. Some patients have sensory or motor defects, in addition. It is important that the physician have some knowledge of the modern theory of pain and of how it can be applied to treat the patient.

All pain is real. We tend to think that when we can identify a lesion in the spine, the pain is "real" and that when we cannot do this, the pain is psychological. It is closer to the truth to say that in nearly all patients, pain has both psychological and physical aspects, that both are "real," and that sometimes one and sometimes the other predominates. At the present time, our knowledge of the way in which pain is perceived is mainly theoretical. Fortunately, we can use both fact and theory to alleviate a patient's pain.

It is reasonable for the clinician to inquire if the pain is mainly of physical origin, if it is chiefly of psychological origin (due to the personality of the patient), or if it results from a combination of physical and psychological causes.

Every patient with low back pain of physical origin undergoes a secondary change in personality. The patient with an acute low back strain or a disc herniation is under stress until the condition that produces the pain is resolved. This presents a relatively simple problem. Even here, the help of an experienced psychologist is often invaluable. The patient who has endured pain for months or years presents a much more difficult problem. This becomes still more difficult when the patient has had one, two, three, or more operations and still has pain. Each episode of pain and operative trauma affects not only the nerves supplying the joints and overlying muscles but also the entire nervous system and thus the entire personality of the patient.

Two further aspects of the problem must be considered. First, for psychological reasons the patient may present with a "chronic psychosomatic pain syndrome" that includes symptoms of low back pain among other symptoms. In this case the physician should seek help from the psychologist and allied personnel in a pain clinic. Second, as a result of long-standing back pain and several operations, the psychological and physical status of the patient may be so poor that it is beyond the power of the physician or surgeon to alleviate the pain. In this instance, it is better to tell the patient frankly that we are not clever enough to be of help. Assistance can be obtained from the psychologist, from the pain clinic, and sometimes, with careful selection, from neuro-augmentive surgery (see Chapter 24).

THE GATE CONTROL THEORY OF PAIN

The Gate Control Theory was first propounded by Melzack and Wall in 1965.[1] It has since undergone some modification. Although still a theory it can be used in practice both to increase our understanding of the perception of pain, and to enable us to plan management of lesions of the lumbar spine in such a way that pain is inhibited.

Summation of Impulses

Pain is not perceived through direct stimulation of free nerve endings in the tissues supplied by small-diameter fibers that pass directly to a pain center in the brain. It is perceived because of the summation of impulses from both large(L)- and small(S)-diameter nerve fibers that activate transmission (T) cells in the dorsal horns of the spinal cord. When the threshold for pain is reached in the dorsal horn, impulses stimulate the T cells and this initiates the central transmission of pain (the action system). Impulses pass to the reticular formation in the brain stem, to the midbrain, and to the cerebral cortex, with resultant perception of pain. This summation of impulses may be accompanied by prolonged activity in the cells of the nervous system and by spread of pain to other body areas.

The Substantia Gelatinosa

The substantia gelatinosa (SG) is situated in the dorsal horns of the spinal cord. It contains cells that exert an inhibitory effect on the transmission of impulses leading to the perception of pain. Impulses passing along the large (L) fibers stimulate the SG cells and increase inhibition of pain. Impulses passing along the small(S) fibers decrease the inhibitory effect of the SC cells and facilitate central pain transmission.

The Gate

Activity in the SG cells closes or opens the gate. Impulses travelling along the L fibers close the gate. Those in the S fibers open the gate so that impulses that lead to pain perception can pass through.

Modulation of Pain Perception

The activity of the gate formed by the SG cells is modulated not only by impulses from the L and S fibers but also by descending feedback from the reticular system, the thalamus, and the cerebral cortex (Fig. 5-1).

PERIPHERAL MODULATION OF PAIN

Mechanoreceptors

Mechanoreceptors, encapsulated corpuscles supplied by large- and medium-sized nerve fibers, are found in the articular capsule, the ligaments, and the fat pads of the posterior joints. These fibers produce information about static joint position, pressure changes in the joints, joint movement (acceleration and deceleration), and stresses that develop in the joint at the extreme point of movement. We have already seen that stimulating L fibers tends to close the gate and inhibit pain perception.[2]

Pain Receptors

Pain receptors, free nerve endings and plexuses that are supplied by S fibers, are found in the articular capsule, the fat pads, the ligaments, and the walls of blood vessels. These receptors become activated by mechanical deformation of joint structures and by mechanical and chemical irritation. Stimulating the S fibers tends to open the gate and to enhance the perception of pain.

Inhibition of Pain

Inhibition of pain is increased by stimulating the mechanoreceptors (L fibers) in two ways: by movement and activity of muscles and joints and manipulation of the joints.

Enhancement of Pain

Pain is enhanced by inactivity and immobilization, by injury to peripheral nerves with loss of L fibers, and by degeneration of peripheral nerves with loss of L fibers.

The physician, therefore, can control pain considerably by therapy that promotes activity and movement. The tempo of such activity must not be so great that it produces pain. Manipulation tends to inhibit pain by stimulating the L fibers. On the other hand, immobilization either from inactivity or produced by segmental muscle hypertonic contraction—often reflex to a posterior joint dysfunction—tends to enhance the perception of pain.

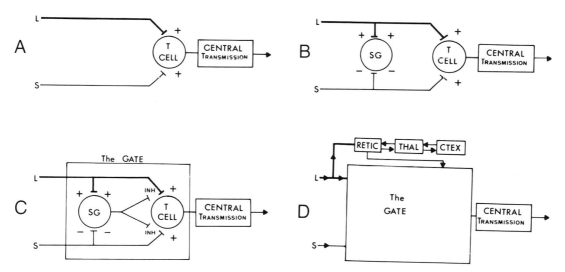

Fig. 5-1. The gate control theory. **(A)** Summation of impulses from large fibers (L) and small fibers (S). Excitatory effect (+) on transmission cell (T). **(B)** Addition of substantia gelatinosa (SG) cell. Impulses from large fibers (L) have an excitatory effect on the SG cell (+), whereas those from the small fibers (S) have an inhibitory effect (−). **(C)** Stimulating the SG cell produces an inhibitory effect (INH) on the T cell, and pain perception is decreased. **(D)** Impulses from large fibers (L) also ascend directly in the dorsal columns to the reticular formation (Retic), the thalamus (Thal), and the cerebral cortex (Ctex), which in turn feed back to modulate activity in the cells of the dorsal horn (the Gate). (Adapted from Melzack R, Wall PD: Pain mechanisms: a new theory. Science 150: 971, 1965. Copyright 1965 by the American Association for the Advancement of Science.)

The painfree intervertebral three-joint complex is one in which normal movement and rhythm take place.

Treating a lesion of this complex necessitates a careful balance between activity and the avoidance of pain. As the lesion heals, the tempo of activity can be increased. Complete healing implies a return to normal activity and movement.

CENTRAL MODULATION OF PAIN

Reticular Formation

The reticular formation in the brain stem discharges impulses continually and exerts an inhibitory effect on pain by closing the gate in the SG via the reticulospinal tract. This inhibitory effect is augmented by the following:

1. Distracting attention from the site of pain
2. Concentrating on work or other activity
3. Sleep
4. Hypnosis
5. Emotional states that increase blood catecholamines
6. Drugs such as largactyl, valium, and morphine

Reticular activity is depressed and pain is enhanced by (1) concentrating attention on the pain and (2) barbiturates.

Cerebral Cortex

The cerebral cortex regulates the activity of the reticular formation. Reticular activity is increased and the perception of pain is inhibited, via depression of cortical activity, by the following four factors: emotional tranquility, sleep, hyperventilation leading to hypocarbia, and ingestion of large amounts of alcohol. The following emotions and substances depress reticular activity by increasing cortical activity: anxiety, uncertainty, and fear; ingesting benzedrine, marijuana, and LSD; *small* amounts of alcohol; coffee; and tea.

Central Control Trigger

Melzack and Wall[1] postulate the existence of a central control trigger in the nervous system that activates the brain processes controlling the sensory input. In this way memory of previous experiences and response to pain impulses may affect the transmission of impulses from the action system.

The Central Biasing Mechanism

It is proposed that the reticular formation in the brain stem acts as a central biasing mechanism that exerts a tonic inhibitory influence on the transmission of impulses leading to pain perception at all levels. Thus, activity in the reticular formation tends to reduce pain perception.

Peripheral and Central Modulation of Pain

Consideration of peripheral and central modulation of pain enables the physician to influence both the process of healing of a lumbar spine lesion and the inhibition of pain. The author is indebted to Leriche[3] for concepts expressed in his book *The Surgery of Pain,* to Melzack and Wall for their explanation of the Gate Control Theory of Pain[1] and to Sandoz[4] for his comments on reflex phenomena associated with spinal derangements and adjustments.

HOW THE PATIENT DESCRIBES PAIN

The Meaning of the Patient's Description

Much has been written about the way in which patients describe their pain. With the few exceptions discussed below, the writer has been disappointed at the lack of help obtained by asking the patient to describe the pain experienced. When pressed to describe the pain, the patient often replies, "I can't describe it but the pain that I have in my back and in my leg is unpleasant," or "makes my life miserable," or "is almost unbearable." The degree of pain felt seems more important than the kind of pain experienced.

Repeated Observation of the Patient

Repeated observation is essential and of great value to the physician. As the physician sees the patient on several occasions, he or she begins to sense the degree to which the patient is troubled by pain. Further help is obtained from the opinion of the psychologist (see Chapter 8). Observing the way in which the patient responds to stress is also of value. The writer obtains a good deal of help from observing the reaction of the patient to a posterior joint injection (see Chapter 10). It is only as the physician begins to know and understand the patient that he or she can assess the degree of pain of which the patient complains.

TYPES OF PAIN

Aching in the Legs

When the patient complains of leg pain, it is necessary to inquire whether this is in fact pain or aching. Aching in posterior thigh or calf is usually due to tightness of the hamstring or gastrocnemii muscles, a common feature of chronic low back pain, and is relieved by exercises to stretch these muscles.

Burning Pain

The distribution of this type of pain is often diffuse and vague. It does not usually conform to one or more dermatomes. It is sympathetic in origin. The sympathetic nervous system takes part in the innervation of the structures within the spinal canal via the recurrent nerve of Luschka and is stimulated in both arachnoiditis and postoperative fibrosis. The diffuse nature of the pain is due to the fact that sympathetic fibers run distally in the adventitia of the arteries rather than with the main nerves supplying the limb.

Unusual Sensations

In central spinal stenosis the blood supply to the nerves of the cauda equina is impaired. One result is the presence of abnormal sensations, bizarre in nature, that may affect the whole of one or both lower limbs. The patient may complain of an unpleasant feeling in the legs that is not pain but may be as disturbing as pain. He may say that the legs feel as though they do not belong to him. The legs may feel as though they are going to let the patient fall, they are made of rubber, or they are surrounded by a tight bandage. Before spinal stenosis was well recognized, the patient with these symptoms was thought to have a psychological problem. Now the presence of such abnormal sensations alerts the physician to the possibility of spinal stenosis.

THE APPRECIATION OF PAIN PERCEPTION

Pain perception takes place in four areas of the brain: the thalamus, the first level of perception; the postcentral cerebral cortex, the site at which the exact location and nature of pain is interpreted; the frontal cerebral cortex, the affective component, i.e., the area in which the experience of pain is associated with the site where it hurts; and the temporal cerebral cortex, the memory component, i.e., the site at which the memory of previous pain experience is stored.

As stated by Wyke,[2] pain is not a primary sensation such as vision or hearing but an abnormal emotional state produced by activating specific afferent pathways (the nociceptive system).

CONCLUSIONS

1. Pain is a complex neurological phenomenon involving polysynaptic pathways that interact at several levels.
2. Pain can be modulated both peripherally and centrally.
3. The treatment of low back pain includes dealing with both the spinal lesion and the patient's pain.
4. The physician can use his knowledge of the pain-modulating factors—peripheral, reticular, and cortical—to stimulate inhibition of pain.

REFERENCES

1. Melzack R, Wall PD: Pain mechanisms: a new theory. Science 150: 971, 1965
2. Wyke B: Neurological aspects of low back pain. In Jayson M (ed): The Lumbar Spine and Back Pain. Grune & Stratton, Orlando, 1976
3. Leriche R: The Surgery of Pain. Ballière, Tindall, & Cox, London, 1939
4. Sandoz RW: Some reflex phenomena associated with spinal derangements and adjustments. Ann Swiss Chiropractors Assoc 7: 45, 1981

6
The Perception of Pain

James N. Weinstein

THE PROBLEM

Why the most common symptom in the field of medicine is the most difficult to understand remains a mystery. This chapter provides a sense of security in the basic understanding of our perception of back pain. To do that we will travel across disciplines to relate the perception of back pain to the anatomical pathways by which these perceptions traverse. We will travel from the surrounding soft tissues to the peripheral nerve and the dorsal horn of the spinal cord and then up to the brain. This will not be a simple, uninterrupted voyage but the obstacles will be identified and we will proceed. Communication is necessary to understand from where we start and is critical between patient and physician. With this in mind our journey toward the understanding of back pain begins.

Many prominent investigators have been unable to communicate a good understanding of their patients' back pain. To this end several investigators of pain have themselves submitted to having their own nerves crushed, cut, or resutured in order to observe and describe their sensory experiences; but none of these investigators have ever agreed with each other.

One must remain optimistic as our knowledge base regarding back pain continues to increase. However, as long as one person has back pain and is without help, our knowledge of back pain remains inadequate.

DEFINITION OF PAIN

The taxonomy committee of the International Association for the Study of Pain (1979) defined pain as "an unpleasant sensory and emotional experience associated with actual or potential tissue damage, or described in terms of such damage."[2] The committee went on to say that pain is always subjective. Each individual learns the application of the word through experiences related to injury in early life. Pain often occurs in the absence of tissue damage and may in some instances be an emotional experience. If one regards his or her experience as painful and reports it in the same ways as pain caused by tissue damage then, it should be accepted as pain. Thus, pain does not always have to be tied to a damaging stimulus.

BACK PAIN

To understand back pain there must be framework from which to work. The main aim should be understanding of the mechanisms, the nature of the back pain, and the rationale for treatment. When one understands the mechanisms, one can begin to institute rational treatment with predictable results. Unfortunately, back pain is what the patient feels and how he expresses these feelings to us. The limitations of the verbalization of these painful experiences are, as we know, restricted. The very nature of back pain and its impact on industrialized countries imposes a sense of urgency; thus, if one method of treatment fails, another is tried, and it is hard to study the natural history of any one condition or the result of a specific treatment.

To understand the basic mechanism by which one perceives back pain, we must begin by knowing the composite parts that bring these perceptions to consciousness.

THE THREE-JOINT COMPLEX (HOUSE)

Each vertebral body within each motion segment is much like a house (Fig. 6-1A). As described in Chapter 4, each vertebral body is connected by an intervertebral disc in front and two posterior facet joints (Fig. 6-1B). The vertebral body is the foundation of the house, whereas the pedicles depict the

HOUSING

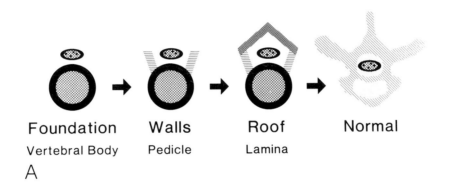

Foundation — Vertebral Body
Walls — Pedicle
Roof — Lamina
Normal

A

THREE-JOINT COMPLEX (HOUSE)

LATERAL VIEW

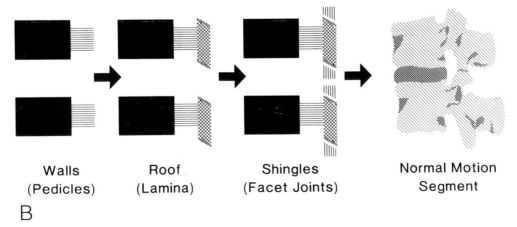

Walls (Pedicles)
Roof (Lamina)
Shingles (Facet Joints)
Normal Motion Segment

B

Fig. 6-1 (A) Each vertebral body within each motion segment is like a house (foundation, walls, roof). **(B)** Each vertebral body (house) is connected to its neighbor by the intervertebral disc in the front and facet joints in the back (shingles). (*Figure continues.*)

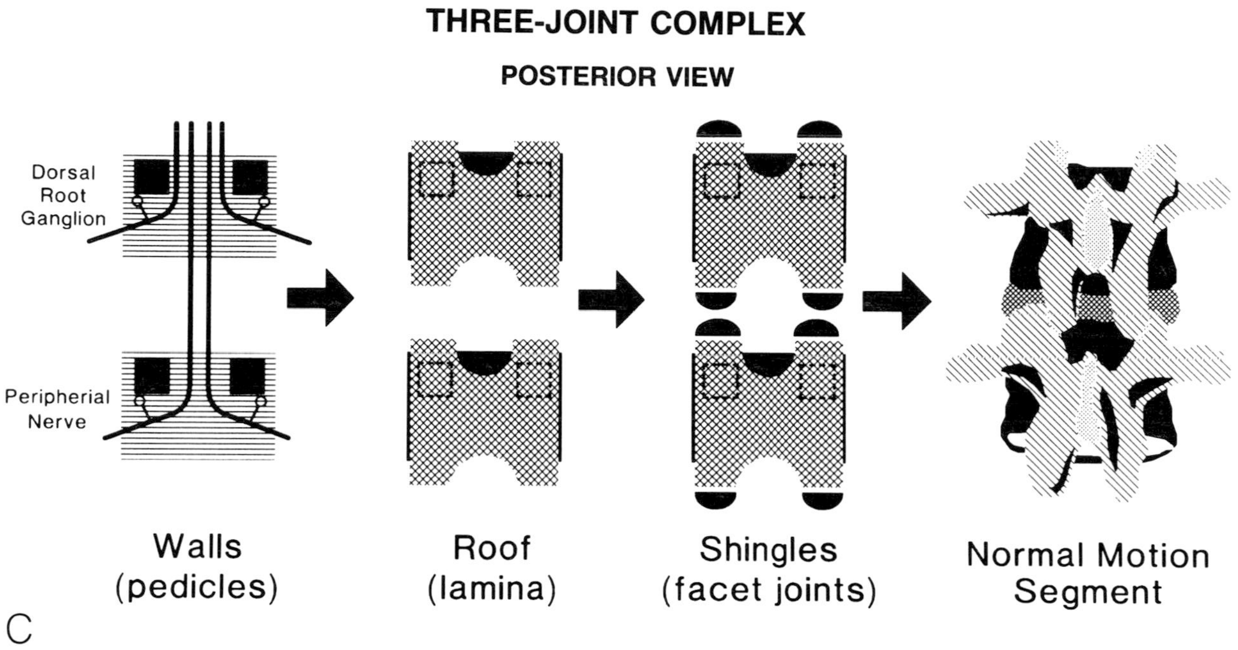

THREE-JOINT COMPLEX

POSTERIOR VIEW

Walls
(pedicles)

Roof
(lamina)

Shingles
(facet joints)

Normal Motion
Segment

C

Fig. 6-1 (*Continued*). **(C)** Beneath the walls of each house the dorsal root ganglion and peripheral nerves associated with that particular motion segment.

walls of the house and the lamina represent the roof of each house. Each roof (lamina) is connected to its neighbors roof by shingles (facet joints). Inside the house lives the spinal cord and nerves. Beneath the pedicles run the peripheral nerves and dorsal root ganglion, which supply information to and from our musculoskeletal system for the necessary communication between our external and internal environment (Fig. 6-1C). The dorsal root ganglion is critically located at each spinal motion segment just beneath the pedicles and in front of the superior facets (shingles) of the neighboring house below. The ganglion serves as modulator (brain) of low back pain, and it may be responsible for the modulation of several known causes of mechanical low back pain.[3] The ganglion is mechanically sensitive and contains many pain transmitters (modulators, neuropeptides) such as substance P, vasoactive intestinal peptide, and calcitonin gene-related peptide.[4] The cells of the DRG terminate mainly in the substantia gelatinosa, Lamina II of the spinal cord, where the gate of Melzack and Wall is located.[5] The three-joint complex (house) and its adjacent tissues (ligaments, joint capsules, disc and muscles) receive their innervation by a pleurisegmen-

tal group of nerves (sinuvertebral) with both sympathetic and dorsal rami components (Fig. 6-2).

NERVES

Accurate diagnosis of back pain rests in understanding the neurological mechanisms producing the pain. To this end there have been numerous investigations of the type and the distribution of peripheral nerves to and within the spinal tissues around the three-joint complex (Table 6-1.)[6–18] Three types of myelinated nerve endings have been identified[8,10,19]: (1) free nerve endings terminating as single tapered tips, (2) complex unencapsulated endings usually terminating in multiple branches with expanded tips, and (3) encapsulated nerve endings of the Vater–Pacini type. Unmyelinated perivascular nerve networks have also been described. Malinsky[10] identified two types of perivascular nerve endings in the immature annulus fibrosus: (1) simple, free termination of a thin nerve fiber along a capillary wall; and (2) more complex branching of a thicker nerve fiber in a blood vessel wall. In addition, plexiform and free unmyeli-

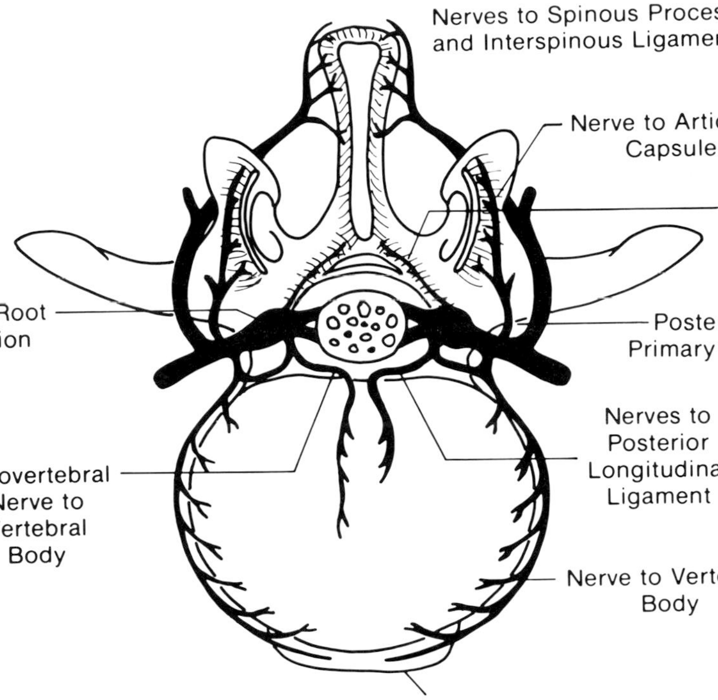

Fig. 6-2 The three-joint complex receives pleuri-segmental innervation by a combination of nerves (sinuvertebral).

nated nerve fiber terminals, not associated with blood vessels, are present. The structure of these various nerve endings significantly influences the type of sensation perceived as well as its intensity.[20] Plexiform and freely ending unmyelinated nerve fibers respond to chemical or mechanical abnormalities and form the pain or nociceptive receptor system. A nociceptor is a receptor sensitive to a noxious or potentially noxious stimulus. These nociceptors, once fired, change their properties; some become more sensitive and some less sensitive. Complex unencapsulated endings are thought to be sensitive to tissue or joint position and encapsulated endings respond to pressure. Perivascular endings have vasomotor or vasosensory functions as well as a nociceptor system.[18,20]

Encapsulated endings appear to be located primarily in the facet joint capsules and in the soft tissues along the anterior or lateral surfaces of the annulus fibrosus.[8,10] The joint capsules also have free nerve endings and complex unencapsulated endings. The

anterior and posterior longitudinal ligaments, the supraspinous ligaments, and the intraspinous ligaments contain free nerve fiber endings and complex unencapsulated endings.[8,9] The posterior longitudinal ligament appears to have the greatest density of nerve endings.[18] The cartilage endplates have perivascular nerves only.[9] The vertebral periosteum is supplied with free nerve endings and complex encapsulated nerve endings,[21] and the vertebrae have perivascular nerves as well as occasional solitary nerves.[22] A number of investigators have reported that the peripheral layers of the annulus fibrosus have free fiber endings, but they did not find nerves in the inner regions of the annulus fibrosus or nucleus pulposus.[8-10,13] However, Shinohara[14] reported free fiber endings in the inner regions of the annulus and the nucleus pulposus of degenerated disc. Other authors[18] indicate that although unmyelinated nerves are present in fetal and neonatal disc, these nerves rapidly disappear with growth. Thus, no nerves are present in the substances

Table 6-1 Distribution of Peripheral Nerves to the Three-Joint Complex and Surrounding Soft Tissues

Fiber Type	Function	Location
Myelinated		
Free	Tissue or joint position	Facet joint capsules; anterior and lateral surfaces of annulus fibrosus; anterior/posterior longitudinal ligaments; supraspinous/intraspinous ligaments; periosteum
Complex unencapsulated	Tissue or joint position	Same as listed above
Encapsulated	Pressure	Facet joint capsules; anterior and lateral surfaces of annulus fibrosus; periosteum
Unmyelinated		
Perivascular	Vasomotor	Cartilage endplates; vertebrae; blood vessels
Simple	Vasosensory	
Complex	Nociceptor	
Free	Chemical	Annulus fibrosus; facet joint capsules; ligaments
	Mechanical	
Plexiform	Nociceptor	

of the mature human intervertebral disc. Ultrastructural investigations have failed to identify nerves in the disc (Fig. 6-2).

RELATIONSHIP OF INJURY TO PAIN

When a nerve is injured the dorsal root ganglion cells send an afferent barrage of signals to the CNS.[23] How the CNS handles these messages is critical to our understanding of the relationship of pain to injury. Realizing that these nerve receptors can send false signals when they receive unusual messages from damaged peripheral tissues further confounds the problem. To this end, Melzack and Wall[5] produced the gate control theory (Fig. 6-3). Messages concerned with pain are transmitted via central cells in the dorsal horn of the spinal cord. This painful transmission within the spinal cord depends on three factors: (1) the arrival of nociceptive messages; (2) the convergent effect of other peripheral afferents, which may exaggerate or diminish the effects of the nociceptive message; and (3) the presence of control systems within the CNS, which influence the central cells. Melzack

and Wall[5] emphasize that convergent controls decide the fate of the arriving messages as they pass through every level of the CNS and eventually produce reaction, sensation, and movement. From the dorsal horn of the spinal cord, the message ascends to its first level of consciousness, the thalamus. Then, the message ascends to the postcentral gyrus of the brain wherein the nature and location of the pain is interpreted. The frontal lobe provides an affective component, whereas the temporal lobe provides stored memories from previous painful experiences. Some cells within the dorsal horn of the spinal cord (substantia gelatinosa) learn to respond not only to a painful stimulus but also to an alerting signal that says a noxious stimulus is about to happen. Thus, the signalling of injury by the central cells in the dorsal horn of the spinal cord are dependent not only on the arrival of a nociceptive afferent impulse but on other peripheral events and the thermostatic setting of excitability by the various central nervous system mechanisms. These controls are contingent on one another and help to explain our variable responses to injury. The presence of such controls means that they themselves may become locked into a pathological position and exaggerate or create pain.

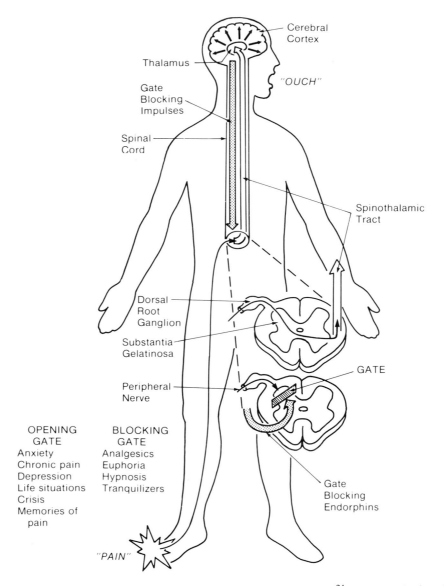

Fig. 6-3 A diagramatic sketch of the gate control theory of pain. Descartes[24] first described such a pathway in 1664. (1) First a toe is injured; this causes a release of various pain modulators, such as substance P, and other chemicals are released. This starts the pain signal on its way as an electrical impulse. (2) The message reaches the dorsal horn of the spinal cord (substantia gelatinosa). (3) It is relayed via the spinothalamic tract to the thalamus, the area of the brain where the painful stimulus first becomes conscious. (4) The message then reaches the cerebral cortex, where the location of pain and its intensity are perceived. (5) Transmission of gate blocking impulses descend from the brain via the spinal cord to provide pain relief. (6) In the dorsal horn, chemicals like endorphins are released to diminish the pain message from the injured toe.

It is through these control systems that various therapeutic modalities have been used in the treatment of back pain (electrical stimulations, acupuncture, analgesias, manipulation). The challenge is to have a better understanding of this complicated system and its peripheral influences (Fig. 6-3).

REFERRED PAIN AND RADICULAR PAIN

The pain originating from a motion segment may be felt at a site far removed from its origin. Deep tenderness of muscles and altered sensation, usually hyperalgesia, occurs in an area of referred pain.[25] In the lumbar spine, pain is often referred to the groin, lower abdomen, and foot. Kellgren's classic studies[24] showed that pain referral to the region of the groin was predominantly from upper lumbar segments. McCall[26] also indicates that groin pain can result from the lower lumbar facets. The facets may also be responsible for buttock and greater trochanteric pain. Pain down the back of the thigh and to the knee and occasionally down the posterior or lateral calf may also emanate from the posterior facet joints. The difficulty in identifying the source of the pain is made greater not only because of overlap of innervation at each level but also because of overlap of pain patterns.[27]

Radicular pain due to nerve root compression is experienced in a dermatome, sclerotome, or myotome because of direct involvement of a lumbar spinal nerve. It is characterized by a detectable sensory, motor, or reflex change. The spinal nerve emerging through the intervertebral foramen is susceptible to compression or irritation by the disc anteriorly and the facet joint complex posteriorly. The intensity of the pain and its radicular nature are dependent on the strength of the stimulus, that is, the amount of tension or compression on the sensitive nerve root. Admittedly, some pain associated with root compression is referred from distortions of neighboring tissues, muscle insertions, joint capsules, and ligaments; but the pain that radiates into the extremities is best produced by stimulation of the root itself.[28]

TYPES OF PAIN

When a patient describes aching in their legs, it is necessary to know whether this is in fact pain or aching. Aching is usually muscular in nature and is often relieved by stretching and/or short periods of rest. Pain, on the other hand, is often associated with a vascular or neurogenic etiology. Spinal stenosis, for example, will impair the blood supply to the nerves of the cauda equina causing pseudoclaudication. On the other hand, vascular, or true claudication may also cause leg pain.

Burning pain is often vague in distribution and does not follow a dermatomal distribution. It is usually of sympathetic origin, and its diffuse nature is related to the fact that the sympathetic fibers run

within the adventitia of the arteries rather than the main peripheral nerves supplying the legs.

SUMMARY

No matter where it occurs in the body and no matter from what cause the unpleasant emotional experience of pain is always an expression of some neurological dysfunction. The central nervous system is not a series of separate parts, each designed to handle a different problem. The perception of pain and its modulation occurs through a complex integrated system that receives messages and reacts to them. The reactions are not always of a "fight or flight" nature but are an attempt to respond to an unpleasant experience, pain. The intricacies of the central nervous system as related to low back pain are far from being understood. Work among different disciplines must continue to put the parts of the puzzle together so that one can remain optimistic about the future of caring for those with back pain.

REFERENCES

1. Denny-Brown, D: The release of deep pain by nerve injury. Brain 88: 725, 1965
2. Merskey H: Pain terms: a list with definitions and notes on usage. Recommended by the IASP Subcommittee on Taxonomy. Pain 6: 249, 1979
3. Weinstein JN: The dorsal root ganglion as a mediator of low back pain. Spine (Accepted for publication)
4. Lieberman AR: Sensory ganglion. p. 182. In London DN: The Peripheral Nerve. Chapman & Hall, London, 1976
5. Melzack R, Wall PD: Pain mechanisms: a new theory. Science 150: 971, 1965
6. Bogduk N, Tynan W, Wilson AS: The nerve supply to the human lumbar intervertebral discs. J Anat 132: 39, 1981
7. Ehrenhaft JL: Development of the vertebral column as related to certain congenital and pathological changes. Surg Gynecol Obstet 76: 282, 1943
8. Hirsch C, Ingelmark B, Miller M: The anatomical basis for low back pain. Acta Orthop Scand 33: 2, 1963
9. Jackson HC, Winkelmann RK, Bickel WH: Nerve endings in the human lumbar spinal column and related structures. J Bone Joint Surg 48A: 1272, 1966
10. Malinsky J: The ontogenetic development of nerve terminations in the intervertebral discs of man. Acta Anat 38: 96, 1959

11. Parke WW, Schiff DCM: The applied anatomy of the intervertebral disc. Orthop Clin North Am 2: 309, 1971

12. Pedersen HS, Blunck CFJ, Gardner E: The anatomy of the lumbosacral posterior rami and meningeal branches of spinal nerves (sinu-vertebral nerves). J Bone Joint Surg 38A: 377, 1956

13. Roofe PG: Innervation of the annulus fibrosus and posterior longitudinal ligament. Arch Neurol Psych 44: 100, 1940

14. Shinohara H: Lumbar disc lesion with special reference to the histological significance of nerve endings of the lumbar discs. J Jap Orthop Assoc 44: 553–570, 1970

15. Wiberg G: Back pain in relation to the nerve supply of the intervertebral disc. Acta Orthop Scand 19: 211, 1949–50

16. Wyke BD: Articular neurology: a review. Physiotherapy 58: 94, 1972

17. Wyke BD: Neurology of the cervical spinal joints. Physiotherapy 65: 72, 1979

18. Wyke BD: The neurology of low back pain. p. 265. In Jayson MIV (ed): The Lumbar Spine and Back Pain. 2nd Ed. Pitman Medical Publishing Co, Kent, 1980

19. Ralston HJ, Miller MR, Kasahara M: Nerve endings in human fasciae, tendons, ligaments, periosteum, and joint synovial membrane. Anat Rec 136: 137, 1960

20. Sunderland S: Nerve and nerve injuries. p. 343. In Peripheral Sensory Mechanism. 2nd Ed. Churchill Livingstone, New York, 1978

21. Ikari C: A study of the mechanisms of low back pain. The neurohistological examination of disease. J Bone Joint Surg 36A: 195, 1954

22. Sherman MS: The nerves of bone. J Bone Joint Surg 45A: 522, 1963

23. Wall PD: Alterations in the central nervous system after deafferentation. Advances in Pain Research 5. Raven, New York, 1983

24. Descartes E: L'Homme, C Angot, Paris, 1664

25. Kellgren JH: On the distribution of pain arising from deep somatic structures with charts of segmental pain areas. Clin Sci 4: 35, 1939

26. McCall IW, Park WM, O-Brien JP: Induced pain referral from posterior elements in normal subjects. Spine 4: 441, 1979

27. Foerster D: The dermatomes in Man. Brain 56: 1, 1933

28. Frykholm R: Cervical nerve root compression resulting from disc degeneration and root sleeve fibroses. Acta Chir Scand, Suppl., 160: 1, 1951

29. Hokfelt T, Johanson O, Ljungdahl A, et al: Peptideric neurons. Nature 284: 515, 1980

THE CLINICAL PICTURE

7

Introduction

William H. Kirkaldy-Willis

With the knowledge and understanding gained from the first part of this book we turn together now to consideration of the clinical picture. This is no easy task.

A SCIENTIFIC APPROACH

A nonscientific approach is all too common. It is tempting for the surgeon to say to himself, "This patient has a disc herniation, demonstrated by the myelogram or the CT scan. The lesion occupies space. An operation is required to remove the lump." Such an attitude is wrong for many reasons, in the first place because we know that 75% of disc herniations resolve and become symptom free in 3 months with conservative care (Nachemson, personal communication). Another example—the surgeon reasons in this way: "This patient has had two disc explorations and a posterior fusion and still has severe low back pain. I will recommend an anterior-interbody fusion because I do not know what else to do and because a small percentage of such patients are relieved of their pain by this procedure."

There is no place in the management of low back pain for any approach other than one that starts by the physician using the most precise and scientific methods available to him. The approach should be as logical and well reasoned as possible.

The scientific approach demands the following of the physician or surgeon:

1. An exact and precise diagnosis of the clinical lesion
2. Knowledge of the nature, site, and level of the lesion
3. Assessment of the phase, dysfunction, the unstable phase, or stabilization, the framework in which the lesion occurs
4. Understanding of the natural history of the disease process
5. Some comprehension of pathomechanics and pathology

The wise physician knows that in practice it is not always possible to be as scientific as one wishes. We make mistakes. We are often uncertain. This does not excuse us from failure to employ an outlook that is as highly scientific and factual as we can make it at this stage in our investigation (Table 7-1).

BEYOND SCIENCE

A Definition

We come to a point in our study of the patient at which perforce we are compelled to go beyond the realm of science into that of metaphysics. This means no more than that we have to move into the realm beyond (meta)factual knowledge of the physical nature of things (physikos). The implication is that the physician moves on from the process of reasoning to one no less real but beyond and above that of

93

Table 7-1 Four Aspects of Diagnosis

Personality	Phase	Site and Nature of Lesion	Differential Diagnosis
The past	Dysfunction	Posterior facets	Extrinsic lesions
Upbringing	Unstable	Sacroiliac joints	Congenital/developmental
Culture	Stabilization	Disc herniation	Trauma
Experiences		Lateral stenosis	Infections
The present		Central stenosis	Rheumatoid
Intelligence		Spondylolisthesis	Neoplastic
Attitudes		Posterior muscles	Metabolic
Hopes, fears		Piriformis syndrome	Vascular
Satisfaction		Quadratus lumborum syndrome	
Resentment		Other muscle syndromes	
Disappointment			
Compensation			
Depression			
Hypochondriasis			
Hysteria			
The future			
Goals			
Hopes			
Fears			

reasoning with the mind. This is a natural transition but one that many of us fear to make.

The Early Stage

As we begin to give consideration to the personality of the patient suffering from low back pain, we are still in the realm of science. A psychological assessment starts by being scientific. It is nearly always qualitative rather than quantitative. As we try to measure the amount of the pain experienced we are mainly guessing.

The Metaphysical Realm

In their interaction the physician or surgeon and the patient soon move together into this realm. The transition takes place gradually but inexorably as the physician seeks to understand (1) the patient's past: his upbringing at home and at school, his cultural background, and any past experiences that color his reaction to pain; (2) what is going on in the patient's mind at the present time: his intelligence, his emotions, his hopes and fears, his satisfaction at home and at work, his feelings of resentment, his disappointments, his desire for compensation, his feelings of depression, and the presence or absence of hypochondriasis or hysteria; (3) the patient's attitude to the future: his goals, hopes, and fears.

The Effect of Personality on Pain Perception

The impact of personality has been considered to some extent in Chapter 5. Each patient reacts differently to pain. Chronic pain has a marked and deep effect on every patient. The patient is not usually aware of this. During the course of several interviews the physician can begin to make a reasonable assessment.

Repeated Trauma and Multiple Operations

Each episode of trauma and each operation, in itself an episode of trauma, has profound effects on the patient's tolerance to pain. Recent research suggests that biochemical changes take place in the nervous system as a result of injury to a spinal nerve and that these extend far beyond the original site of trauma. It is likely that some of these reactions are mediated via the sympathetic nervous system.

The Process of Assessment

This process is initiated by the physician or surgeon. When managing a simple or straightforward problem, he may well be able to complete the assessment of the patient's personality on his own. Simple measures render the patient free from pain in a short period of time. The patient's confidence is restored. With a little help he is back at home and at work and once again in the normal rhythm of life. In dealing with more complex or longstanding problems, help is sought from a psychologist who has an understanding of and interest in managing problems that arise in the patient with low back pain. This matter is dealt with in some detail in Chapter 8.

It is essential that the physician and the psychologist sit down together to decide if the problem is mainly psychological and should be managed by the psychologist, if it is mainly physical and should be treated conservatively or by operation by the surgeon, or if it is a combined problem that requires help from both psychologist and surgeon. There are several other possibilities. (1) Objective data may clearly indicate that the results of an operation will be uncertain; nonetheless, sometimes it is right to take a chance and operate. (2) Surgery may be indicated from a physical standpoint, but for other reasons it appears unlikely to help the patient; in that case it is contraindicated. (3) The situation is so bad that the surgeon can do no more to help. The patient should be told this in a kindly, frank, and open way. (4) Neuroaugmentive surgery may offer a good chance of relief of pain. That subject is considered in Chapter 24.

THE PHYSICIAN AND THE PATIENT

Rapport between physician and patient is built as a result of several interviews. During the course of these the physician tells the patient (1) what is wrong with his back, (2) how this can be put right, (3) the chances of success, (4) the problems and difficulties that lie ahead, and (5) what the future holds. Will the patient return to a normal home life? Will he be able to return to previous work? Will he need to look for lighter work?

Be Good to Your Back and It Will Be Good to You

It is essential for the patient to learn, through an understanding of his condition and through trust in his physician, to work first with the doctor and then on his own to complete the cure for himself. At some stage, and probably more than once, the physician needs to say, "I cannot cure your back pain. I can help you with advice, with various methods of treatment, possibly by an operation. It is up to you, with my help, to cure yourself. I and others will show you how to do this. But you yourself will have to make a big effort."

Referral to Another Physician

None of us should be reluctant to refer a patient to another physician (1) when the nature of the problem is beyond our particular knowledge and skill—not infrequently I refer patients to the pain clinic, the neurologist, or the rheumatologist; (2) when we realize that the patient is not satisfied with our management of his case; and (3) when it has not been possible to build the necessary rapport with the patient.

Kindness and Toughness

It goes without saying that patients with low back pain need a great deal of kindly and sympathetic understanding from their physician. When the patient is not making the necessary effort to help himself, it is kind to be tough. The patient sometimes needs to be told quite frankly that he will not improve until he makes an attempt to follow instructions given in the Back Class, to lose weight, and to do exercises regularly. The patient in this category who returns to the physician complaining that the pain is as bad as ever needs to be told, "Your back is no better because you have not followed my instructions. Go away and carry out what I've told you."

The Value of the Truth

Sometimes the physician has great difficulty in telling the truth to the patient. An example will make this clear. The patient with severe arachnoiditis needs to be told, "This is the serious nature of your trouble. I myself can do no more to help you. Another operation will only make things worse. It is possible that the doctor in the pain clinic can help you or refer you to someone else who can. You may well have to put up with pain for the rest of your life."

On other occasions, for example, when the patient, not really suffering much pain, has returned seeking more compensation, it gets the physician off the hook to say, "You are receiving a reasonable amount of compensation. I am sorry that I am not clever enough to be of any further help to you."

Make Haste Slowly

Except in dealing with a rare condition, such as a central disc herniation at L5-S1 in the presence of an acute chorda equina syndrome, it is never wise to rush to operation. Even when the surgeon considers that an operation will be necessary, it is wise to lead the patient slowly to this decision. The following approach is a good one, "I will try to help you without performing surgery. If at any time you feel that you cannot bear the pain any longer or that the treatment you are having is unbearable, tell me so, and if you ask me, I will be prepared to operate then." The onus of the decision is on the patient.

THE PATIENT'S RESOURCES

Each of us has resources for healing within the body. Every doctor is well aware of this but patients are often quite unconscious of this important fact. It is relatively easy for them to understand that the cells of the body are active in healing a cut finger or in fighting an infection. It is more difficult to get across to them that they have resources in the body to heal a lesion in the low back. For example, the patient who is contented and relaxed, who has confidence in the physician, and who can smile and laugh will get well more quickly than one who is anxious and afraid. An important part of the doctor's task is to help the patient to mobilize these inner resources. In doing this he may work with the patient himself; may seek help from the family and friends; may ask the psychologist for help; may get the social worker on the job; or when appropriate, talk to the

minister, rabbi, or priest of the patient's church and ask for his help with the patient.[1]

OTHER RESOURCES

In treating an acute illness (common cold, appendicitis) little supportive help is needed to supplement the correct treatment for the condition. In managing a chronic condition (peptic ulcer, ulcerative colitis, low back pain) many other factors have to be considered in addition to the regime of treatment.

Figure 7-1 shows that each person can be considered a circle with four quadrants representing the physical, mental, emotional, and spiritual aspects of his or her personality. In the management of low back pain the physician has to try to determine how much each of these four factors is responsible for the predicament of the patient. It has been said that 75% to 90% of all physical ills arise from emotional or spiritual problems. All patients with a physical problem also have an emotional one. In some people the emotional problem is by far the greater one.

The Environment

We need also to consider the way in which the patient reacts to the environment. Figure 7-2 demon-

FOUR ASPECTS IN EACH INDIVIDUAL

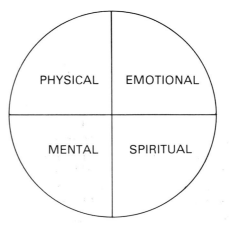

Fig. 7-1 The four aspects in each individual (after Arthur Bell.)

THE INDIVIDUAL AND
THE ENVIRONMENT

Fig. 7-2 The individual and the environment.

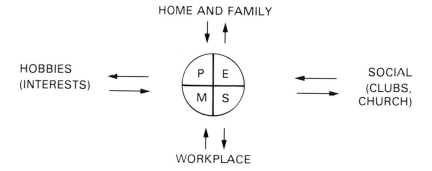

strates the four main components of the environment: home, workplace, hobbies, and contacts with other people. We need to think not only of the ways in which we can help the patient to adjust to home, work, and society but also how, on occasion, we can change these for the benefit of the patient.

Goals

The happy, healthy person is one who has satisfying goals. Our aim as physicians and therapists should be to help the patient back to a point at which he or she can again pursue the goals he or she finds satisfying. We all need both short and long term goals. Lenin wrote about religion, "It is the opiate of the people, designed to distract their attention from present ills to think of pie in the sky when they die." To this the physician who is a realist can reply, "We like pie. We believe that people need pie both now in this world and later on as well."

THE PAIN DRAWING

Psychological assessment of the patient is considered at some length in Chapter 8. It is not possible to do this type of assessment in more than a small percentage of patients.

All patients are required to complete a pain drawing on their first visit to our clinic. The drawing can be done and assessed quickly. It gives a good deal of valuable information about both physical and psycho-

logical problems and enables the physician or surgeon to decide which patients should be referred for a full psychological assessment. The clinician uses the scoring sheet drawn up by Wiltse (personal communication) (Table 7-2).

Mechanical Causes of Pain

THE POSTERIOR JOINT SYNDROME

Figure 7-3 is a pain drawing made by a patient with a posterior joint syndrome. The distribution of pain is characteristic. Only one type of pain is recorded. The score is 0.

THE SACROILIAC SYNDROME

Figure 7-4 is from a patient with the sacroiliac syndrome. Stabbing pain in buttock, posterior thigh, and groin is one characteristic picture for this condi-

Table 7-2 Scoring Sheet for Pain Drawing

Writing anywhere	1
Unphysiological pain pattern	1
Unphysiological sensory change	1
More than one type of pain	1
Both upper and lower areas of body involved	1
Markings outside body	1
Unspecified symbols	1

Score: 1 = Normal. 5 or more = Very bad.
(Courtesy of L. L. Wiltse.)

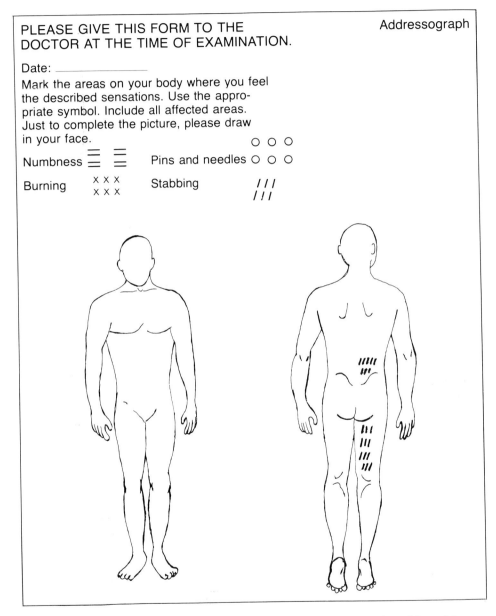

Fig. 7-3 Pain drawing by a patient with posterior joint syndrome. (Adapted from Mooney V, Robertson J: The facet syndrome. Clin Orthop 115: 149, 1976.)

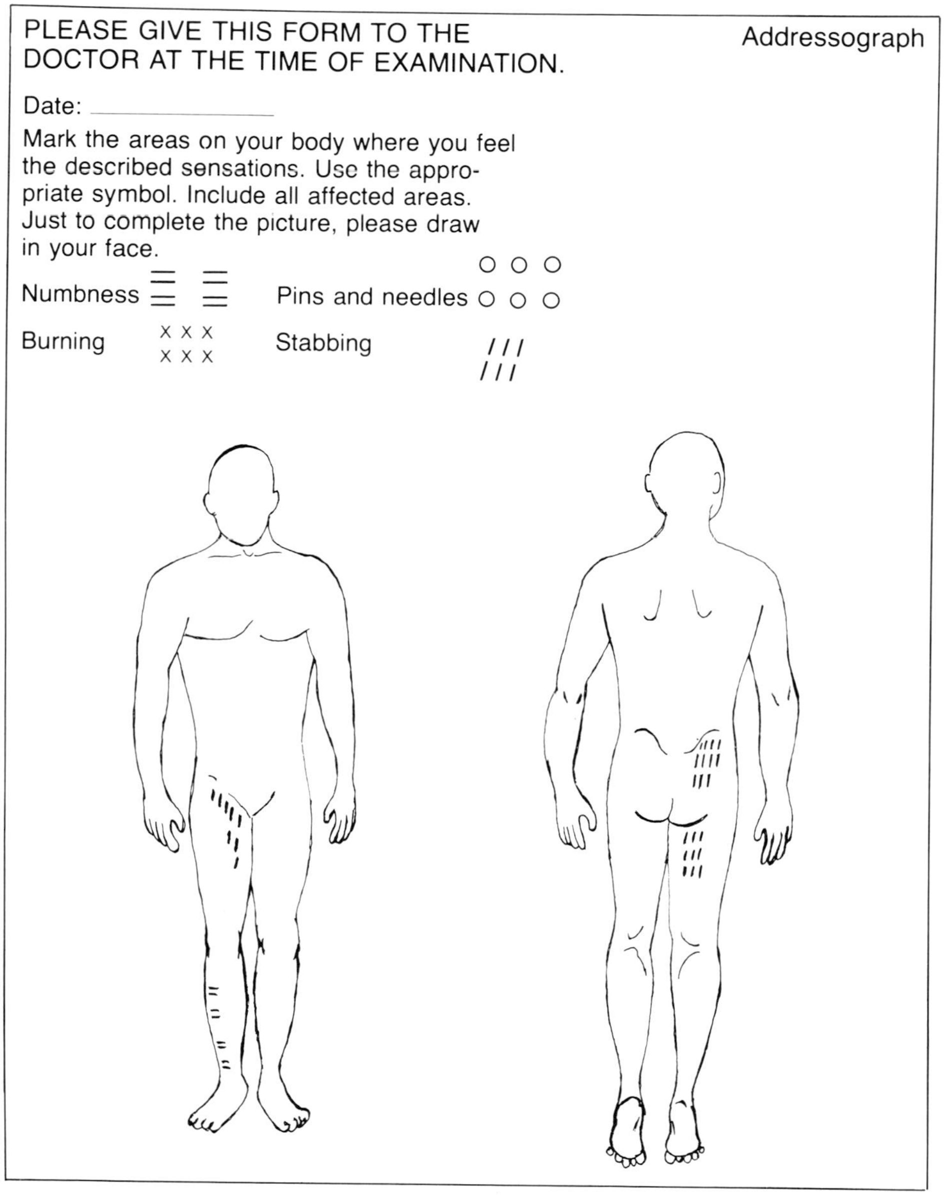

PLEASE GIVE THIS FORM TO THE
DOCTOR AT THE TIME OF EXAMINATION.

Addressograph

Date: _____

Mark the areas on your body where you feel
the described sensations. Use the appropriate symbol. Include all affected areas.
Just to complete the picture, please draw
in your face.

Numbness = =   Pins and needles O O O
                                           O O O

Burning   x x x   Stabbing   / / /
          x x x   / / /

Fig. 7-4 Pain drawing by a patient with sacroiliac syndrome. (Adapted from Mooney V, Robertson J: The facet syndrome. Clin Orthop 115: 149, 1976.)

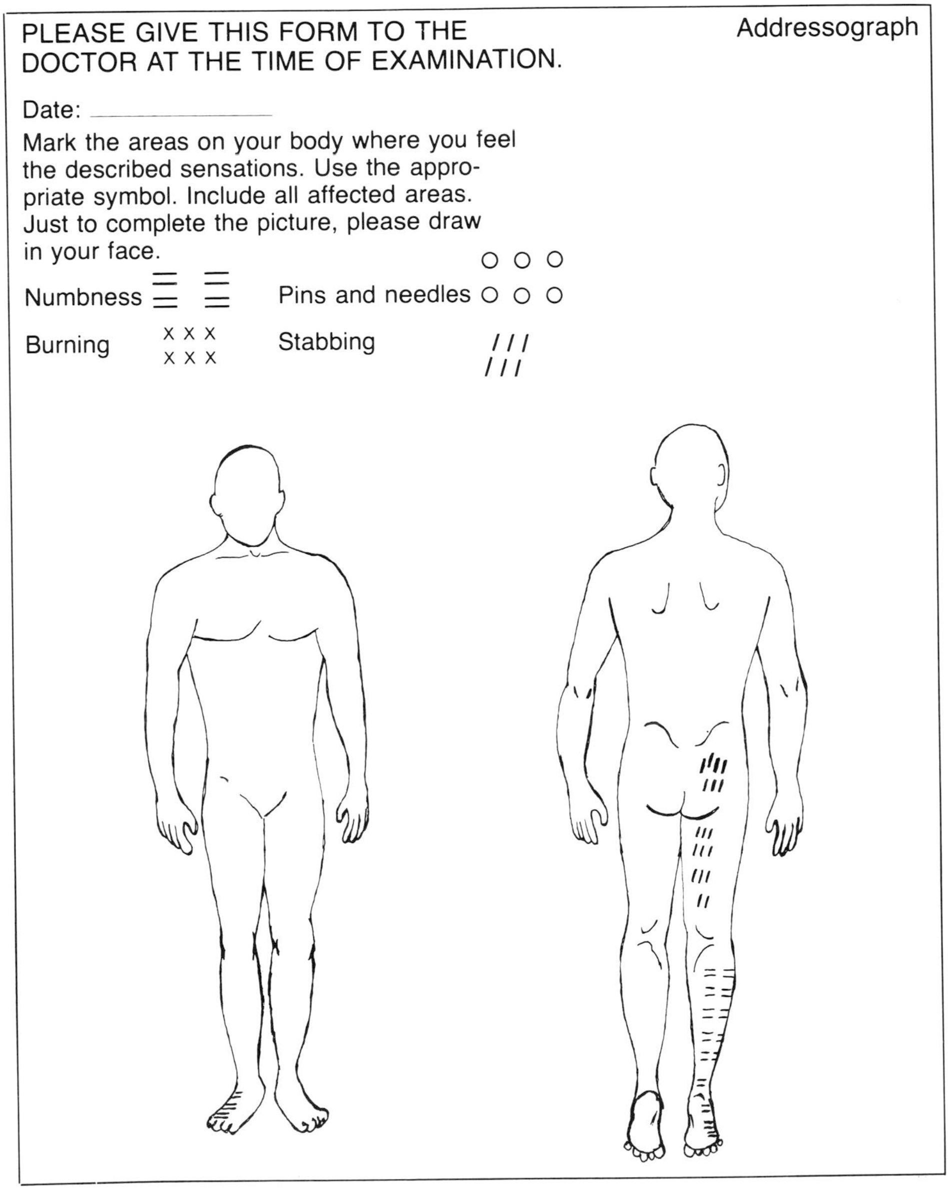

Fig. 7–5 Pain drawing by a patient with an L5–S1 disc herniation. (Adapted from Mooney V, Robertson J: The facet syndrome. Clin Orthop 115: 149, 1976.)

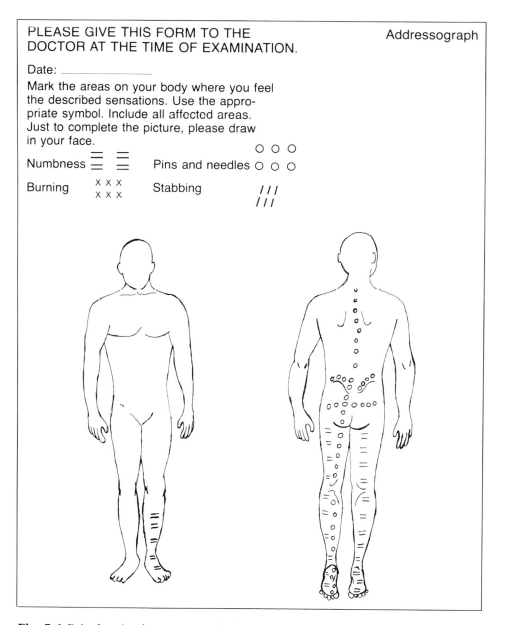

Fig. 7-6 Pain drawing by a patient who has pain with psychological overlay following a disc herniation. (Adapted from Mooney V, Robertson J: The facet syndrome. Clin Orthop 115: 149, 1976.)

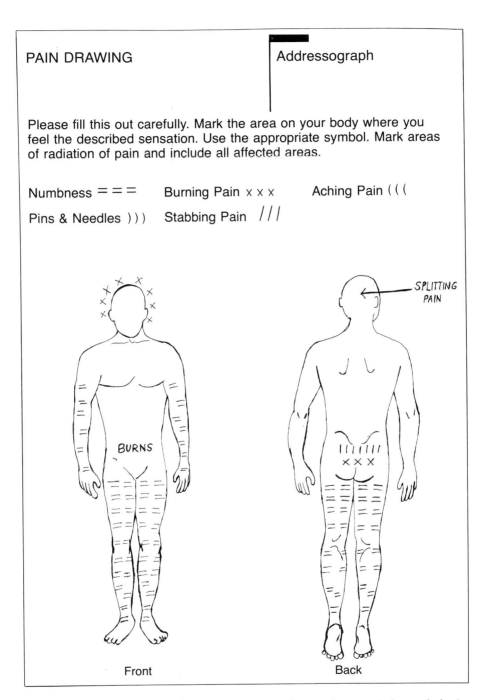

Fig. 7-7 Pain drawing by a patient with symptoms that are almost entirely psychological in origin. (Adapted from Mooney V, Robertson J: The facet syndrome. Clin Orthop 115: 149, 1976.)

tion. Numbness along the lateral calf is also recorded. The score is 1.

AN L5-S1 DISC HERNIATION

Figure 7-5 gives the classical distribution of pain and numbness resulting from a herniation at the L5-S1 level. The score is 1.

Pain of Psychological Origin

Figure 7-6 is a drawing made by a patient who 1 year previously had a discotomy for an L5-S1 disc herniation. The pain pattern is not physiological; the sensory change is not physiological; more than one type of painful sensation is recorded; both the upper trunk and the legs are involved. The score is 4. The pain has a marked psychological overlay.

Pain of Mechanical and Psychological Origin

Figure 7-7 is a drawing by a patient whose symptoms are almost entirely psychological. The pain pattern and the sensory change are both nonphysiological. The chart contains writing. Both upper and lower limbs are involved. There are markings outside the body. The score is 5. The patient requires help from a psychologist in a pain clinic.

REFERENCES

1. Cassel EJ: The nature of suffering and the goals of medicine. N Engl J Med 306: 639, 1982
2. Mooney V, Robertson J: The facet syndrome. Clin Orthop 115: 149, 1976

8
Psychological Assessment

A. J. Roy Cameron
Larry F. Shepel

Psychological factors may markedly affect the way people experience and express pain.[1] The mounting evidence supporting this proposition has caused greater attention to be paid to the psychological assessment and management of pain patients.

Our objective in this chapter is to describe psychological assessment procedures that may be useful in evaluating patients with back pain. We have tried to describe our approach in concrete, practical terms in the hope that physicians and surgeons will find some useful suggestions for screening and referring patients, and develop a clearer understanding of how a psychologist might assess patients who are referred for evaluation.

THE PURPOSE OF THE PSYCHOLOGICAL ASSESSMENT

The purpose of the evaluation is to understand the patient's problem from a social and psychological perspective. Chronic back problems often result in secondary personal difficulties; conversely, psychological factors may give rise to or exacerbate complaints of pain and disability.[2] In the interests of formulating a sound, comprehensive treatment plan, it is useful to know how the back problem has affected the person's life or if psychological factors may be compounding the presenting complaint. *The ultimate objective, always, is to find ways to work with the patient or family to reduce distress and disability.*

Avoid Diagnostic Labels

Terms such as "hysterical," "hypochondriacal," and "regressed" often result in miscommunication, since their meanings are vague and they tend to engender negative perceptions of the patient and a sense of pessimism regarding the prognosis. Rather than falling back on such terms, it is important to identify as specifically as possible the environmental, behavioral, cognitive, and emotional factors that are relevant to the problem and its amelioration.

Distinguishing between "organic" and "functional" problems is of dubious value from the present point of view. Physical and psychological difficulties are not mutually exclusive. Nor can one type of difficulty be inferred from the presumed absence of the other. Regardless of the results of physical investigations, it seems prudent to try to understand what social or psychological difficulties (if any) exist, and how these might be resolved.

INDICATIONS FOR PSYCHOLOGICAL ASSESSMENT

In most settings it is neither feasible nor necessary to conduct a formal, complete psychological assessment of all patients who have back pain. It seems reasonable to consider referral with patients who meet any of the following criteria:

1. Evidence of significant psychological distress (e.g., anxiety, depression, irritability)
2. Evidence of a stressful life situation; e.g., a major life change such as bereavement or occupational change or the presence of chronic tensions such as notable vocational or family dissatisfaction
3. Complaints that appear disproportionate to organic findings
4. Social isolation
5. Evidence of drug abuse
6. A problem that is chronic or becoming so

Patients meeting one or more of these criteria may have complex problems and warrant careful evaluation including, perhaps, a referral for a formal psychological assessment.

THE REFERRAL PROCESS

The way the referral is conducted can dramatically affect the quality of the evaluation. Patients who are comfortable and confident about participating in the assessment are likely to be more candid than those who are defensive and wary. A careful referral process increases the probability that the patient will cooperate.

The basic problem is that pain patients quite understandably (and usually quite correctly) believe that their problems have a physical basis. The relevance of a psychological referral is unclear to the patient. So is its meaning. The patient may infer that the referring physician or surgeon believes that the problem is somehow less than real or that the patient is psychologically unstable. If so, the patient is almost certain to be quite guarded with the psychologist. The defensiveness may be expressed in the form of reticence, hostility, or a Pollyanna presentation, with the patient trying to project an image of robust psychological health by denying even mundane difficul-

ties. The likely result is that the psychologist develops an incomplete or distorted view of the patient and his circumstances.

Clinical experience suggests that the following guidelines may help to circumvent or reduce defensiveness among patients who are referred to a psychologist.

1. Acknowledge the legitimacy of the problem. Patients are less likely to be defensive if they know that the referral does not imply that they are suspected of malingering or exaggerating. They may be reassured by unequivocal recognition that the pain is considered real. It is usually easy for physicians to give this reassurance, and for patients to accept it, when there are significant physical findings. The credibility of the verbal reassurance may be enhanced if the psychological referral is scheduled concurrently with ongoing physical investigations.

Potential problems arise when complaints seem disproportionate to organic findings. Even then, reassurance that the physician recognizes the genuine distress of the patient appears to be in order in most instances. For these patients usually do appear to be experiencing pain, whatever the origin. In any case, since we lack both objective measures of pain and a definitive understanding of pain mechanisms, the patient's self-report cannot be dismissed lightly regardless of hard findings.

2. Provide a positive rationale for the referral. If the patient misconstrues the psychologist as an adversary who is likely to discredit him or his problem, it is difficult for the psychologist to win his confidence. It is important that the psychologist be introduced as an ally who is concerned with finding solutions to problems rather than with passing judgment on the patient or the problem. For instance, if surgery is planned, it might be noted that to ensure the best possible result, it is important to investigate secondary difficulties that may have arisen because of the pain and to make sure that they are understood and dealt with appropriately. If surgery is not contemplated, the psychologist may be presented as someone who is often able to help patients find ways to ease discomfort and reestablish normal activities. The rationale should be honest and positive, should reflect respect for the legitimacy of the problem, and should make sense to the patient.

3. Inform other staff members of the general rationale. Persons other than the referring doctor often influence the patient's perception of the psychological referral. Skeptical patients may ask different clinical and clerical staff members about the consultation. If everyone offers a similar reassuring rationale, the patient is likely to be put at ease. But if explanations conflict or some staff members seem uncomfortable or evasive (because they don't know how to respond), the patient may become increasingly wary. It is therefore helpful if all staff members who have contact with patients are prepared to discuss the referral with the patient in an informed, matter-of-fact, reassuring way.

4. *Let the patient know that the referral is routine.* In some settings, psychological evaluations are routine. If the assessment is routine, the patient may be reassured by knowing this. Of course, if the referral is not at all routine, the patient should not be misled into believing it is: Such deception is not only distasteful but is also readily detected through conversations with other patients and staff and may undermine trust. For the same reason, a statement that the referral is routine should be qualified as appropriate (e.g., "I routinely refer patients who have longstanding, perplexing problems like yours to make sure we don't overlook anything that might be helpful.")

5. *Personalize discussion of the referral.* Personalized discussion can both help to explain the referral and contribute to a comfortable, friendly tone. Three types of personalized comments may be useful.

First, the referring doctor might talk in a hypothetical way about his or her own probable reactions to a problem similar to the patient's. For instance, in suggesting that chronic pain often creates secondary personal problems, the doctor might say something like this: "A problem like you've been living with almost always wears a person down. I know that if I had to live with the sort of difficulty you've had, for as long as you've had it, it would certainly create a strain and take a toll." This sort of statement may help to normalize psychological or interpersonal problems associated with pain.

Second, the psychologist may be described in a personal way. Apprehensions may be reduced if the psychologist can be described as a helpful, friendly sort of person. (It is to be hoped that the psychologist has *some* redeeming personal qualities that can be mentioned!) If most patients have found that they enjoyed their contacts with the psychologist, it wouldn't hurt to note that.

Third, it may help to describe briefly specific instances in which the psychologist was able to assist people who had problems similar to that of the patient. If it's convenient, or if a patient is especially wary, it may also be useful to arrange for the patient to talk with previous patients who benefitted from working with the psychologist.

6. *Make it clear that the referral does not imply a transfer.* If patients mistakenly believe that they are being "dumped," they are likely to be resentful. They may have a more positive attitude toward the psychological assessment if they understand clearly that the physician or surgeon will continue to arrange any further tests or consultations required to ensure a thorough physical investigation, and maintain contact and review the patient's records regularly to monitor developments and progress.

We have discussed the referral process and related consultation issues in more detail elsewhere.[3]

STRUCTURED TESTS AND QUESTIONNAIRES

Minnesota Multiphasic Personality Inventory

The Minnesota Multiphasic Personality Inventory (MMPI) is the psychological test most commonly used to assess pain patients. It consists of some 550 true/false questions and yields scores on 10 clinical scales. Although all scales may be diagnostically useful, scales 1 and 3—also known as the Hypochondriasis (Hs) and Hysteria (Hy) scales, respectively—are particularly noteworthy. A high score on scale 1 indicates that the patient has reported experiencing a wide range of somatic complaints involving various physical functions and body areas. A high score on scale 3 results when the patient has reported some combination of physical complaints, superior adjustment, and sadness and lack of satisfaction with life.[4]

THE MMPI AS A PREDICTOR OF TREATMENT RESPONSE

High pretreatment scores on MMPI scales 1 and 3 have been associated with poor response to surgical procedures[5–7] and conservative treatment[8] (only scale 1 scores were predictive in the latter study). Pretreatment scores on a number of MMPI scales have been found to correlate with response to anesthesiologic and psychiatric interventions.[9] Results of these studies suggest that the MMPI may be useful in helping to identify patients who have a poor prognosis in response to a variety of common treatments.

A NOTE OF CAUTION IN USING THE MMPI

It is prudent to use the MMPI cautiously. In some studies, no significant relationship was found between pretreatment MMPI scores and response to surgical[10] and rehabilitative[11,12] treatment. Moreover, in studies where a statistically significant association has been found between MMPI scores and treatment response, the relationship has sometimes been so modest as to be of limited clinical value.[6] As a final caveat, it is noteworthy that empirical study of the "Low Back Pain" and "Dorsal" scales (derived from the MMPI) has raised serious doubts about the validity of these particular scales.[13–15]

PRACTICAL ISSUES IN USING THE MMPI

There are practical as well as empirical grounds for using the MMPI judiciously. Patients sometimes resent taking the test. Some are overwhelmed by its length. (Although preliminary evidence suggests that shorter versions of the MMPI may be useful for assessing back patients,[16] additional investigations, especially prospective treatment outcome studies, are required to evaluate the predictive validity of these abbreviated tests.) Other patients object to the MMPI because, as a general psychiatric screening test, it includes questions about serious psychiatric symptoms that are usually irrelevant to the patient's situation; these questions may imply that the assessor believes the patient to have gross psychological problems. Still other patients are offended at being asked to spend time answering questions that may seem trivial, intrusive, or redundant.

Hence, the test must be introduced in a sensitive way so that negative reactions are minimized or circumvented. Part of the introduction may emphasize that the test helps us understand in a more precise way how the patient is feeling both physically and psychologically. We often note, for instance, that depression is common among people with chronic

pain and that the test provides a standardized way of measuring the degree of depression. If the patient seems to resent a psychological evaluation, it may be best to omit the MMPI or to postpone it until rapport is established.

Serious misinterpretation of test results may occur. *The profile must be interpreted by someone familiar with MMPI interpretation and current MMPI research.*

THE MMPI AS A GROSS SCREENING INSTRUMENT

Elevations on scales 1 and 3 have been associated with less favorable response to common treatments, as noted above. Our evaluation of patients who have t-scores greater than 70 on either of these scales, or whose test profile is otherwise abnormal, is especially thorough. We assume that these people may be at above-average risk for poor response to physical treatments and we want to ensure that from a psychological point of view everything possible is done to secure a good outcome.

McGill Pain Questionnaire

The McGill questionnaire was developed by Melzack[17] to provide detailed information about both the intensity and the quality of pain. The central part of the questionnaire (Fig. 8-1) lists three classes of adjectives that may be used to describe pain: *sensory* adjectives focus on temporal, spatial, pressure, thermal, and other sensory qualities; *affective* adjectives refer to the emotional (tension, fear) and autonomic properties of the experience; *evaluative* words allow the patient to report the overall subjective intensity of the total pain experience.

The questionnaire yields scores (described in Melzack's paper) that provide a number of quantitative indexes of the patient's discomfort. These may be useful both for monitoring progress and for understanding in a more fine-grained way what the patient is experiencing.

THE INTERVIEW

The MMPI and other structured tests may help to identify patients whose problems are complicated by psychological factors. But they provide little information about what might be done to resolve the

What Does Your Pain Feel Like?

Some of the words I will read to you describe your *present* pain. Tell me which words best describe it. Leave out any word-group that is not suitable. Use only a single word in each appropriate group—the one that applies *best*.

1	2	3	4
1 Flickering	1 Jumping	1 Pricking	1 Sharp
2 Quivering	2 Flashing	2 Boring	2 Cutting
3 Pulsing	3 Shooting	3 Drilling	3 Lacerating
4 Throbbing		4 Stabbing	
5 Beating		5 Lancinating	
6 Pounding			

5	6	7	8
1 Pinching	1 Tugging	1 Hot	1 Tingling
2 Pressing	2 Pulling	2 Burning	2 Itchy
3 Gnawing	3 Wrenching	3 Scalding	3 Smarting
4 Cramping		4 Searing	4 Stinging
5 Crushing			

9	10	11	12
1 Dull	1 Tender	1 Tiring	1 Sickening
2 Sore	2 Taut	2 Exhausting	2 Suffocating
3 Hurting	3 Rasping		
4 Aching	4 Splitting		
5 Heavy			

13	14	15	16
1 Fearful	1 Punishing	1 Wretched	1 Annoying
2 Frightful	2 Gruelling	2 Blinding	2 Troublesome
3 Terrifying	3 Cruel		3 Miserable
	4 Vicious		4 Intense
	5 Killing		5 Unbearable

17	18	19	20
1 Spreading	1 Tight	1 Cool	1 Nagging
2 Radiating	2 Numb	2 Cold	2 Nauseating
3 Penetrating	3 Drawing	3 Freezing	3 Agonizing
4 Piercing	4 Squeezing		4 Dreadful
	5 Tearing		5 Torturing

Fig. 8–1 Adjective checklist section of the McGill Pain Questionnaire. (Reprinted by permission of the publisher from Melzack R: The McGill Pain Questionnaire: major properties and scoring methods. Pain 1:277, 1975, by Elsevier Science Publishing Company Inc.)

problem. Information required to formulate a treatment plan is obtained by interviewing and observing the patient and, if possible, the family. We shall discuss interviewing and behavioral observations separately, although they may overlap considerably.

During the interview we try to get a *general* picture of patients and their circumstances. We want to know what their day-to-day lives are like, who are the significant people in their lives and what sort of relationships they have with them, what interests them, what they worry about, how they see themselves and others, what important experiences they've had, and what sorts of things they would like to accomplish in life.

We also want to get a very *specific* picture of the pain problem, and we'll limit the present discussion

to this aspect of the interview. By the time the interview is complete, we want to know as much as we can about (1) the history of the problem from the point of view of the patient, (2) situational fluctuations in pain, (3) secondary problems that have arisen because of the pain, (4) how the patient expresses pain, (5) how others react to the patient's pain and disability, (6) what effect the patient believes the problem is having on others, (7) if the patient derives important benefits from having pain and disability, (8) how the patient thinks about the problem, (9) patterns of medication use, (10) the patient's mood, (11) what the patient has tried to do to alleviate the pain, and (12) if the patient would have any interest in working with a psychologist. We'll comment briefly on each of these issues in turn.

Problem History

Beginning the interview by asking about the history of the problem helps put patients at ease by allowing them to start with material that is usually well rehearsed and not emotionally charged. It also helps to establish a clear sense that we are interested in focusing on the pain problem and its resolution and are not conducting a psychiatrically oriented interview.

It is important to note discrepancies between the patient's report and the written record. Misunderstandings may give rise to unnecessary worry. We also note comments the patient makes about care received in the past; this information clarifies the patient's preferences and may therefore enable current staff to relate to the patient more effectively. Complaints or concerns about current care are solicited and the patient is encouraged to let us know if we are doing things that are annoying.

Situational Fluctuations

Under what conditions is the pain better or worse? What activities or situations are avoided because of pain? Under what circumstances is the pain either reduced or largely ignored because of compelling diversions? Has the patient explored ways to minimize the impact of situations that trigger pain (e.g., by experimenting with different positions if sexual intercourse is painful)?

Most patients report that pain fluctuates with activity. Few indicate spontaneously that pain varies with mood or stress. To elicit such information we note that many patients find that their mood affects their ability to tolerate pain, and we encourage the patient to discuss fluctuations in *pain tolerance* as a function of mood or external stresses. We are careful to avoid implying that the negative mood or stress is the presumed primary cause of the pain.

Secondary Problems

"What effects has the pain had on you and your relationships?" This open-ended question helps to establish which effects are most salient for the patient. Common problems include difficulties at work (including household chores), sleep disturbance, tension (irritability, "bad nerves"), depression, strained family relationships, financial worries, disruption of sexual interest and activities, and restriction of recreational pursuits. If the patient omits any of these areas, we make specific inquiries.

Problems attributed to pain are explored in detail to determine if they are in fact secondary problems. It is crucial to know, for instance, how things were before the pain began. This is diagnostically significant since one might expect secondary problems to dissipate spontaneously in many (though not all) cases if the back problem can be resolved. However, if the patient attributes an independent problem (e.g., chronic relationship difficulties, primary depression) to the back problem, one would not expect this "secondary" problem to be relieved through physical treatment.

Expression of Pain

Pain may be expressed in many ways. These include verbal reporting, complaining, crying, taking medication, sighing, grimacing, reclining, rubbing the affected area, limping, and inactivity. It is useful to know how the patient expresses pain and how patterns of expression vary across situations.

The way the patient expresses pain may have either adaptive or maladaptive consequences. For instance, a person who attempts to be stoical and inhibit any acknowledgment of pain may be seen as inexplicably "moody" by others: in this case, letting others know about the problem may help to avoid misunderstanding and strained relationships. Conversely, a patient who exhibits persistent, theatrical pain displays may elicit resentment and/or excessive nurturance that undermines the patient's independence. If a person must live with a chronic or recurrent problem, the quality of the person's life will be determined to a considerable extent by the adaptiveness of the pain expression.

Reactions of Others

Ideally, families and coworkers should make necessary allowances for the patient's pain and disability while doing everything possible to encourage independence and normal activities. Difficulties arise if others become (1) resentful, impatient, and antagonistic; (2) excessively solicitous in a way that keeps attention focussed on the pain and discourages independence; or (3) overbearing or condescending in encouraging the patient's progress. Many patients are reluctant to say negative things about the significant people in their lives, and sensitivity is required to elicit candid information.

Effects of the Problem on Others

Does the patient's back problem create serious difficulties for others? Patients sometimes have a sense of guilt that their problem causes hardship for others. Their specific concerns may or may not be realistic. If they are unfounded, it is important to clarify this. If it appears that others are indeed affected as adversely as the patient imagines, attention can be focussed on attempting to reduce these problems.

Benefits from Pain

Patients may receive psychological or financial benefits from pain or disability. Such benefits can represent impediments to rehabilitation. However, identification of payoffs for pain is a difficult, complex process.

The basic diagnostic problem stems from the fact that back problems almost always result in some life changes that *could* be construed as beneficial from the patient's point of view. For instance, back problems commonly result in sympathetic attention, decreased vocational responsibility, and financial compensation. Even people who normally get all the attention they want, sincerely enjoy their work, and are unquestionably highly motivated to get back to normal find themselves receiving such "benefits." Hence the simple observation that the presenting problem results in "benefits" does not justify a conclusion that the patient is relying on the back problem to secure psychological or financial advantages.

On the other hand, it would seem naive to overlook the possibility that such benefits might undermine the patient's response to treatment. It seems prudent to investigate very carefully those patients who have been dissatisfied with their work or personal lives. The person who has been dissatisfied but has lacked the skill or courage to make changes may discover that the back problem makes it possible to alter or avoid unpleasant vocational or personal situations.

To say that the symptoms may be yielding important benefits does not necessarily imply that the patient is deliberately manipulative. Consider, for instance, a man who has felt progressively inadequate in his work and in his sexual relationship. He develops a back problem and finds that he has a legitimate reason to avoid both work and sex. This man may be less likely to resume work and sexual relations than another patient who has the same organic problem but who thrives on his work and thoroughly enjoys sexual relations. It is not that the first man consciously decides to keep complaining of pain to avoid stressful activities; he is just less likely than the second man to disregard continuing discomfort, because he lacks the zest for living that pulls the second man back into a normal routine.

In a situation like this, a key diagnostic task is to determine the feasibility of helping the patient find solutions to the background problems. If our hypothetical man is able to find ways to improve vocational satisfaction and to establish a gratifying, comfortable sexual relationship with his wife, one would expect his prognosis to be improved.

The Patient's Thoughts about the Problem

The way the patient thinks about the problem may influence the degree of subjective discomfort and "pain behavior." We try to get an idea of the extent to which the patient is *preoccupied* with pain and related problems. A number of indicators suggest preoccupation. Patients may acknowledge that the problem is so bad that they often have difficulty getting their minds off it. Or they may demonstrate preoccupation by continually bringing conversations back to their complaints. Elevation on MMPI scale 1 and evidence that the patient's life is largely devoid of satisfying, absorbing activities suggest indirectly that preoccupation may be a problem.

It is also instructive to notice how patients *label* their pain. There is evidence that the same aversive stimulus may be experienced as more or less painful depending on how it has been labeled.[18] It seems plausible to hypothesize that patients who have developed a habit of regularly thinking and talking about their pain as "excruciating," "unbearable," etc., may thereby exacerbate their discomfort. This is not to deny that some pain is indeed excruciatingly intense, but merely to suggest that loose usage of such extreme labels may magnify perceptions of the pain.

Finally, we try to determine if patients have specific *fears or misconceptions*. Fears of cancer and progressive degenerative conditions are the most common fears we see in patients with back pain. Such fears may be engendered or intensified by diagnostic investigations: patients going for tests in nuclear medicine, for instance, have sometimes inferred that a diagnosis of cancer was being considered.

Patients with catastrophic fears may be reluctant to voice them. They may be inhibited by a foreboding sense that a feared diagnosis will be confirmed if investigated or by a concern about appearing hypochondriacal. If patients are simply asked what they think is causing their pain, they often merely repeat opinions of physicians as if these opinions are their own. And, indeed, they may genuinely believe that these explanations are rational. However, this does not necessarily mean that they do not at the same time harbor fears that something more sinister is wrong. To overcome inhibitions about reporting catastrophic fears, it may be useful to say something like this: "Sometimes the people we see have private fears about what is wrong with them. If you have any nagging fears in the back of your mind, even fears you've hesitated to express because you know they're probably groundless, it's important that we know about them. Some of the people who come to us have been worrying needlessly for a long time and have found it helpful to bring their concerns out in the open so they could be discussed with the doctors on our team."

Medication Use

It is important to identify patients who are overusing analgesic medications. We also explore the use of psychotropic drugs. Some patients take substantial amounts of either analgesics or psychoactive drugs in response to problems (e.g., irritability, tension, depression, insomnia) that may be relieved, partially if not wholly, through psychological means.

Mood

Pain patients are sometimes depressed. The relationship between pain and depression is not clearly understood and is undoubtedly complex.[19] Whether a primary or secondary problem, depression may require direct treatment.

The diagnosis of depression is described in detail elsewhere.[20] In brief, it is noteworthy that some patients who deny depression are manifestly depressed

according to psychiatric criteria; conversely, not all who describe themselves as depressed would be diagnosed as clinically depressed using the same criteria. Therefore, it is hazardous to rely solely on the patient's self-reported mood (although this is obviously important) in assessing depression. Other commonly used indicators of depression include elevation on scale 2 (Depression) of the MMPI and psychiatric criteria; the following list of indicators is abbreviated from the Research Diagnostic Criteria for Major Depressive Disorders:[21]

1. Increased or poor appetite; weight gain or loss (change of at least .5 kg/week for several weeks or 4.5 kg/year, not dieting)
2. Sleep difficulty, including too much
3. Reduced energy, tiredness
4. Psychomotor retardation or agitation
5. Loss of interest or pleasure in sex, social contact, or other usual activities
6. Self-reproach, excessive guilt
7. Diminished capacity to concentrate or think—e.g., indecisiveness, slowed thinking
8. Recurring thoughts of death or suicide; any suicidal behavior

Full psychiatric diagnostic criteria are described by Spitzer and his colleagues.[21]

In addition to assessing depression, it is important to consider the extent to which the person may be experiencing stress or anxiety. Patients may report being anxious (edgy, jumpy, nervous, highstrung, worried, etc.), experiencing chronic tensions, or undergoing major adjustments in their lives. Physical agitation or evidence of notable muscle tension is also noteworthy.

It is assumed that negative mood reduces pain tolerance. Depression and anxiety may also contribute directly to the sense of subjective distress that the patient labels pain.

The Patient's Attempt to Cope with Pain

Most patients attempt to reduce their pain and attendant problems in a variety of ways. It is informative to explore the range of strategies they use. Some have extensive repertoires of coping behaviors, while others rely almost wholly on activity restriction, medication, and medical or chiropractic treatments. It is important to identify patients who lack personal strategies for reducing discomfort and instances where patients may have prematurely given up a potentially useful strategy; e.g., some patients report unsuccessful attempts at self-relaxation (see Chapter 22), but inquiry suggests that training in or application of relaxation procedures is inadequate.

Interest in Working with a Psychologist

Not all patients whom we think might benefit from working with a psychologist are prepared to do so. Practical restrictions or personal reservations that would preclude psychological treatment need to be investigated before such treatment is recommended.

Interviewing the Family

Whenever possible, interviews with family members or others who know the patient well are conducted with the patient's knowledge and permission. It is easier for others to provide independent opinions and points of view if they are interviewed alone. We solicit their observations and impressions regarding the problem and its effect on both the patient and other family members. Apparent discrepancies between accounts given by the patient and others need to be explored carefully; it can be misleading to discount either version out of hand.

BEHAVIORAL DATA

Specific information about the patient's behavior patterns is extremely informative. Fordyce[22] has published a number of very simple record forms that yield detailed information about the patient's activity level (Fig. 8-2). Developing a treatment plan and monitoring treatment progress may be greatly facilitated by having patients maintain such records during evaluation periods. The Psychosocial Pain Inventory[23] is also designed to systematize collection of pertinent data.

Behavioral tests may be undertaken to establish the patient's tolerance for normal activities. For example, if a patient complains that walking is painful, it is helpful to determine exactly how long or how far the person can walk under various conditions (e.g., walking continuously, pausing for brief rests). This information is of practical value for planning a treatment program, establishing concrete treatment goals, and evaluating treatment progress.

Simple behavioral experiments may also be conducted to examine the extent to which the patient's pain-related behaviors are responsive to environmental changes. For instance, the patient's expressions of pain might be monitored during staff-initiated conversations that focus on pleasant topics having nothing to do with the patient's distress. If one can show that pain expression is reliably less frequent under the influence of such commonly available distracting activities, it suggests that the patient might benefit from a treatment plan that promotes increased involvement in diverting activities. In an analogous way, it is possible to conduct similar experiments designed to identify environmental factors (e.g., conversations focusing on pain, disability, and hardships) that may increase pain expression in order to pinpoint conditions that the patient and family should attempt to reduce (e.g., unnecessary conversations about pain). Evidence that pain expression fluctuates depending on such environmental shifts does not, of course, rule out an organic basis for the problem.

Fordyce's book[22] presents an extended discussion of the behavioral analysis of pain problems and includes many valuable practical clinical suggestions.

THE UPSHOT OF THE ASSESSMENT

It would be nice if psychologists could predict with confidence each patient's response to surgery or other physical treatments. Unfortunately, that is not possible. The results of the psychological assessment may influence one's general level of optimism or pessimism about probable response to treatment. The MMPI research for instance, provides some evidence that gross predictions may be possible in at least some settings. But precise predictions are hazardous: Some patients who seem to be high risks from a psychological point of view respond well; others whose cases seem straightforward have disappointing outcomes. The psychologist's findings may be taken into account by a surgeon who has to make a judgment about whether or not to proceed with surgery. But it is

Please check each day which of the activities listed you engaged in.

Week of _____ , 19 ____

	MON	TUES	WED	THURS	FRI	SAT	SUN
1. VISITING – – – – – – – – –							
Came to visit:							
Relative(s)							√
Others	√						
None							
Went out to visit:							
Relative(s)						√	
Others							
None							
2. OUTSIDE HOME TRIPS – – – –							
Sight-seeing excursion			√				
Movie, ballgame, concert, etc.							
Attended meeting							
Shopping					√		
Other							
None							
3. INSIDE HOME ACTIVITIES – – –							
Calls made to relative(s) friends/neighbors				√			
Calls you received from relatives, friends, neighbors				√		√	
Reading							
Television							
Radio/records/tape							
Hobbies/handicrafts		√					
Others							
None							
4. WALKING QUOTA – – – – – –	√	√	√	√	√	√	√

Fig. 8–2 Activity diary. (Adapted from Fordyce W: Behavioral Methods for Chronic Pain and Illness. CV Mosby, St Louis, 1976.)

hard to imagine a case where surgery would be withheld on psychological grounds in the face of compelling physical indications for an operation.

In practice, we find our post-assessment discussions with the surgeon extremely valuable in formulating a treatment plan. These meetings provide an opportunity to integrate information and to develop a treatment strategy and rationale that can be shared with the patient.

If there is evidence of psychological difficulty, an appropriate treatment plan is formulated (in consultation with other members of the team) and presented to the patient for consideration. Common psychological treatment strategies are considered in Chapter 22. In cases where indications for surgery are also present, the goal of the psychological treatment is to maximize the probability of a good surgical result. In the absence of remarkable physical findings, the goal is to do everything possible to resolve psychological difficulties, subjective discomfort, and physical disability in the hope that this, coupled with other rehabilitative efforts, will improve the quality of the patient's life and reduce distress.

ACKNOWLEDGMENT

We are grateful to Myles Genest, Donald Meichenbaum, Kenneth Prkachin, Barr Taylor, Dennis Turk, and Carl von Baeyer for comments on previous drafts of this material.

1. Melzack R: The Puzzle of Pain. Penguin, Harmondsworth, 1973
2. Mersky H, Boyd D: Emotional adjustment and chronic pain. Pain 5: 173, 1978
3. Cameron R, Shepel LF: The process of psychological consultation in pain management. In Holzman AD, Turk DC (eds): Pain Management: A Handbook of Psychological Treatment Approaches. Pergamon, New York, 1986
4. Marks PA, Seeman W: Actuarial Description of Abnormal Personality. Williams & Wilkins, Baltimore, 1963
5. Blumetti AE, Modesti LM: Psychological predictors of success or failure of surgical intervention for intractable back pain. In Bonica JJ, Albe-Fessard D (eds): Advances in Pain Research and Therapy. Vol. 1. Raven Press, New York, 1976
6. Pheasant HC, Gilbert D, Goldfarb J, Herron L: The MMPI as a predictor of outcome in low-back surgery. Spine 4: 78, 1979
7. Wiltse LL, Rocchio PD: Preoperative psychological tests as predictors of success of chemonucleolysis in the treatment of the low-back syndrome. J Bone Joint Surg 57A: 478, 1975
8. McCreary C, Turner J, Dawson E: The MMPI as a predictor of response to conservative treatment for low back pain. J Clin Psychol 35: 278, 1979
9. Strassberg DS, Reimherr F, Ward M, et al: The MMPI and chronic pain. J Consult Clin Psychol 49: 220, 1981
10. Waring EM, Weisz GM, Bailey SI: Predictive factors in the treatment of low back pain by surgical intervention. In Bonica JJ, Albe-Fessard D (eds): Advances in Pain Research and Therapy. Vol. 1. Raven Press, New York, 1976
11. Cummings C, Evanski PM, Debenedetti MJ, et al: Use of the MMPI to predict outcome of treatment for chronic pain. In Bonica JJ (ed): Advances in Pain Research and Therapy. Vol. 3. Raven Press, New York, 1979
12. Moore JE, Armentrout DP, Parker JC, Kivlahan DR: Empirically derived pain patient MMPI subgroups: prediction of treatment outcome. J Behav Med 9: 51, 1986
13. Rosen JC, Frymoyer JW, Clements JH: A further look at validity of the MMPI with low back patients. J Clin Psychol 36: 994, 1980
14. Towne WS, Tsushima WT: The use of the low back and dorsal scales in the identification of functional low back patients. J Clin Psychol 34: 88, 1978
15. Tsushima WT, Towne WS: Clinical limitations of the low back scale. J Clin Psychol 35: 306, 1979
16. Turner J, McCreary C: Short forms of the MMPI with back pain patients. J Consult Clin Psychol 46: 354, 1978
17. Melzack R: The McGill Pain Questionnaire: major properties and scoring methods. Pain 1: 277, 1975
18. Hall KRL, Stride E: The varying response to pain in psychiatric disorders. Br J Med Psychol 27: 48, 1954
19. Romano JM, Turner JA: Chronic pain and depression: Does the evidence support a relationship? Psychol Bull 97: 18, 1985
20. Lewinsohn PM, Lee WML: Assessment of affective disorders. In Barlow DH (ed): Behavioral Assessment of Adult Disorders. Guilford, New York, 1981
21. Spitzer RL, Endicott J, Robins E: Research diagnostic criteria: rationale and reliability. Arch Gen Psychiatry 35: 773, 1978
22. Fordyce WE: Behavioral Methods for Chronic Pain and Illness. CV Mosby, St Louis, 1976
23. Heaton RK, Getto CJ, Lehman RAW, et al: A standardized evaluation of psychosocial factors in chronic pain. Pain 12: 165, 1982

9

The Three Phases of the Spectrum of Degenerative Disease

William H. Kirkaldy-Willis

The three phases of the degenerative process—dysfunction, the unstable phase, stabilization—are schematized in Figure 9-1. For clarity these three are separated into well-defined horizontal bars. In fact no such clear-cut distinction between them exists. The patient may pass gradually from one phase to the next. Following a recurrent episode of trauma the patient may pass from dysfunction to the unstable phase. During recovery he may pass back to dysfunction. As seen in Chapter 1, the tendency over a period of years is that the patient's symptoms increase so that he passes from dysfunction to the unstable phase and on to stabilization, but this does not invariably occur.

DYSFUNCTION

The majority of patients seen in a low-back-pain clinic suffer from dysfunction. During this phase the pathological changes are relatively minor and perhaps reversible. For this reason such changes are more difficult to demonstrate. The term dysfunction implies that at one anatomical level (usually L4–5 or L5–S1) the three components of the joint are not functioning normally. The early pathological changes in the posterior facet joints and the disc are described and illustrated in Chapter 4. Following injury these changes produce symptoms as discussed below. After recovery from injury the symptoms may cease. Further injury results in reappearance of symptoms.

Presentation

The presentation varies considerably. For convenience it can be divided into three types: rotational or compressive strain, sometimes due to a major but more often to a minor episode of trauma; pain that occurs after activity that is unusual for the patient, for example, the sedentary worker who gardens vigorously all weekend in early summer and some hours or 1 to 2 days later complains of severe low back pain of sudden onset for no clear reason; and recurrence of pain due to a very minor episode of trauma.

Mechanisms

The mechanisms involved are shown in Figure 9-2. The episode of trauma results in posterior joint (and annular) strain. Because of small capsular (and

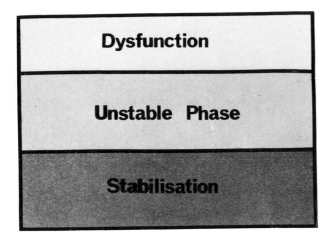

Fig. 9-1 The three states (phases of the degenerative process.

annular) tears, a small degree of joint subluxation takes place. The posterior joint synovium is injured, leading to synovitis. The posterior segmental muscles protect the joint by sustained hypertonic contraction. The muscle becomes ischemic and this causes more pain. Accumulation of metabolites in muscle further aggravates the pain and sustains the hypertonic state of contraction. The posterior joints continue to be

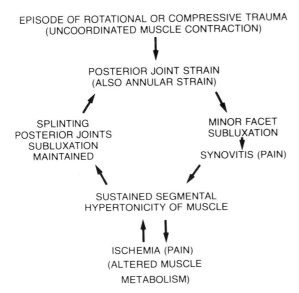

Fig. 9-2 Mechanics of dysfunction. (Courtesy of S. V. Paris.)

splinted and the minor subluxation is maintained. These changes later lead to fibrosis.

Symptoms

The symptoms are those of acute, subacute, or chronic low back pain. Pain is often localized to one area and to one side. Pain may be referred to the groin, to the region of the greater trochanter, and to the posterior thigh as far as the knee; it rarely passes below the knee. The pain is relieved by rest and made worse by movement. One or more particular movements "catch" the patient and aggravate the pain.

Signs

There are multiple signs. Tenderness to pressure is present, usually on one side and at one level over the sacrospinalis and multifidus muscle. The muscle at this site is in a state of sustained contraction (hypertonic). Lateral bending is abnormal; i.e., the patient bends more to one side than to the other (hypomobility). Muscle activity is abnormal. For example, normally the muscle on the right contracts when the patient bends to the left; however, this pattern may be altered. All movements are restricted, especially extension. Some degree of functional scoliosis, seen more clearly on forward flexion, may be present. Palpation at the level of the lesion may demonstrate that one spinous process is out of line with the next.

Radiographic Changes

Anteroposterior stress radiographs demonstrate several abnormalities. Movement is decreased asymmetrically; i.e., the spine bends more to one side than to the other. The spinous processes may be out of line at one level. Normally, when the spine is bent laterally, the spinous processes rotate slightly to the side of bending. In dysfunction the spinous processes may not move (rotate) to the side to which the patient has bent. Normally, with lateral bending the disc height is reduced on the concave side. In dysfunction the space on the concave side may remain open.

Oblique views may show irregularity of posterior facets.

Lateral stress radiographs are rarely abnormal. In longstanding dysfunction they may reveal that small osteophytes are present at the anterior surface of the vertebral bodies and that the disc is slightly reduced in height. Figure 9-3 demonstrates radiographic changes seen in the anteroposterior view. Figure 9-3A shows a high riding L5 vertebra with the L5–S1 level at risk. Figure 7-3B shows a low riding L5 vertebra with the L4–5 level at risk. In normal lateral bending the disc closes on the concave side and the whole spine rotates so that the spinous processes shift to the concave side (Type I). During dysfunction hypertonic muscles restrict rotation as the spine bends to the opposite side and may progress to the point at which the disc fails to close or even opens on the opposite side. Malalignment of spinous processes suggests rotational deformity, which can be confirmed by lateral bending views. These changes are demonstrated in Figures 9-3C to J. Table 9-1 sets out in tabular form the symptoms, signs, and radiographic changes found in dysfunction.

Two problems arise. First, as we have seen in discussing the pathology of low back pain (Chapter 4), changes affecting the facet joints also affect the disc and vice versa. In dysfunction the changes chiefly affect the facet joints, but small annular tears are also present. Sometimes a disc herniation is present as well. Therefore it is necessary to exclude this condition. This point will be discussed as we turn to consider herniation of the nucleus pulposus. Second, dysfunction at one level may complicate the unstable phase at another, usually lower, level as the lesion spreads to involve more than the original level.

THE UNSTABLE PHASE

With each successive episode of trauma, healing of capsular tears of the posterior joint and annular tears of the disc is less complete because the collagen of scar tissue is not as strong as normal collagen. The three parts of the joint complex are thus increasingly at risk. Early in Phase I the patient is more likely to develop recurrent dysfunction. Toward the end of this phase it becomes likely that the patient will pass into Phase II. Throughout Phase II there is a tendency for the problem to recur, and on each occasion the instability becomes more marked.

Presentation

The presentation may either be similar to that described above for dysfunction or chronic and insidious without any recorded history of minor trauma.

Mechanisms

The mechanisms involved are twofold: a further episode of trauma and continuing stress. Either or both of these result in increased dysfunction. Progressive changes seen in the facet joints are degeneration of cartilage, stretching or attenuation of the capsule, and laxity of the capsule. Changes in the disc are coalescence of tears, loss of nuclear substance with internal disruption, and bulging of the annulus around the circumference of the disc. The result is detectable increased abnormal movement in the three-joint complex. The patient has entered the unstable phase (Fig. 9-4).

Symptoms

The symptoms may be no more than those seen in severe dysfunction. The patient may complain that his back feels weak, that it feels as though it is going to give way, or that certain movements, coming upright again after bending forwards, produce a "catch" in his back.

Signs

The signs are twofold. Increased abnormal movement between one vertebra and the next may be detected by inspecting or palpating the spinous processes when the patient moves or lies on one side. A "catch," a sway, or a shift at one level may be observed as the patient returns to the standing position after bending forward. The patient may not be able to do this without supporting himself by placing his hands on knees or thighs.

Radiographic Changes

Changes seen on x-ray confirm the diagnosis. Anteroposterior lateral bending radiographs may show that one vertebral body shifts to one side on the body

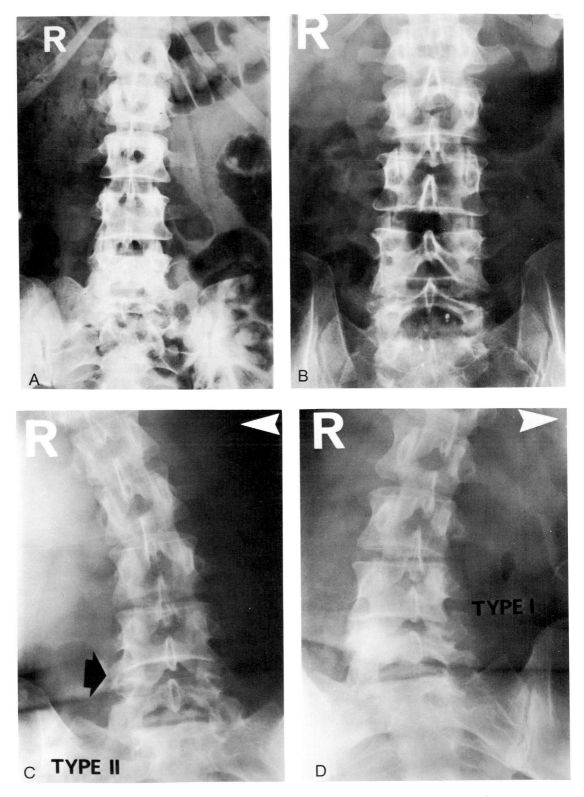

Fig. 9-3. The radiological changes seen in dysfunction. (*Figure continues.*)

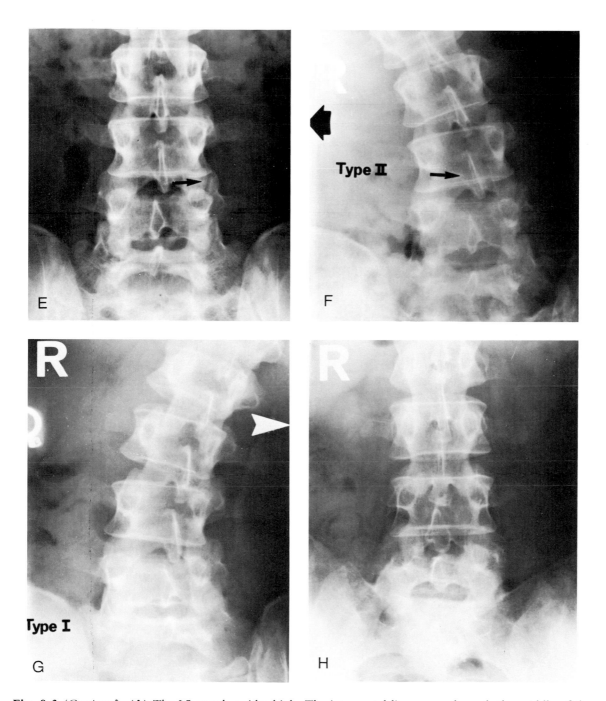

Fig. 9-3 (*Continued*). **(A)** The L5 vertebra rides high. The intercrestal line passes through the middle of the L5 body. The L5–S1 joint is at risk. **(B)** The L5 vertebra is low in the pelvis. The intercrestal line passes through the upper part of the L4 body. The L4–5 joint is at risk. **(C)** When the spine is bent laterally to the right the spinous processes do not move in that direction. This lack of movement is characteristic of a Type II change (dysfunction). **(D)** Radiograph from the same patient as in (C). When the spine is bent laterally to the left, the spinous processes move to the left. Such movement is normal and is called a Type I movement. **(E)** Standing erect (AP) view. The L4 spinous process (opposite the arrow) is to the left of that of L5. This indicates dysfunction with rotation. **(F)** The same patient as in (E). When the spine is bent laterally to the right, the spinous process fails to move to the right. The L4 and L5 processes are malaligned. Dysfunction is confirmed. **(G)** The same patient as in (E) and (F). When the spine is bent laterally to the left, the spinous processes move normally to the left. They are normally aligned. **(H)** Standing erect AP view. L4 vertebra is slightly tilted on L5. (*Figure continues.*)

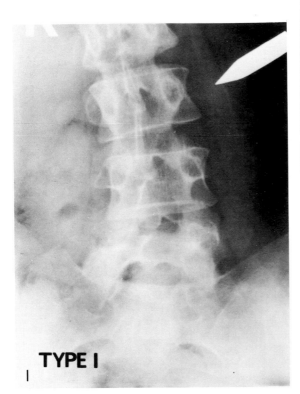

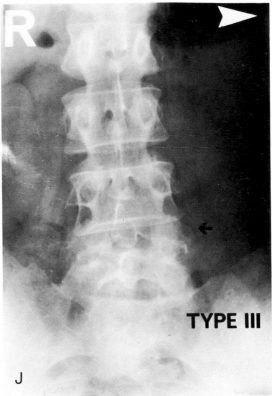

Fig. 9-3 (*Continued*). **(I)** The same patient as in (H). On lateral bending to the right the spinous processes moves to the right in a normal way (Type I). **(J)** The same patient as in (H) and (I). On attempted lateral bending to the left, the spine remains erect. The disc space opens on the left, a Type III change indicative of marked dysfunction.

Table 9-1 The Symptoms, Signs, and Radiological Changes Seen in Dysfunction

Symptoms
    Low back pain
        Often localized
        Sometimes referred
    Movement painful

Signs
    Local tenderness
    Muscle contracted
    Hypomobility
    Extension painful
    Neurological exam usually normal

Radiographs
    Abnormal decreased movement
    Spinous processes malaligned
    Irregular facets
    Early disc changes

below it—usually L4 or L5—and/or that a spinous process rotates on the one below, resulting in malalignment. This malalignment may be reduced on flexion to one side and increased on flexion to the other. One body may tilt abnormally on another.

Oblique views may demonstrate that the facet joints have opened and are malaligned.

Lateral radiographs in both flexion and extension frequently show increased movement. In degenerative spondylolisthesis the upper vertebra moves forward on the lower in flexion (because of erosion of the superior facets) and back toward the normal position in extension. More commonly a small degree of retrospondylolisthesis seen in flexion becomes greater in extension. Extension may cause increased narrowing of the intervertebral foramen. The disc may open to an abnormal degree, at its anterior aspect during extension and at its posterior aspect during

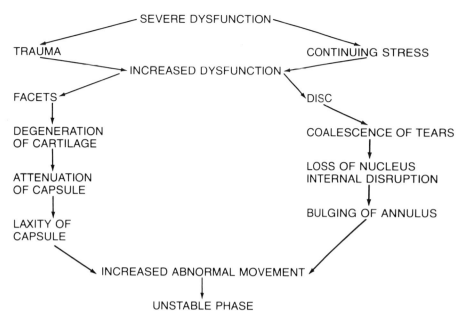

Fig. 9-4 Mechanisms of the unstable phase.

flexion. There may be an abrupt change in pedicle height at one level because one vertebra has rotated on another. CT scan images may show abnormal opening and closing of posterior joints on rotation to both left and right.

A summary of the clinical and radiological findings is shown in Table 9-2. Radiographs demonstrating some of the features of the unstable phase are shown in Figure 9-5.

Two points should be noted. First, in a patient with instability at the L4–5 level concomitant dysfunction may be present at the L3–4 or L5–S1 level. Second, the patient may shift from Phase II back to Phase I. For example, minor trauma may produce enough added capsular and annular laxity in a case of severe dysfunction so that the physician can detect, clinically and radiologically, the presence of increased abnormal movement and place the patient in Phase II. Adequate treatment may result in sufficient healing by scar formation in the posterior joint capsule and the annulus so that the increased movement disappears and the patient is once again in Phase I. But the condition may be so severe that no treatment other than fusion can deal with the instability.

Table 9-2 The Symptoms, Signs, and Radiological Changes Seen in the Unstable Stage

Symptoms
    Those of dysfunction
    Giving way of back: "catch" in back (on movement)
    Pain on coming to standing position after flexion

Signs
    Detection of abnormal movement (inspection, palpation)
    Observation of "catch," sway, or shift when coming erect after flexion

Radiographs
    Anteroposterior
        Lateral shift
        Rotation
        Abnormal tilt
        Malaligned spinous processes
    Oblique
        Opening facets
    Lateral
        Spondylolisthesis (in flexion)
        Retrospondylolisthesis (in extension)
        Narrowing foramen (in extension)
        Abnormal opening of disc
        Abrupt change in pedicle height
    CT changes

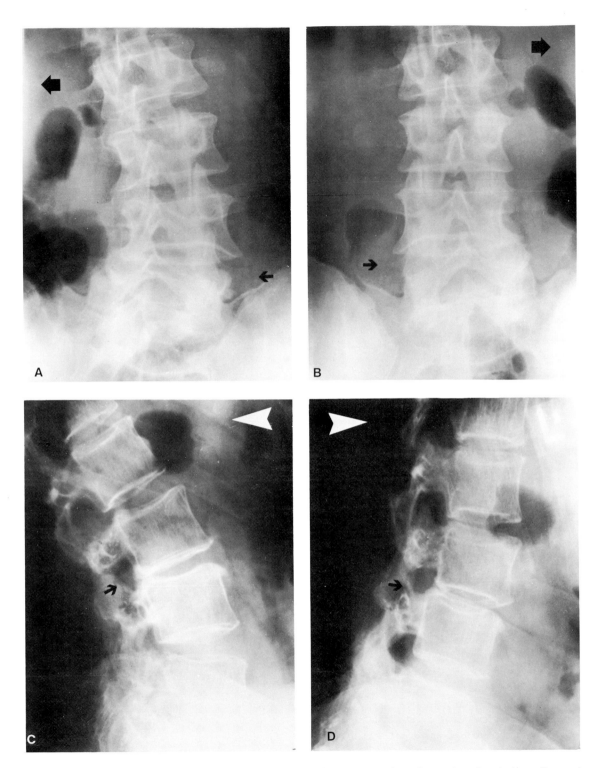

Fig. 9-5 The radiological changes seen in the unstable phase. **(A)** When the patient bends laterally to the right (viewer's left), the body of L4 moves laterally to the left relative to the body of L5 (arrow). **(B)** The same patient as in (A). On attempted lateral bending to the left (viewer's right), the spine remains erect. The body of L4 shifts to the right (arrow). Instability is seen at L4–5. **(C)** In this lateral view in extension the body of L3 is displaced slightly forward on that of L4 (arrow). **(D)** The same patient as in (C). In flexion the body of L3 is further displaced forward on that of L4 (arrow). Instability is due to degenerative spondylolisthesis. (*Figure continues.*)

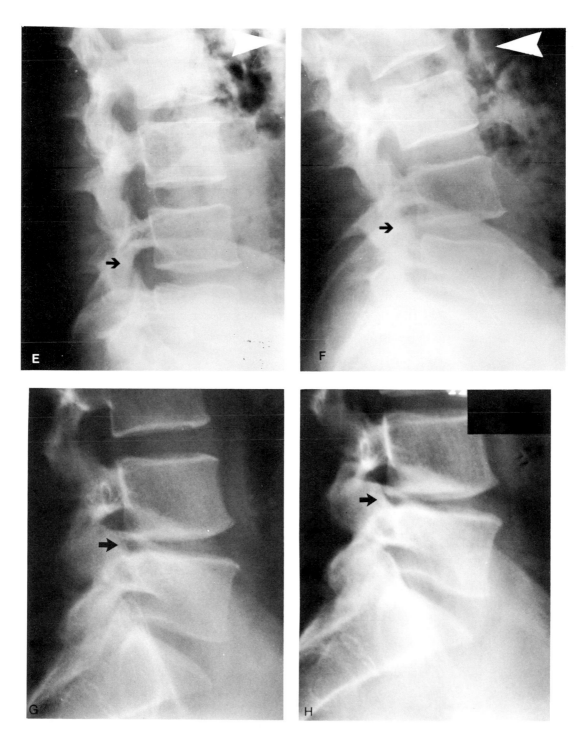

Fig. 9-5 (*Continued*). **(E)** Lateral view in flexion. Posterior aspects of the vertebral bodies (arrow) are aligned normally. **(F)** The same patient as in (E). In extension the body of L4 is displaced posteriorly on that of L5 (arrow). Retrospondylolisthesis is indicative of instability of minor degree. **(G)** Lateral view in flexion. The vertebral body of L4 is displaced posteriorly on that of L5 (arrow). **(H)** The same patient as in (G). In extension the body of L4 is further displaced posteriorly on that of L5. The anterior aspect of the L4–5 disc has opened. Marked retrospondylolisthesis indicates gross instability. (*Figure continues.*)

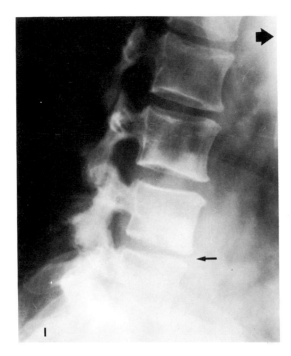

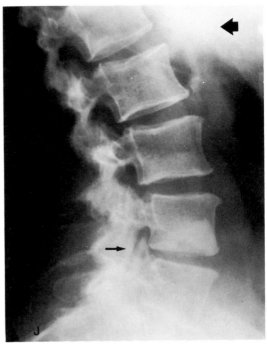

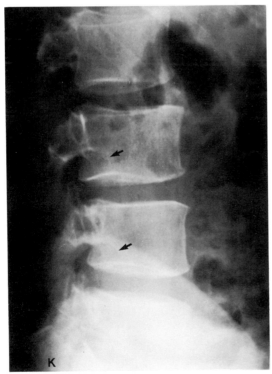

Fig. 9-5 (*Continued*). **(I)** Lateral view in flexion. Loss of disc height at L4–5 (arrow). On either side of the disc the anterior aspects of the bodies are closely approximated (instability). **(J)** The same patient as in (I). In extension retrospondylolisthesis of L4 on L5 (arrow) is present. Thus signs of instability in both flexion and extension are present in this patient. **(K)** At the L3 and L4 levels abrupt loss of pedicle height (arrow) is apparent compared with that at L2 (above the arrow). At L3 and L4 the base of the pedicles lies over and not behind the vertebral bodies. This change is caused by rotation of L3 on L2 and indicates instability in this case. (*Figure continues.*)

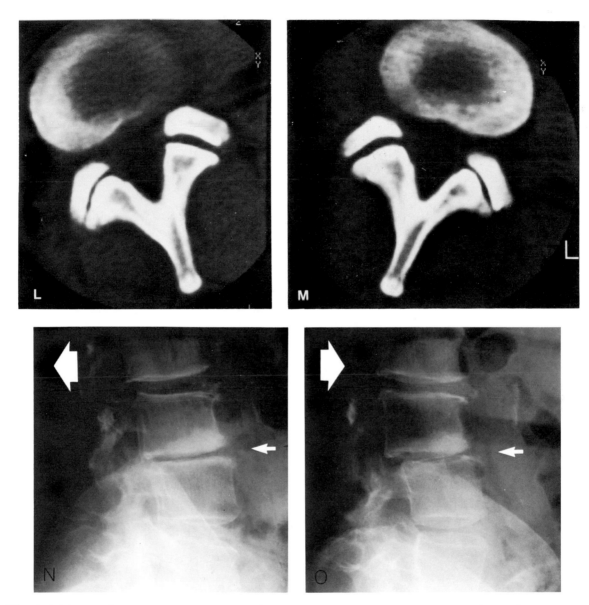

Fig. 9-5 (*Continued*). **(L)** CT scan at L4–5. When the spinous process rotates to the left, the left posterior joint opens widely. **(M)** CT scan of the same patient at L4–5. When the spinous process rotates to the right, the right posterior joint opens. Instability is seen at L4–5. **(N)** Lateral view in extension showing marked L3–4 disc resorption. L3 is slightly displaced backwards on L4. **(O)** In the same patient a lateral view is shown in flexion. L3 is markedly displaced backwards on L4, which is an unusual type of instability.

STABILIZATION

The patient enters Phase III as a result of increasing stiffness of a spine that was previously unstable.

Presentation

Phase III disease presents in two ways. In the older patient, there is a long history of low back pain. Back pain is commonly associated with a degenerative scoliosis and abnormal muscle action. Leg pain is often the predominant feature. This will be discussed more fully when we consider central and lateral spinal stenosis. More rarely, in younger patients, the back pain decreases and leg pain is the most pronounced feature.

Mechanisms

Three mechanisms are at work. Stiffness of the posterior joints is increased because of destruction of articular cartilage, fibrosis within the joint, enlargement and locking of the facets, and periarticular fibrosis. Similar changes occur in the disc, with loss of nuclear material, approximation of vertebral bodies, destruction of the cartilage plates, fibrosis within the disc and osteophyte formation around the periphery of the disc. Occasionally a bony ankylosis joins two vertebrae together. These changes often cause entrapment of spinal nerves as discussed in Chapter 10 (Fig. 9-6).

Symptoms and Signs

Frequently low back pain that was severe over past years becomes less incapacitating. This in fact may be the most common occurrence rather than the exception. Painful episodes may occur from time to time. These are often muscular in origin and can be relieved by xylocaine (Lidocaine) injections and/or by wearing an Elasticon garment.

Signs

Commonly seen signs are tenderness to pressure over several areas; marked stiffness of the spine, with

Table 9-3 The Signs, Symptoms, and Radiological Changes Seen in Stabilization

Symptoms
    Low back pain of decreasing severity

Signs
    Muscle tenderness
    Stiffness
    Reduced movement
    Scoliosis

Radiographs
    Enlarged facets
    Loss of disc height
    Osteophytes
    Small foramina
    Reduced movement
    Scoliosis

FACETS

DESTRUCTION OF CARTILAGE
↓
FIBROSIS IN JOINT
↓
ENLARGEMENT OF FACETS
↓
LOCKING FACETS
↓
FIBROSIS AROUND JOINT

DISK

LOSS OF NUCLEUS
↓
APPROXIMATION OF BODIES
↓
DESTRUCTION OF PLATES
↓
FIBROSIS IN DISK
↓
OSTEOPHYTES

INCREASED STIFFNESS
↓
STABILIZATION

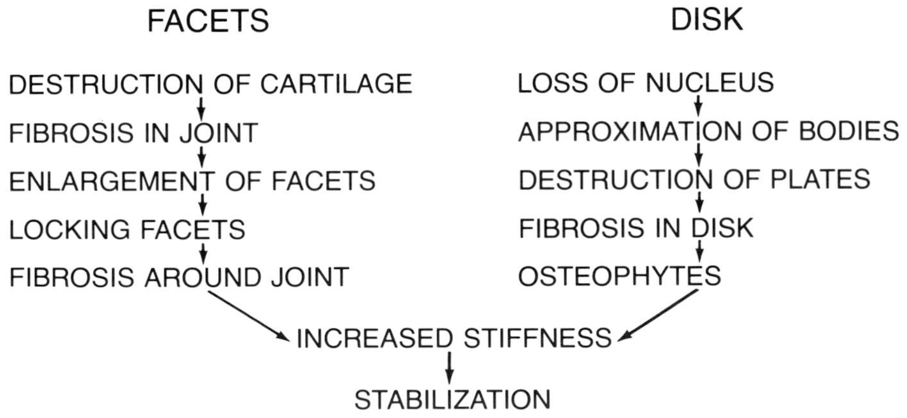

Fig. 9-6 Mechanisms of stabilization.

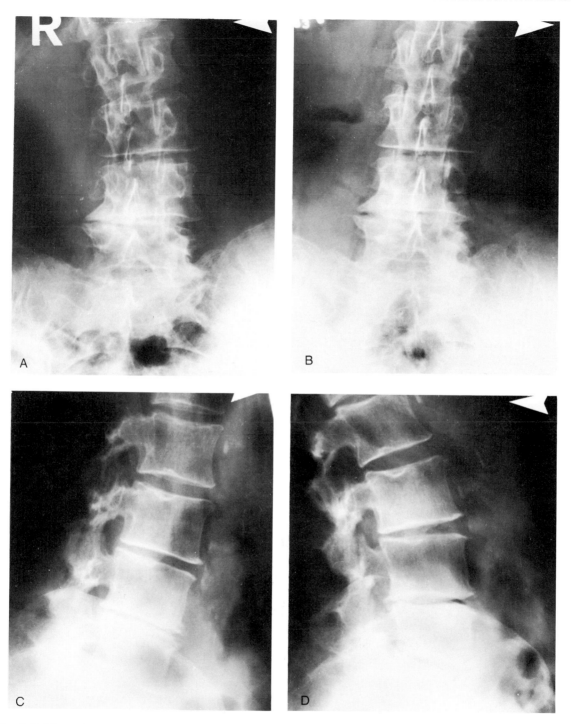

Fig. 9-7 The radiological changes seen in Phase III, stabilization. **(A)** When the patient bends to the right, little or no movement of L4 on L5 or of L5 to the sacrum is evident. **(B)** The same patient as in (A). Lateral bending to the left also does not produce movement of L4 on L5 or of L5 on sacrum. **(C)** The same patient as in (A) and (B). This lateral view in flexion further confirms that no movement occurs at L4–5 or at L5–S1. **(D)** The same patient as in (A), (B), and (C). This lateral view in extension further confirms that no movement is present at the lower two levels. The degenerative changes in this patient's lower lumbar spine have advanced to the point of stabilization. (*Figure continues.*)

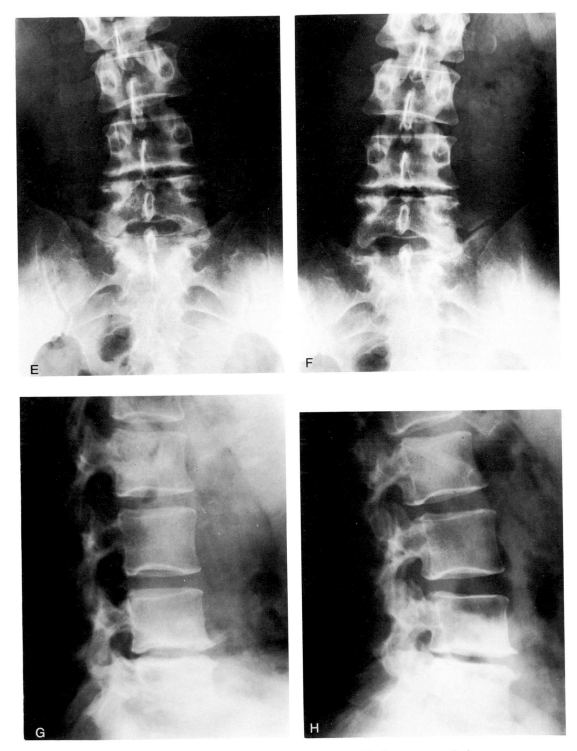

Fig. 9-7 (*Continued*). **(E)** Lateral bending to the right (viewer's left) demonstrates little or no movement at the L4–5 level. **(F)** The same patient as in (E). Lateral bending to the left (viewer's right) shows no movement at the L4–5 level. **(G)** The same patient as in (E) and (F). Lateral view in flexion shows that the L4–5 disc is markedly narrowed. **(H)** The same patient as in (E), (F), and (G). Lateral view in extension confirms the absence of movement at the L4–5 level. Stabilization at this level is due to advanced degenerative change.

reduction of movement in all directions; and a scoliosis, often with a rotational component. Neurological signs indicating nerve entrapment are sometimes elicited.

Radiographic Changes

Radiographs show marked degenerative spondylosis at one or at several levels, with enlarged and irregular posterior facets, loss of disc height, osteophytes that arise from the vertebral bodies, marked loss of movement (anteroposterior and lateral stress radiographs), marked reduction in the size of the foramina, and scoliosis.

It is important to remember that, with few exceptions, during Phase III back pain is not usually a serious problem, but leg pain with altered sensation and muscle weakness may be severe when the spondylotic changes have produced stenosis. Rarely, the resulting scoliosis may cause severe back pain.

The clinical and radiological findings are presented in Table 9-3, and radiographs showing typical changes in Figure 9-7.

CONCLUSIONS

It is important to assess as accurately as possible the stage (Phase) reached in the spectrum of degenerative disease of the lumbar spine because the treatment differs depending on the phase. This will be discussed in a later chapter. In brief, it is likely that conservative measures will be adequate during dysfunction; during the unstable phase a decompression may be required to treat a disc herniation or central or lateral stenosis and a fusion may be necessary to treat instability; in the final phase (stabilization) decompression may be indicated for central and/or lateral stenosis, but fusion is very seldom required.

ACKNOWLEDGMENTS

The author wishes to record his thanks to Dr. J. D. Cassidy for the illustrations of dysfunction and to Dr. H. F. Farfan for his help with the definition of instability.

SUGGESTED READINGS

Cassidy JD, Potter GE: Motion examination of the lumbar spine, J Manip Physiol Therapeut 2: 151, 1979

Dupuis PR, Yong-Hing K, Cassidy DJ, Kirkaldy-Willis WH: Radiologic diagnosis of degenerative lumbar spinal instability. Spine 10: 262, 1985

Frymoyer JW: The role of spinal fusion. Spine 6: 284, 1981

Helfet AI, Gruebel DM, Segmental Intervertebral Instability and Its Treatment: Disorders of the Lumbar Spine. Philadelphia, JD Lipincott, 1978

Hirsch C, Nachemson A: The reliability of lumbar disc suyrgery. Clin Orthop 29: 189, 1963

Kirkaldy-Willis WH, Farfan HF, Instability of the lumbar spine. Clin Orthop Rel Res, 165: 110, 1982

Nachemson A: The role of spinal fusion. Spine 6: 306, 1981

10

The Site and Nature of the Lesion

William H. Kirkaldy-Willis

We turn now to consider the site and nature of specific clinical lesions. Table 10-1 demonstrates first the phase (the framework in which the lesion is seen) and then the lesion by name. Three points must be borne in mind. First, a specific lesion can be identified in more than one phase. For example a disc herniation may occur at the end of Phase I, during Phase II, and, rarely, during Phase III. Second, for clarity, lesions will be described as single discrete processes. Often more than one lesion is present at any given time. This we know from our study of pathology in Chapter 4. For example, we shall describe the posterior facet syndrome and disc herniation separately. In practice, trauma to the facet is nearly always accompanied by trauma affecting the annulus. Compression injuries to the disc result in posterior facet degeneration at a later date. The condition called degenerative disc disease probably implies an equal amount of destruction of both facets and disc.

Third, one specific lesion may set the stage for the development of another. For example, the posterior facet syndrome may be complicated by the sacroiliac syndrome at a later date.[1] The clinical lesions will be considered in the following order:

1. Posterior facet syndrome
2. Sacroiliac joint syndrome
3. Maigne's syndrome
4. Myofascial syndromes
5. Herniation of the nucleus pulposus
6. Combined degenerative changes in posterior joint and disc
7. Lateral lumbar spinal nerve entrapment (lateral stenosis)
   - (a) General considerations
   - (b) During Phase II (instability)
   - (c) During Phase III (stabilization)
8. Referred and radicular pain
9. Central spinal stenosis
10. Degenerative spondylolisthesis
11. Isthmic spondylolisthesis

THE POSTERIOR FACET SYNDROME

The pathological lesions seen in the posterior facet joints have already been reviewed (Ch. 4). The presentation of this syndrome, the mechanisms, involved, the symptoms and signs, and radiological changes have been discussed in Ch. 9 under the heading Dysfunction and will not be repeated here. The presenting symptoms and signs during Phase I come chiefly from the posterior joints and the segmental

133

Table 10-1 Specific Clinical Lesions

Dysfunction	Posterior facet syndrome
	Sacroiliac syndrome
	Maigne's syndrome
	Myofascial syndromes
	Gluteus maximus
	Gluteus medius
	Gluteus minimus
	Quadratus lumborum
	Piriformis
	Tensor fasciae latae
	Hamstring
	Disc herniation
Unstable Phase	Facet and disc degeneration
	Lateral stenosis
	Central stenosis
	Disc herniation
Stabilization	Lateral stenosis
	Central stenosis
	Multilevel stenosis
	Disc herniation

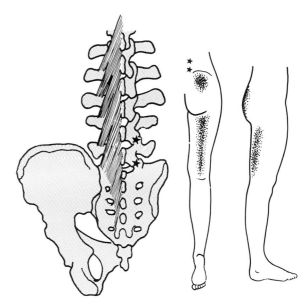

Fig. 10-1 Posterior facet (joint) syndrome. Star shows site of local pain over facet joint. Shaded areas shows referred pain to knee.

muscles posterior to them. Symptoms arise from the posterior joints in several different ways (Figs. 10-1 and 10-2).

Phase I, Dysfunction

In Phase I the patient may present with the symptoms and signs characteristic of the posterior facet syndrome or with a combination of the symptoms and signs of that syndrome and those of a disc herniation. In the case of a central disc herniation the clinical findings may be masked by those arising from the facet syndrome. When the herniation is more lateral, a careful clinical examination and CT scan images make the diagnosis more obvious. In addition, the symptoms and signs of a posterior facet syndrome may be complicated by those of a sacroiliac syndrome (see below).[2,3]

Phase II, The Unstable Phase

During Phase II a part of the symptom complex arises from changes in the posterior joints and a part comes from pathology in the disc. As seen in Chapter 4 the cause of instability is marked laxity of both the capsule of the posterior joints and the annulus fibrosus. As in Phase I most of the symptoms arise

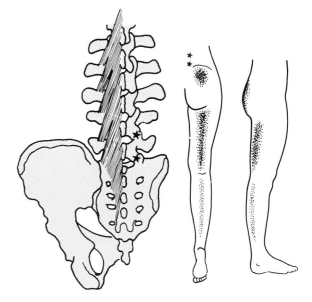

Fig. 10-2 Posterior facet (joint) syndrome. Star shows site of local pain over facet joint. Shaded areas shows referred pain, which sometimes passes below the knee to calf, ankle, foot, and even to the toes. (Bernard TN, Kirkaldy-Willis WH: Recognizing specific characteristics of nonspecific low back pain. Clin Orthop Rel Res 217: 96, 1987.)

from changes in the facet joints to which, as seen in Chapter 9, must be added the rather vague symptoms that suggest the presence of instability. Fortunately stress radiographs demonstrate the presence of increased abnormal movement in both posterior joints and disc.

Degenerative Disc Disease

The term "degenerative disc disease" is misleading. Degeneration of the annulus is present in Phase I. It is of minor degree until a disc herniation occurs. In Phase II the disc degeneration is of major degree, a sign that instability is present. In Phase III degeneration of the disc (and of the posterior facet joints) is advanced. Thus radiological findings tell us whether we are dealing with a problem in Phase I, Phase II, or Phase III. It is this interpretation that matters when we turn to consider treatment.

Multiple Lesions

Recurrent rotational trauma most commonly affects the L4–5 joint. Frequently such a lesion spreads to an adjacent level at a later date. A simple example makes this clear. The initial trauma results in dysfunction at the L4–5 level. Recurrent trauma may produce increased dysfunction and eventually the patient enters the unstable phase. Further trauma may lead to dysfunction at the L3–4 level. In this instance we are dealing with posterior joint symptoms at two levels. To recognize this and to appreciate the different nature of the two lesions is vital in managing the problem.

THE SACROILIAC SYNDROME

Structure and Function of the Joint

The sacroiliac joint has well-developed cartilage surfaces, a synovial membrane, strong anterior and posterior ligaments, and a large internal sacroiliac ligament. After the fifth decade of life fibrosis takes place between the cartilage surfaces. By the sixth or seventh decade the joint has usually undergone fibrous ankylosis. Bony ankylosis is a rare phenomenon late in life. The joint surfaces can rotate 3° to 5° in the

younger symptom-free patient. The joint has two functions: to provide elasticity to the pelvic ring and to serve as a buffer between the lumbosacral and the hip joints.[4]

Presentation

The syndrome presents with pain over one sacroiliac joint in the region of the posterior superior iliac spine. This may be accompanied by referred pain in the leg.

Mechanism

The mechanism of injury is not well understood. Until late in middle age a small amount of movement (3° to 5°) is usually present in the sacroiliac joint. After that age, movement is reduced by articular cartilage degeneration, by fibrosis, and rarely by bony ankylosis. It is possible that minor dysfunction in this joint leads to pain. It seems more reasonable to suppose that pain results from sustained contraction of muscle overlying the joint. This hypertonicity may accompany dysfunction in the sacroiliac or in the L4–5 or L5–S1 posterior joint.

Symptoms

Typical symptoms are pain over the back of the sacroiliac joint that varies in its degree of severity and referred pain in the groin, over the greater trochanter, down the back of the thigh to the knee, and, occasionally, down the lateral or posterior calf to ankle, foot, and toes (Figs. 10-3 to 10-5).

Signs

The signs include tenderness on pressure over the posterior superior iliac spine, in the region of the sacroiliac joint, or in the buttock. Movement of the joint is usually reduced. Normally the joint moves by rotating in the sagittal plane. Restricted movement can be detected in two ways.

In the first, the patient stands with one hand resting to support himself on the couch. To examine the left joint the examiner places the thumb of his or her right hand over the spinous process of L5 and the thumb of his or her left hand over the left posterior

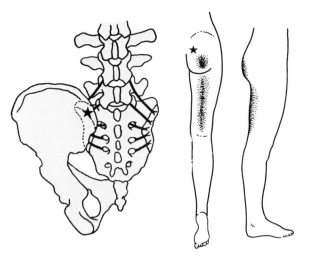

Fig. 10-3 Sacroiliac joint syndrome. Star show site of local pain. Shaded areas show referred pain to knee.

superior iliac spine. The patient then flexes both left hip and left knee and lifts up the knee toward the chest. As this is done, the examiner can detect a small but definite amount of movement. Rotation in the joint causes the iliac spine to move downward in relation to the spinous process of L5. When the sacro-

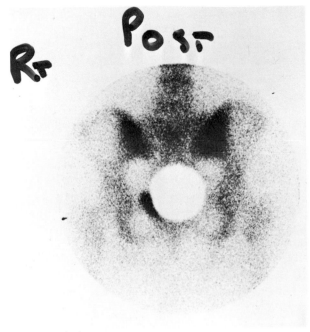

Fig. 10-5 Bone scan in a patient with a sacroiliac syndrome. Sometimes, as seen here in the joint on the left, there is an increased uptake of the isotope in the affected joint.

iliac joint is "fixed," this movement of the iliac spine relative to the spinous process is reduced or absent.

Confirmation can be obtained by the second test. To examine the left joint the examiner places the right thumb over the apex of the sacrum and the left thumb over the ischial tuberosity. In a normal joint, flexing the left knee and hip and bringing the knee toward the chest causes the ischial tuberosity to move laterally away from the apex of the sacrum. When the joint is "fixed," the lateral movement does not take place (Fig. 10-6). The joint on the right is examined in a similar way. Additional tests are illustrated in Figures 10-7 to 10-9.

Radiographic Changes

Usually no changes can be detected in the sacroiliac joint. Later in life small osteophytes can be seen at the lower margins of the joint. Radiographs do not assist the clinician to make the diagnosis but they do help to exclude other conditions such as early ankylosing spondylitis.

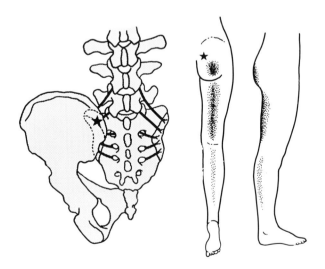

Fig. 10-4 Sacroiliac syndrome. Star shows site of local pain. Ahaded areas show referred pain. Sometimes the pain is referred to the groin, lateral or posterior calf, ankle and occasionally to foot and toes. (Bernard TN, Kirkaldy-Willis WH: Recognizing specific characteristics of nonspecific low back pain. Clin Orthop Rel Res 217: 96, 1987.)

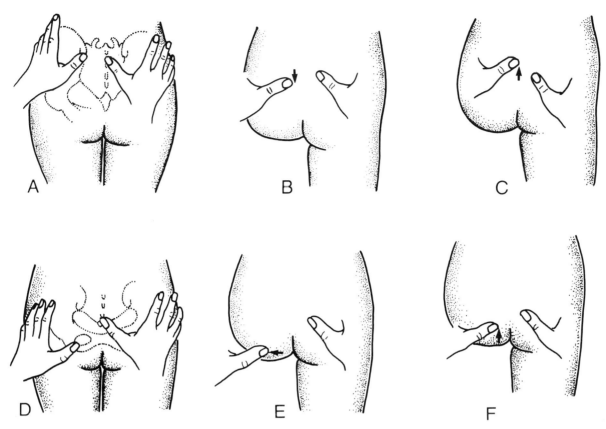

Fig. 10-6 Tests to demonstrate left sacroiliac fixation. Tests for upper part of joint in **(A)**, **(B)**, and **(C)** and for lower part in **(D)**, **(E)**, and **(F)**. **(A)** The examiner places the left thumb on the posterior superior iliac spine and the right thumb over one of the sacral spinous processes. **(B)** When movement is normal, the examiner's left thumb moves downward as the patient raises the left leg. **(C)** When the joint is fixed, the examiner's left thumb moves upward as the patient raises the left leg. **(D)** The examiner places the left thumb over the ischial tuberosity and the right thumb over the apex of the sacrum. **(E)** When movement is normal, the examiner's left thumb moves laterally as the patient raises the left leg. **(F)** When the joint is fixed, the examiner's left thumb moves slightly upward as the patient raises the left leg.

Comments

The sacroiliac syndrome is a well-defined syndrome. The physician who is cognizant of it and who looks for it will find that it is a commonly seen type of dysfunction. The exact nature of the lesion is not known. This syndrome usually responds well to manipulation or to injection of 1% lidocaine or 0.25% bupivacaine (Marcaine) into the joint or into the ligaments and fascia posterior to the joint. Often the same symptoms and signs are present with a posterior joint syndrome. Sometimes the pain in a patient with spondylolisthesis or in a patient who has had a fusion from L4 to the sacrum is caused by the sacroiliac syndrome and responds to treatment for it. Awareness that the syndrome exists, detecting its presence, and instituting the appropriate treatment enable the physician to relieve the pain in many patients who have previously responded poorly to treatment for what were thought to be other low back lesions.

MAIGNE'S SYNDROME

This syndrome, described by Maigne of Paris, is a lesion of the T12–L1 posterior joint. The pathogenesis, symptoms, and signs are similar to those previ-

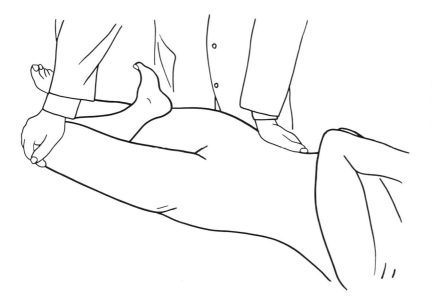

Fig. 10-7 Faber Patrick's test. The patient lies on the back in a supine position. In this case the pain is over the left sacroiliac joint. The left leg near the ankle is placed in front of the right thigh above the knee. The examiner places his left hand over the patient's right iliac crest, and his right hand pushes downward over the medial aspect of the left knee. This may elicit pain in the sacroiliac joint region.

ously described for the posterior facet syndrome—pain and tenderness over the affected joint.

Referred pain is mediated via the cluneal nerves, the posterior rami of the T12 or L1 spinal nerves. These nerves pass downward and outward on each side to supply the skin at the level of the iliac crest. The referred pain is experienced at this level. Pinching the skin and rolling the skin between thumb, and index finger cause pain (Fig. 10-10).

THE MYOFASCIAL SYNDROMES

Six different syndromes are associated with low back pain. The pathophysiology has been discussed in Chapter 4. There is pain and local tenderness in an area characteristic for each muscle, and often there is referred pain in a distribution specific for each muscle. The affected area of muscle is firm or hard to

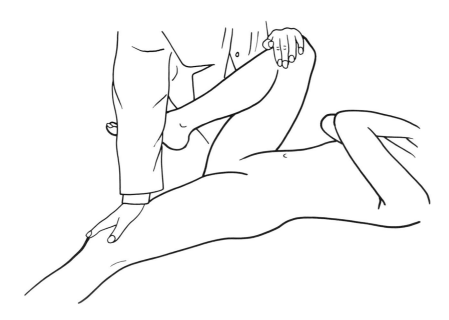

Fig. 10-8 Gaenslen's test. The patient lies supine on the couch in this test for left sacroiliac joint. The examiner flexes the patient's right knee and hip and presses downward over the left thigh to hyperextend the hip. This may elicit pain in the sacroiliac joint region on the left.

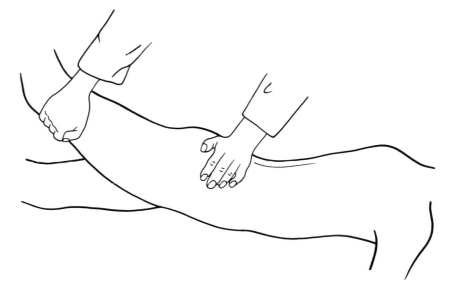

Fig. 10-9 Extension test. The patient is placed prone on the couch. The examiner places one hand under the thigh above the knee on the affected side. With the other hand he presses downward over the crest of the ilium to elicit pain in the sacroiliac joint. This is the most specific and reliable test.

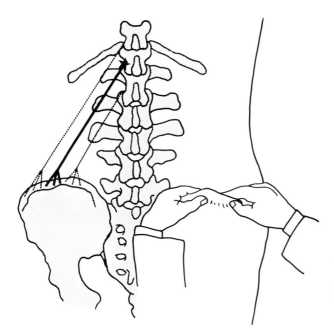

Fig. 10-10 Maigne's syndrome. The star indicates the site of posterior facet pain and tenderness. The cluneal nerves supply the skin near the iliac crest. Rolling and pinching the skin at this level is painful. (Bernard TN, Kirkaldy-Willis WH: Recognizing specific characteristics of nonspecific low back pain. Clin Orthop Rel Res 217: 96, 1987.)

palpation; sometimes it has a "ropey" consistency and may appear to be contracted or in spasm.

The Gluteus Medius Syndrome

The site of local pain and tenderness is shown by the star in Figure 10-11 A and B. The referred pain may pass down the back of the thigh and calf almost to the ankle or down lateral thigh and calf, as in Figure 10-11 B. Stretching the muscle by abducting and externally rotating the hip is often painful.

The Gluteus Maximus Syndrome

The site of local pain and tenderness is indicated by the stars and that of referred pain by the shaded areas in Figure 10-12. This lesion is often associated with a sacroiliac syndrome.

The Quadratus Lumborum Syndrome

The site of local pain and tenderness is shown by the star and the distribution of the referred pain by the shaded areas in Figure 10-13. On occasion the

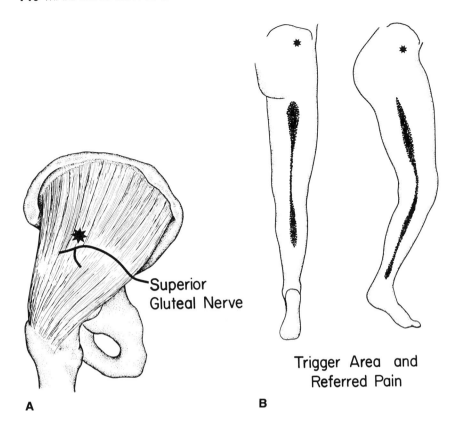

Trigger Area and
Referred Pain

A   B

Fig. 10-11 Gluteus medius syndrome. **(A)** The star demonstrates the site of local pain and tenderness. **(B)** The shaded areas show the distribution of referred pain. (Bernard TN, Kirkaldy-Willis WH: Recognizing specific characteristics of nonspecific low back pain. Clin Orthop Rel Res 217: 96, 1987.)

local pain is over an area higher or lower than shown here. Stretching the muscle by bending to the opposite side may exacerbate the symptoms.

The Piriformis Syndrome

The piriformis syndrome presents as a twisting injury of one leg while the patient is carrying or lifting in an awkward position. The pain, often deep-seated in rectum or vagina, may be severe and incapacitating. The referred pain is down the back of the thigh to the knee and sometimes to the ankle as in Figure 10-14. Pain on muscle contraction may be demonstrated by asking the patient to sit on the examining table with knees apart and ankles together and to resist the attempt of the physician to bring the knees together. On rectal or vaginal examination pressure with the finger tip over the muscle just medial to the ischial spine may be intensely painful.

The Tensor Fasciae Latae Syndrome

The local and the referred pain is indicated by the stars and by the shaded areas, respectively, in Figure 10-15.

The Hamstring Syndrome

In the hamstring syndrome there is local pain and tenderness over the hamstring origin from the ischial tuberosity.

Further Comments about Myofascial Syndromes

It is important to recognize and diagnose these syndromes because they can easily be confused with other conditions such as a disc herniation or lateral

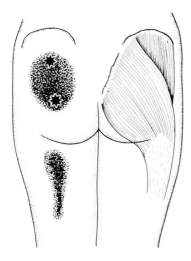

Trigger Areas and Referred Pain

Fig. 10-12 Gluteus maximus syndrome. The two stars demonstrate the sites of local pain and tenderness and the shaded areas show the referred pain. (Bernard TN, Kirkaldy-Willis WH: Recognizing specific characteristics of nonspecific low back pain. Clin Orthop Rel Res 217: 96, 1987.)

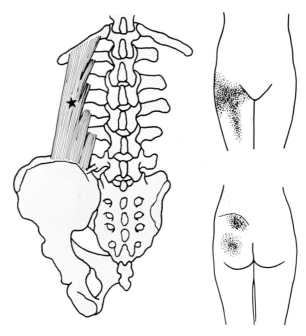

Fig. 10-13 Quadratus lumborum syndrome. The star (left) indicates the common site of local pain and tenderness. The shaded areas (right) show the distribution of referred pain. (Bernard TN, Kirkaldy-Willis WH: Recognizing specific characteristics of nonspecific low back pain. Clin Orthop Rel Res 217: 96, 1987.)

stenosis. The diagnosis can be confirmed by treatment. Spraying the affected area of muscle with fluorimethane and then stretching it manually or alternatively injecting it with 0.25% bupivacaine (Marcaine) solution often results in complete pain relief.

HERNIATION OF THE NUCLEUS POLPOSUS

Herniation of the nucleus pulposus can be of two kinds. A localized protrusion into the spinal canal, known as a "disc protrusion," may be present. The annular fibers are thinned, allowing nuclear material to move posteriorly, but are not completely ruptured. Alternatively, the posterior annulus may be completely ruptured, which allows the nucleus to extrude into the canal. This is called an "extrusion" of the disc. The circumferential bulging of the annulus right around the disc, which is seen in Phase II, is not a herniation and must not be confused with it. The

place of the disc herniation in the overall scheme of degernation is discussed in Chapter 4. This lesion occurs most often at the end of Phase I or early in Phase II. Later in Phase II loss of nuclear material results in lower pressures in the disc and the likelihood of herniation is less. Rarely, for reasons not well understood a disc herniation occurs in Phase III.

Presentation

The patient, usually between the ages of 30 and 50 years, recounts pain in the back and leg after lifting or after twisting and moving a heavy object. The symptoms and signs of disc herniation at different levels ar clearly outlined in Figure 10-16.

Mechanism

The most common mechanism of injury is a series of recurrent rotational injuries that produce circumferential and radial tears and finally, with further

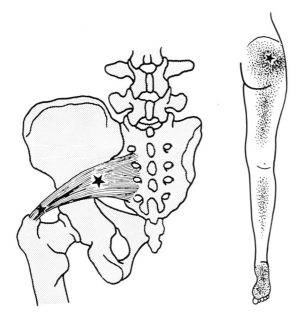

Fig. 10-14 Piriformis syndrome. The large star (left) and the small star demonstrate the sites of local pain and tenderness. Its most common site is in the center of the muscle just medial to the ischial spine. The shaded areas (right) indicate the site of referred pain. (Bernard TN, Kirkaldy-Willis WH: Recognizing specific characteristics of nonspecific low back pain. Clin Orthop Rel Res 217: 96, 1987.)

trauma, a yielding of the annulus to produce a localized bulge. In some cases the annulus is completely ruptured. A severe compression injury with the spine flexed may cause a sudden rupture of the annulus.

Symptoms

The patient gives a history of attacks of low back pain over months or years. A relatively minor degree of trauma is followed by acute severe low back and leg pain. Often the back pain disappears with the onset of leg pain. The pain is made worse by forward bending, by coughing and by sneezing. It is relieved by rest with the patient recumbent and the knees flexed. In the case of a small midline protrusion no leg pain may be present. Occasionally the patient complains of muscle weakness, when this is of marked degree. Still more rarely there may be complaints of bladder and bowel dysfunction.

Signs

Commonly the physician can detect numbness over one dermatome (hypoesthesia). Muscle weakness of the quadriceps, of the dorsiflexors of ankles and toes, or of the plantarflexors may be present. The patient

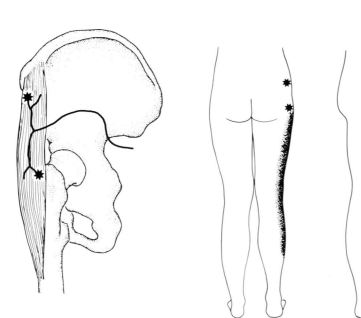

Fig. 10-15 Tensor fasciae latae syndrome. The stars show the sites of local pain and tenderness and the shaded areas the distribution of the referred pain. (Bernard TN, Kirkaldy-Willis WH: Recognizing specific characteristics of nonspecific low back pain. Clin Orthop Rel Res 217: 96, 1987.)

Level of herniation	Pain	Numbness	Weakness	Atrophy	Reflexes
L3–4 disc; 4th lumbar nerve root	Lower back, hip, postero-lateral thigh, anterior leg	Antero-medial thigh and knee	Quadriceps	Quadriceps	Knee jerk diminished
L4–5 disc; 5th lumbar nerve root	Over sacro-iliac joint, hip, lateral thigh and leg	Lateral leg, web of great toe	Dorsifexion of great toe and foot; difficulty walking on heels; foot drop may occur	Minor	Changes uncommon (absent or diminished posterior tibial reflex)
L5–S1 disc; 1st sacral nerve root	Over sacro-iliac joint, hip, postero-lateral thigh and leg to heel	Back of calf; lateral heel, foot and toe	Plantar flexion of foot and great toe may be affected; difficulty walking on toes	Gastrocnemius and soleus	Ankle jerk diminished or absent
Massive midline protrusion	Lower back, thighs, legs and/or perineum depending on level of lesion; may be bilateral	Thighs, legs, feet and/or perineum; variable; may be bilateral	Variable paralysis or paresis of legs and/or bowel and bladder incontinence	May be extensive	Ankle jerk diminished or absent

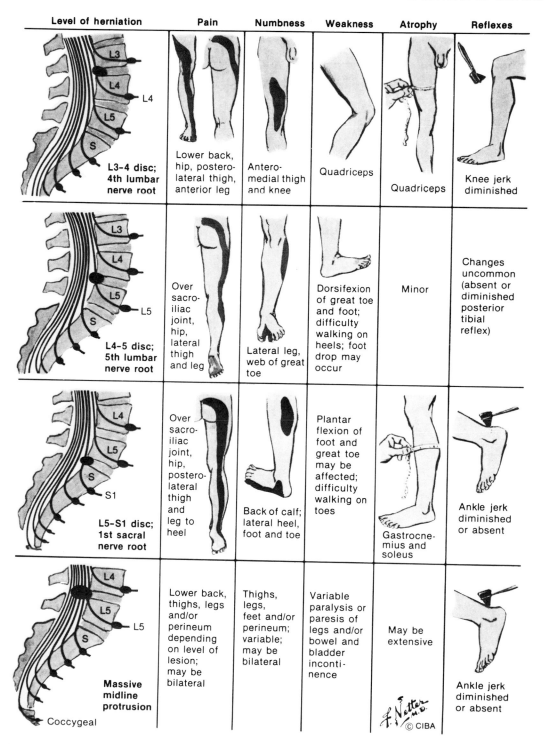

Fig. 10–16 The clinical features of herniated nucleus pulposus. (© 1980 Ciba Pharmaceutical Company, Division of CIBA-GEIGY Corporation. Reprinted with permission from Keim HA, Kirkaldy-Willis WH: Low back pain. Clin Symp 32: 6, 1980. Illustrated by Frank H. Netter, M.D. All rights reserved.)

may not be able to pass urine or to defecate normally. Muscle atrophy of the quadriceps, of the gastrocnemii and soleus, or of the short toe extensors may be detected. The knee or ankle reflex may be absent or diminished. Straight leg raising is often markedly diminished. When the patient is able to stand, it is noted that the normal lumbar lordosis is lost. The back is straight. There may be a list to one or the other side. All movements are restricted. On attempted forward flexion, the list (a functional scoliosis) is increased. The Lasegue and bowstring tests are often positive. Performing the Lasegue test on one side may produce pain in the opposite (the affected) leg. With a small central herniation few signs may be present in the lower limb. In this case the presence of a list and diminished straight leg raising strongly suggest that a small central herniation is present[5] (see Fig. 17-8).

Radiographic Changes

No changes may be present. The lateral view may demonstrate slight reduction of disc height. The changes characteristic of the unstable phase may be seen.

Comments

It is relatively easy to distinguish between a posterior facet syndrome and a classical disc herniation. The patient with a small central herniation is difficult to diagnose. The presenting symptoms and signs may at a glance be those of a facet syndrome. The presence of a list and of marked diminution of straight leg raising strongly suggest that a disc herniation is present. Sometimes the lateral radiograph may reveal the presence of a small area of lucency adjacent to the upper or lower part of a vertebral body. This is a Shmorl's node and is caused by rupture of a cartilage plate with extrusion of disc material into the vertebral body. It usually does not produce symptoms. Diagnostic tests are described in Chapters 11 and 14.

COMBINED POSTERIOR FACET AND DISC DEGENERATION

As outlined in Chapter 4, changes occurring in the posterior facets affect the disc and vice versa. Early changes produce dysfunction. Progressive changes lead to the unstable phase. The result of these changes is often referred to vaguely as "degenerative disc disease." In the author's opinion it is better to think of this lesion as a combined degeneration of all three parts of the joint.

The symptoms and signs are those of the unstable phase.

The radiological changes seen in this phase have been described in Chapter 9.

LATERAL LUMBAR SPINAL NERVE ENTRAPMENT

Presentation

Lateral lumbar spinal serve entrapment (lateral stenosis) has two types of presentations: that seen during Phase II (the unstable phase) and that seen in Phase III (stabilization). The entrapment may be isolated, it may occur with a disc herniation, or it may follow discectomy or chemonucleolysis. At this point the reader is advised to review the section on lateral entrapment (stenosis) in Chapter 4 before proceeding further. The concept of lateral entrapment is difficult to master.

Mechanism

As shown in Chapter 4, the mechanism involves progressive degenerative changes in both facets and disc, loss of disc height, subluxation of facets that allows the superior facet to move upward and forward on the inferior facet and impinge on the pedicle above, and narrowing of the intervertebral foramen and, still more important, of the lateral part of the nerve canal medial to the foramen (Fig. 10-17). The spinal nerve that exits at this level may be entrapped. Osteophytes that form on the medial edge of the superior facet may impinge on the nerve that exits one level lower and cause entrapment. Thus at L4–5 the L4 and/or the L5 nerves may be entrapped. At L5–S1 both the L5 and /or S1 nerves may be involved (Fig. 10-18).

Wiltse et al.[6] have described a "Far Out syndrome" with entrapment of the L5 nerve between the transverse process of L5 and the ala of the sacrum.

Entrapment During Phase II

This is a *recurrent* and *dynamic* type of entrapment. Instability of both disc and posterior facets allows abnormal increased movement both in rotation and

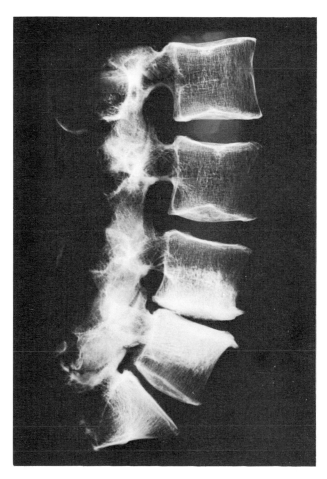

Fig. 10-17 Isolated disc resorption. Lateral radiograph of autopsy specimen of lumbar spine shows that marked resorption of the L4–5 disc has occurred. The vertebral bodies on either side are sclerotic. Retrospondylolisthesis of L4 on L5. The superior articular process of L5 is near the back of the body of L4, narrowing the foramen.

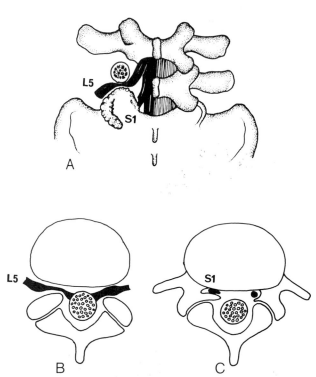

Fig. 10-18 Diagram demonstrating how two nerves are at risk at the L5–S1 level. **(A)** The L5 nerve is entrapped between the pedicle of L5 and the superior facet of the sacrum, and the S1 nerve is entrapped between the enlarged superior facet of the sacrum and the back of the body of the sacrum. **(B)** The cross section shows entrapment of the L5 nerve between the anterior part of the superior sacral facet and the back of the vertebral body of the sacrum on the left side. **(C)** The cross section reveals entrapment of the left S1 nerve in the narrow gutter at the base of the superior sacral facet.

in flexion-extension. With rotation the superior facet moves backward and forward, as the posterior joint opens and closes, and impinges on the spinal nerve. During extension the lateral canal is narrowed and the same kind of impingement occurs. Thus, the causes of this type of entrapment are twofold: structural changes narrow the lateral canal and recurrent dynamic narrowing occurs because the superior articular process moves back and forth (see Chapter 4).

Entrapment During Phase III

By Phase III progressive degenerative changes have led to stabilizing the previously unstable segment. The deformity is fixed, often with some rotation.

No movement occurs at the affected level. The changes are solely structural.

Entrapment Symptoms in Phase II and Phase III

The patient may or may not complain of low back pain. The most common site of the pain is in the buttock, trochanteric region, and posterior thigh to the knee. Sometimes the pain passes further distally down the back of the calf (S1) or down the lateral aspect of the calf (L5) to the ankle and, occasionally, to the foot and toes. The patient may complain of altered sensation or hypoesthesia in the L5 or S1 dermatome. It should be appreciated, first, that these

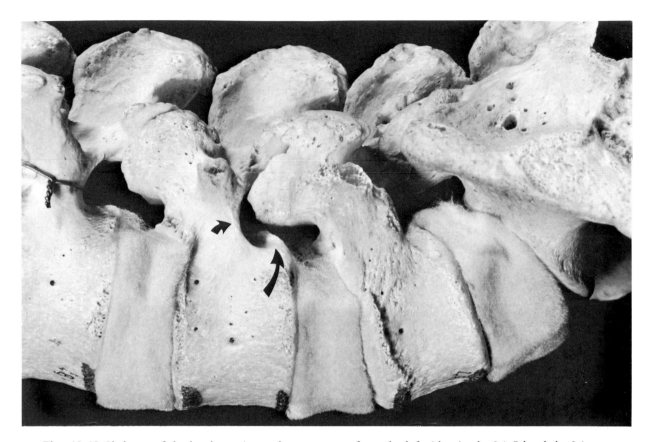

Fig. 10-19 Skeleton of the lumbar spine and sacrum seen from the left side. At the L4–5 level the L4 nerve is entrapped laterally between the pedicle of L4 and the superior articular process of L5 (small arrow) (see Fig. 10-18B). At a slightly lower level the L5 nerve is entrapped more medially between an osteophyte on the posterior aspect of the body of L4 and the anterior aspect of the superior articular process of L5 (large arrow) (see Fig. 10-18C).

symptoms differ little from those of Phase I and those of a posterior facet syndrome and, second, that the symptoms may be the same in both types of entrapment. In recurrent dynamic entrapment the symptoms may be intermittent.

Entrapment Signs in Phase II and Phase III

Movements of the lumbar spine are usually not much restricted. Straight-leg raising may be slightly reduced on the affected side. Neurological findings are usually normal. However, some blunting to touch and pin prick over the L4, L5, or S1 dermatome may be present (Fig. 10-19). Loss of motor power and reflex changes are rare. The Lasegue and Bowstring tests may be positive (see following section, referred and radicular pain).

Additional Signs Observed in the Unstable Phase

The signs indicative of Phase II may be elicited (see Chapter 9, section on the unstable phase). Pain may be elicited with the patient in one of three positions (Fig. 10-20). First, the patient lies on his side with the painful leg on the couch. The examiner stands behind the patient, holds his chest and trunk with one hand, and rotates his pelvis forward toward the other side. This maneuver may move the lower superior facet toward the vertebral body and cause pain by creating pressure on the spinal nerve. The same test can be done with the patient standing. The examiner sits behind the patient and holds the pelvis to prevent movement. An assistant, standing in front of the patient, grasps the chest with both hands and rotates chest and upper trunk first to one side and

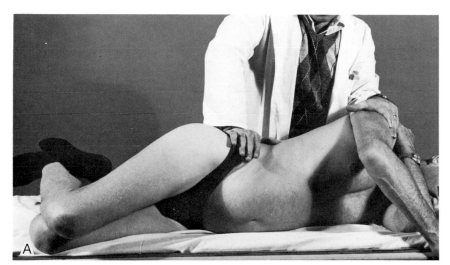

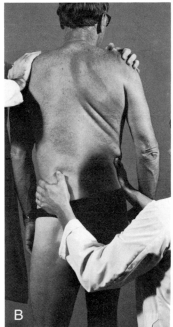

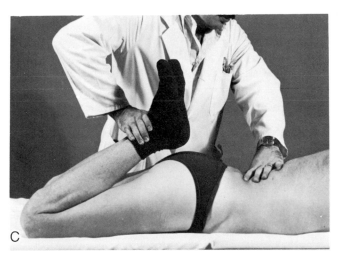

Fig. 10-20 Tests for dynamic lateral entrapment. **(A)** The patient lies on his side with the painful side on the couch. The physician holds the patient's chest with the left hand and rotates the pelvis away from him with the opposite hand. This sometimes accentuates the left pain. **(B)** The patient stands erect. The physician holds the pelvis firmly. An assistant, standing in front of the patient, rotates the turnk first to one side, then to the other. This sometimes reproduces the leg pain. **(C)** The patient lies prone. The examiner presses lightly over the lumbar spine with his left hand and flexes the knees and exteds the hips with his right hand. This produces hyperextension and, in cases of central stenosis and of dynamic lateral stenosis may reproduce the leg pain (Pheasant test).

then to the other. This movement may produce pain in the affected lower limb by shifting one superior articular process nearer to the back of the vertebral body above it. In a third test the patient lies face down. With the left hand the examiner maintains gentle pressure on the back of the lumbar spine. With his right hand, he flexes both the patient's knees until the heels touch the buttocks. The hyperextension produced by this maneuver may result in leg pain that occurs because the lateral canal is narrowed by for-

ward displacement of the superior articular process (Pheasant test). These tests are not always positive even when dynamic lateral stenosis is present.

Radiographic Findings

The disc space at L4–5 or L5–S1 may be reduced in height and the vertebral bodies adjacent to the disc may be sclerotic (see Fig. 10-17). The foramen at one level may be smaller than normal. Lateral stress films may show that in extension the upper body moves backward on the lower retrospondylolisthesis) and that the superior facet shifts toward the back of the vertebral body. The radiographic changes characteristic of the unstable phase may be seen in the dynamic type of lateral entrapment.

Comments

Lateral entrapment is a relatively common syndrome. The symptoms and signs are vague and merely suggest the presence of this lesion. The presence of the typical radiographic changes make the diagnosis more definite. CT scan images that make the diagnosis certain will be discussed in Chapter 11 under the heading Diagnosis.[7]

REFERRED AND RADICULAR PAIN

It is convenient at this point to discuss the symptoms and signs that enable us to differentiate between referred and radicular pain.

Referred pain has the same distribution as the innervation of the affected posterior joint. With a lesion of the L4–5 joint the pain is of L4 and L5 distribution: down the back of the thigh and somtimes to the inner or outer calf. A lesion of the L5–S1 joint gives referred pain down the back of the thigh and sometimes down the back or outside of the calf, i.e., the L5 or S1 dermatomes. Subjective sensory changes in the L4, L5, or S1 dermatomes may be present. Motor and reflex changes are rare.

Radicular pain is due to irritation, inflammation, tension, or compression of the anterior division of a spinal nerve. Sensory, motor, and reflex changes are often present. Frequently, a definite reduction in straight leg raising is present. The Lasegue or Bragard test (dorsiflexion of the foot with maximum straight leg raising) is often positive. The Bowstring test (at maximum straight leg raising, the knee is flexed a few degrees and digital pressure is applied over the posterior tibial and lateral popliteal nerves at knee joint level) may produce pain and tenderness over one or other nerve. Tenderness may be present when pressure is applied over the sciatic notch. These simple tests often help the physician to differentiate between referred and radicular pain. They are particu-

larly helpful in cases of lateral entrapment. They are not infallible. Further examinations such as the electromyogram will be described in Chapter 11 under Diagnosis (Table 10-2).

When injection of 0.25% bupivacaine (Marcaine) to a posterior facet joint or sacroiliac joint abolishes leg pain, it is most likely referred pain. When a selective nerve block of the L4, L5, or S1 nerve at the foramen reproduces and after injection of local anesthetic abolishes the leg pain, the pain is likely due to entrapment of the main anterior branch of the nerve.

CENTRAL SPINAL STENOSIS

Presentation

The condition most commonly presents as pain and altered sensation in one or both lower limbs. Occasionally motor weakness is the predominant symptom.

Mechanism

The posterior facets are enlarged and protrude in a medial and anterior direction so that the central canal is narrowed. Although it is the superior facets that narrow the lateral canals, the inferior facets are chiefly responsible for central canal narrowing. The presence of osteophytes at the back of the vertebral bodies and bulging of the annulus of the disc further narrow the canal. When preexisting developmental narrowing of the canal is present, a small disc herniation and/or some degree of central stenosis can produce severe symptoms. Pressure of these structures on the nerves of the cauda equina produces most of the symptoms and signs. Venous hypertension due to pressure on the veins of the cauda equina or the nerve roots perhaps is responsible for part of the clinical picture. Central stenosis is often accompanied by lateral canal stenosis at one or more levels. Starting at one level, usuallay L4–5, the spondylosis and stenosis can spread to involve several levels.

Symptoms

The clinical picture is bizarre. The usual presenting symptom is pain in one or both legs. It may involve one dermatome in one leg and a different dermatome

Table 10-2 Distinguishing Features of Low Back Syndromes

Syndrome	Back Pain	Leg Pain	Restriction of Movement	Restriction of S.L.R.	Nerve Compression Tests	Neurological Deficit
Posterior facet	Over joint	Referred (post. thigh)	Low back	Moderate	Negative	None
Sacroiliac	Over joint	Referred (anteropost. thigh)	Of joint	Rare	Negative	None
Herniation of nucleus pulposus	Often none	Post. thigh Post. lateral calf to toes	Low back	Marked	Positive	One level
Piriformis	Deep rectal, vaginal	Post. thigh	Hip rotation	Rare	Negative	None
Quadratus lumborum	Lateral to erector spinae	Groin Ant. thigh Post. thigh	Low back	Rare	Negative	None
Other muscle syndromes	Over muscle	Referred	Varies	Rare	Negative	None
Lateral stenosis	Often none	Buttock Trochanter Post. thigh Calf Ankle Toes	Rare	Moderate	Positive	Sometimes present
Central stenosis	Often not severe	Common Bizarre	Varies	Moderate	Positive	Multilevel

in the other. It may involve the whole of one or even both legs. Its nature varies. Often, after walking three or four blocks the patient has to rest because of leg pain. After a few minutes rest the patient can walk the same distance again (neurogenic claudication). Pain in bed during the night is often relieved by walking round the room for a few minutes. This type of pain can be distinguished from that of vascular claudication by the fact that the patient can ride a stationary bicyble (with the lumbar spine in flexion) for several minutes without pain. In vascular claudication the patient quickly develops leg pain.

Sensory changes are common. The patient may complain of numbness in part or the whole of one or both lower limbs. He may say that the legs feel cold (when in fact they are not cold), that they do not belong to him, or that they feel as if made of rubber.

Muscle weakness is not commonly a presenting symptom though the patient may complain that he tires easily. Rarely, muscle weakness is severe.

Signs

Movements of the lumbar spine are only slightly restricted and only mildly painful. Sensory changes differ from those of a disc herniation. In the latter they are usually restricted to one dermatome. In central stenosis sensation may be diminished over several dermatomes in one or both lower limbs. The distribution may be different in one leg from that in the other. Alternatively, the whole of one leg may exhibit altered sensation.

Motor power may be diminished in the distribution of one or two motor nerves in one leg and that of different nerves in the other leg. For example the

Table 10-3 Differential Diagnosis of Central Spinal Stenosis

Vascular claudication
Diabetic neuropathy
Other peripheral neuropathies
Motor neurone disease
Multiple sclerosis
Other lesions of central nervous system
Spinal infections (acute, subacute, chronic)
Neoplasms (involving cauda equina, spinal nerves, or vertebrae)

quadriceps may be weak on the left and the ankle dorsiflexors on the right. It is useful to test muscle power with the spine extended and the patient lying prone with knees flexed (Pheasant test). In this position motor weakness may be more marked. After testing for muscle power in both legs, it is useful to ask the patient to walk briskly for 5 minutes. Retesting after this may reveal increaesd muscle weakness. Occasionally, muscle weakness is so severe that the patient is unable to stand or walk.

Reflexes may be diminished or absent, the quadriceps on one side and the Achilles tendon reflex on the other. The overall picture is usually bizarre, but when the central stenosis involves only one level, the picture may resemble that of a disc herniation and may be mistaken for that (Tables 10-3 and 10-4).

Radiographic Changes

Plain radiographs demonstrate enlarged posterior facets, approximation of one lamina to the next, decreased distances between the articular processes, di-

Table 10-4 Classification of Spinal Stenosis

Congenital/developmental

Acquired
    Degenerative (central, lateral, both of these)
    Combined (with disc herniation, with developmental stenosis, with both)
    After laminectomy (scarring)
    After fusion (above the fusion, beneath the fusion)
    Trauma (early and late changes)
    Paget's disease
    Fluorosis

minished disc height, the presence of osteophytes that arise from vertebral bodies, and decreased size of the foramina. These changes are characteristic of spondylosis and are no more than suggestive of stenosis. Stress anteroposterior and lateral radiographs may reveal that instability is present (Fig. 10-21).

Comments

To the physician who is not aware of central spinal stenosis as a possible diagnosis, the symptoms may suggest a psychoneurosis, a desire for compensation, or a lack of desire to return to work. The physician who is aware that the syndrome exists will find the symptoms, signs, and radiographic changes strongly

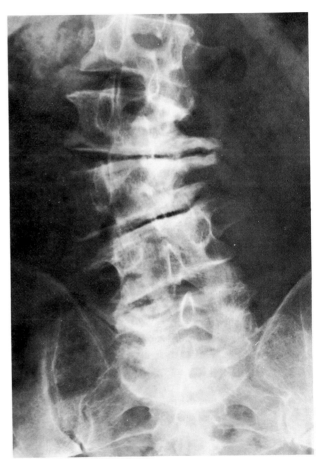

Fig. 10-21 Generalized spondylosis with scoliosis. The patient had symptoms and signs of compression of the L5 nerve on the right.

suggestive of the diagnosis. The diagnosis is made definite by myelography and by CT scan images.[8,9,10]

DEGENERATIVE SPONDYLOLISTHESIS

Presentation

The presentation is very similar to that seen in central spinal stenosis.

Mechanism

The mechanism involves is that of lumbar spondylosis, with marked erosion of posterior articular processes. In this respect degenerative spondylolithesis differs from other types of spondylosis, which produce enlargement of articular processes. The disc yields and the inferior articular process moves forward as the superior process is continually more and more eroded. The upper vertebral body is displaced forward on the lower body. The nerve that exits one level below the lesion is entrapped between the inferior articular process of the upper vertebra and the back of the body of the lower vertebra. At the L4–5 level the L5 nerve is entrapped between the inferior process of L4 and the body of L5. This lesion is most commonly seen at the L4–5 level but is sometimes encountered at the L3–4 or L5–S1 level. Rarely, a slip is seen at two or three levels (see Ch. 4, Fig. 4-18A).

Symptoms and Signs

The symptoms are similar to those of central spinal stenosis.

The signs differ little from those seen in central stenosis. Examination of the lumbar spine may reveal that an upper spinous process is displaced forward on the process that is one below it.

Radiographic Changes

Radiographs show the same changes as for spondylosis. An upper vertebral body has slipped forwards on the one below it. In the presence of instability, the upper vertebral body may be normally aligned

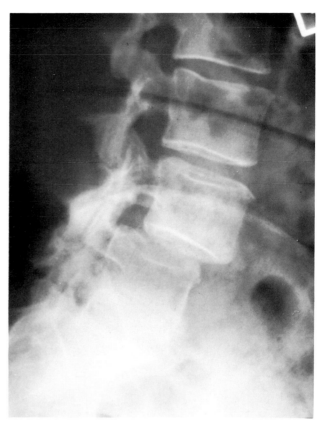

Fig. 10-22 Degenerative spondylolisthesis of the 4th on the 5th lumbar vertebra.

on the lower in the lateral view in extension and displaced forward in the flexion view (Fig. 10-22).

ISTHMIC SPONDYLOLISTHESIS

Presentation

The condition may present with low back pain alone, with a combination of low back and leg pain, or rarely, with leg pain alone.

Mechanism

The mechanism of production of the defect is not well understood. Some writers think it is due to a fall onto the buttocks. Others think that it is a fatigue fracture; still others that it is due to flexion, extension, or rotational trauma.[11] The result is a bilateral fracture

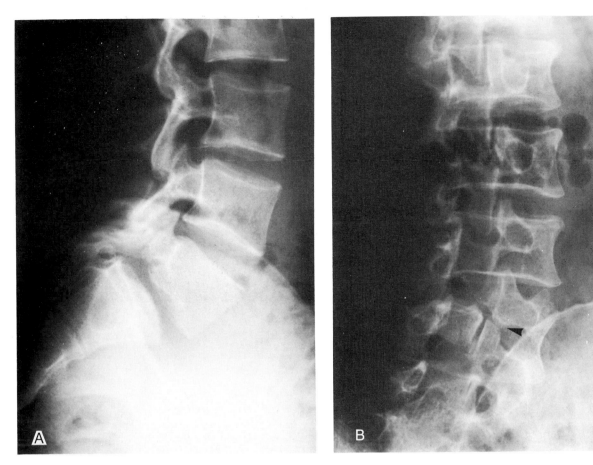

Fig. 10-23 Isthmic spondylolisthesis. **(A)** The body of L5 has slipped forwards on that of the sacrum. **(B)** Oblique radiograph in the same patient. A defect is seen in the pars interarticularis (arrow). (*Figure continues.*)

of the pars interarticularis. It is thought that this usually occurs when the patient is between the ages of 6 and 12 years. Slowly, over subsequent years, the disc yields and the upper vertebra (usually L5) slips forward on the lower (usually S1). The slippage is graded as follows: (1) first degree, less than one third of the distance between the front and the back of the vertebral body; (2) between one third and two thirds of this distance; (3) more than two thirds of this distance; and (4) spondyloptosis, slippage of one body completely forward on the body below with rotation through 90°. At the L5–S1 level, the L5 nerve is entrapped by forward displacement of that part of the pars interarticularis that lies immediately above the defect (the fracture) as it passes laterally to the L5–S1 foramen (see Chapter 4, Fig. 4–18B).

Symptoms

Low back pain, leg pain, or both of these may be present. Occasionally, the leg pain is bilateral. In patients of any age pain may be sufficient to bring the patient to the physician. In children, adolescents, and young adults, the pain is commonly in the back alone. In older patients, often with superadded degenerative disease, the pain is usually in both back and leg. The leg pain is usually in the L5 nerve distribution.

Signs

Movement of the lumbar spine is painful, most marked in extension. Movements are slightly restricted, especially in extension. A step may be felt

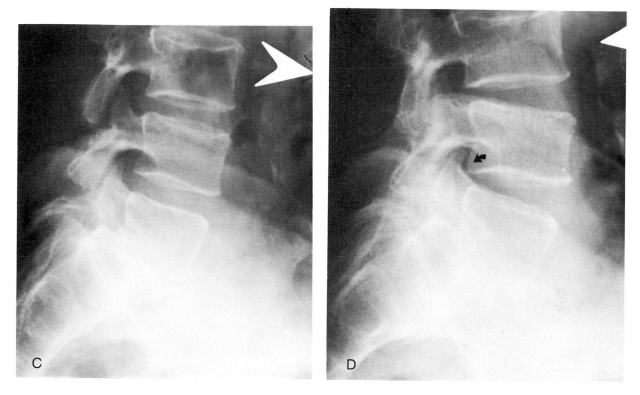

Fig. 10-23 *(Continued)*. **(C)** Another patient. Lateral view in flexion. Note the size of the L4–5 foramen. **(D)** The same patient as in (C). In extension retrospondylolisthesis of L4 on L5 is present and the L4–5 foramen is very narrow. The isthmic spondylolisthesis at L5–S1 is complicated by instability at L4–5.

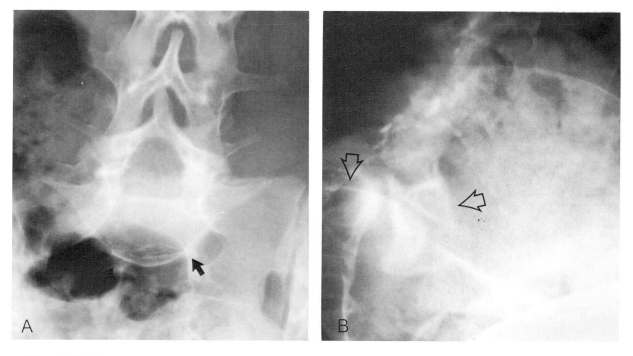

Fig. 10-24 (A) AP radiograph of patient with spondyloptosis. The arrow points to an inverted "Napoleon's hat" characteristic of this lesion. **(B)** Lateral radiograph of the same patient. The arrow on the left points to the upper surface of the sacrum. The arrow on the right points to the upper surface of the body of L5. The body of L5 is displaced completely forwards on that of the sacrum and is rotated 90°.

between the upper and lower spinous processes. When the slippage is at the L5–S1 level, the spinous process of L4 is felt anterior to that of L5. Straight leg raising may be slightly diminished. Sensation is diminished over the L5 dermatome. Muscle weakness occurs in the muscles supplied by the L5 nerve, the dorsiflexors of ankle and toes. In adolescents marked hamstring tightness may be present.

Radiographic Changes

The lateral view shows that the body of L5 is displaced forward on the sacrum. In the oblique view a fracture line (a defect) is demonstrated in the pars interarticularis. When there is instability flexion and extension lateral films sometimes show movement of L5 on the sacrum (Figs. 10–23 and 10–24).

Comment

The radiographic findings are so obvious that the physician is tempted to explain the symptoms and signs on this basis in every patient. There are two pitfalls. The pain may be caused, not by the spondylolisthesis, but by a concomitant sacroiliac syndrome. It is therefore imperative to exclude this. It is advisable to treat the sacroiliac syndrome first. When such treatment does not relieve the pain, attention is given to management of the slippage. In spondylolisthesis strain is thrown on the posterior joints one level higher. This may cause pain and occasionally is responsible for lateral nerve entrapment at this higher level when there is instability at this level.

SUMMARY

In this chapter the different syndromes that are found in the three phases of the degenerative process are reviewed. We turn in the next chapter to consider the diagnostic procedures that are used to make as complete and accurate a diagnosis as possible.

REFERENCES

1. Kirkaldy-Willis WH, Hill R: A more precise diagnosis for low back pain. Spine 4: 102, 1979
2. Cassidy JD, Kirkaldy-Willis WH: The posterior facet joints in low back pain. Presented at the Annual Meeting of the International Society for the Study of the Lumbar Spine, Toronto, June, 1982
3. Mooney V, Robertson J: The facet syndrome. Clin Orthop 115: 149, 1976
4. Bowen V, Cassidy JD: Macroscopic and microscopic anatomy of the Sacroiliac joint from embryonic life until the eighth decade. Spine 6: 620, 1981
5. Keim H, Kirkaldy-Willis WH: Low back pain. Ciba Clin Symposia 32: 6, 1980
6. Wiltse LL, Guyer R, Spence C, et al: Alar transverse process impingement of the L5 spinal nerve: The far out syndrome: Spine 9: 1, 1984
7. Burton CV, Kirkaldy-Willis WH, Yong-Hing K, Heithoff KB: Causes of failure of surgery on the lumbar spine. Clin Orthop 157: 191, 1981
8. Kirkaldy-Willis WH, Paine KWE, Cauchoix J, McIvor GWD: Lumbar spinal stenosis. Clin Orthop 99: 30, 1974
9. Kirkaldy-Willis WH, McIvor GWD (eds): Symposium on spinal stenosis. Clin Orthop 115, 1976
10. Wiltse LL, Kirkaldy-Willis WH, McIvor GWD: The treatment of spinal stenosis. Clin Orthop 115, 83, 1976
11. Wiltse LL, Newman PH, Macnab I: Classification of spondylolysis and spondylolisthesis: Clin Orthop 117: 23, 1976

11

Diagnostic Techniques

William H. Kirkaldy-Willis
Stanley Tchang

It is time to consider how a complete and accurate diagnosis can be made. In doing this we have two different aspects of the problem in mind: the phase in which the lesion exists and the nature and site of the lesion. Before going further, the reader is advised to review the illustrations of radiographs in Chapter 9.

For clarity we will describe one method by which the diagnosis can be made in a spinal unit. In the less severe cases (usually in Phase I, dysfunction) the diagnosis is presumptive and the treatment is simple. Patients in this category make up 90% of the referrals to a bank clinic. Using this method time and expense are saved. An example serves to illustrate our approach.

The patient has been evaluated clinically and radiologically. A presumptive diagnosis of dysfunction that chiefly affects the posterior facet joints has been made. The treatment is to attend the spine education program, to wear a light-weight elastic supporting garment, and to undergo a course of five to ten manipulations. When this treatment regimen is successful, the patient's case is reviewed after 3 months. If treatment fails to relieve the symptoms, the patient is admitted to the hospital overnight for injection of 0.25% bupivacaine (Marcaine) into the posterior joints and overlying muscle. Relief of pain for only a few hours confirms that these joints are the chief

source of the pain. However, long-lasting relief may be obtained. If the injections fail, the patient attends daily for 2 or 3 weeks as an outpatient for physiotherapy and occupational therapy. It is usually thought advisable to admit patients in whom this regimen fails to the hospital so that the nature of the lesion can be defined precisely. It is likely that the patient will require a CT scan, possibly a myelogram, and psychological evaluation.

This approach to diagnosis and treatment is not completely accurate. It does mean that 90% of patients can be relieved of their pain in a simple way at low cost. It allows the physician time to concentrate on other, more difficult problems. No patient is neglected. The patient with severe acute symptoms and signs or with a neurological deficit is admitted to the hospital quickly for diagnosis and treatment.

DIAGNOSTIC TECHNIQUES

Clinical Examination

Careful clinical examination and review of stress radiographs go far toward making the diagnosis. They are in fact essential. Later it is necessary to correlate clinical findings with those obtained from the myelogram or the CT scan (Table 11-1).

Table 11-1 Diagnostic Tests

Dysfunction
    Stress radiographs
    Effect of facet injection
    Effect of manipulation

Unstable phase
    Stress radiographs (to assess the phase)
    CT scan, myelogram, nerve blocks, EMG (to diagnose the lesion)

Stabilization
    Stress radiographs (to assess the phase)
    CT scan, myelogram, nerve blocks, EMG (to diagnose the lesion)

Injection of Posterior Joints

Injection of posterior joints is often most helpful. Our usual custom is first to inject (using 0.25% bupivacaine and fluoroscopic control) the joints at what is considered the affected level—usually L4–5. The patient then stands up, puts his back through a full range of movements, and tells the examiner whether or not he still has pain. If the first injection does not relieve the pain, another level—perhaps L5–S1—is injected. The patient tests the effect of this in the same way. If necessary, on rare occasions, the L3–4 joint may then be injected. This procedure makes it possible to identify the level of the lesion with certainty and to determine if the major source of pain lies in the facet joints.

Manipulation

Benefit from manipulation directed to a specific joint provides evidence of dysfunction of that joint.

Myelography

Until recently, when patients had persistent leg pain, it was the custom in most centers to request a myelogram. Now that third and fourth generation high resolution CT scanners are available in many centers, this diagnostic tool bids high to replace myelography in most patients. Because the CT scan is not universally available, we will discuss myelography first.

In performing a myelogram, the water-soluble contrast medium metrizamide should be used. This medium is absorbed into the blood stream. Complications are few. Headaches, nausea, and vomiting are not as common or as persistent as after myelography done with an oil-based contrast medium. Cases in which the patient becomes disoriented or even psychotic for a few hours have been reported. Seizure is a rare complication following lumbar examination with metrizamide. Up to now no arachnoiditis has been reported in humans following metrizamide myelography.

A disc herniation within the confines of the central spinal canal is usually clearly demonstrated by an anterior or anterolateral defect in the contrast column at the disc space or by the cutting off of one nerve sheath. It is necessary to differentiate the defect caused by the presence of a herniation from that caused by the presence of spinal tumors. A myelographic defect caused by the presence of extradural tumors may simulate that caused by a disc herniation. However, the most common tumor in this group is metastasis, and it is invariably associated with bone destruction. Extradural neurofibroma produces characteristic bony erosion. Intradural tumors are confined within the dural sac, which is not displaced away from bony margins. Extradural abscess may present as an extradural mass, but usually the disc space is narrowed and destruction of the endplate of the adjacent vertebrae is evident. Myelography never demonstrates the presence of a disc herniation in the lateral nerve canal or lateral canal stenosis unless medial enlargement of the superior facet by an osteophyte is present.

Central spinal stenosis is clearly shown. In the degenerative type the canal is small and clover leaf or trefoil in shape because of medial protrusion of enlarged posterior articular processes and backward protrusion of osteophytic outgrowths from the back of the vertebral bodies. In the developmental type the central canal is small in both sagittal and coronal planes. In the combined type the observed changes demonstrate the features of both degenerative and developmental stenosis. The extent of the process—the number of segments involved—is also clearly delineated. It is useful during the course of the examination to ask the patient while he is standing to extend his lumbar spine as much as possible. Stenosis not evident in the neutral position may become evident with the spine extended, or stenosis already noted may become more marked (Figs. 11-1 and 11-2).

The CT Scan

Computerized tomographic scanning is now widely used to diagnose lesions in the lumbar spine. At the start of our experience 5 years ago we soon became aware that for the first time we could see lateral canal stenosis and measure the degree to which it was present. We soon realized that in diagnosing central and lateral stenosis this was the best tool yet available. With the advent of high resolution scanning it is now possible to demonstrate soft tissue shadows. A high window setting is used for bony structures and a low one for soft tissues. With a cursor (a small white rectangle) placed over the soft tissue shadow, a mean density reading can be obtained. In this way the nature of the soft tissue can be assessed with reasonable accuracy. The mean density of disc material is the highest; fibrous tissue is next; then the densities of spinal nerves, of cauda equina, and fat follow in descending order. With the patient's trunk supine on the table and the pelvis rotated first to one side, then to the other using a small pillow or sandbag, it is possible to study the effect of rotation on the facets and lateral canals. The same can be done for flexion—extension movement.

Figures showing CT images illustrate the changes to be seen more clearly than any script. The following lesions are thus described: changes in the facet joints (Fig. 11-3A to F), changes due to disc herniation and fibrosis (Fig. 11-4A to F), and changes due to central and lateral stenosis (Fig. 11-5A to F). Entrapment due to osteophytes is illustrated by Figures 11-6 and 11-7. Disc herniation is documented in greater detail in Figures 11-8 to 11-10, with left lateral (Fig. 11-9) and left central herniation (Fig. 11-10) clearly distinguished. Herniation with right lateral stenosis is seen in Figure 11-11. Additional examples of central and lateral stenosis are illustrated in Figures 11-12 and 11-13 respectively. Changes deriving from spinal fusion are documented in Figure 11-14. A word of caution is necessary. Lesions or bony protuberances demonstrated in the myelogram or by the CT scan may not produce symptoms. It is essential to correlate the clinical symptoms and signs with myelographic and CT findings. In cases when doubt is present, a

selective nerve block and/or electromyelography may be of assistance.

Selective Nerve Blocks

The rationale of this procedure is to identify the spinal nerve at the level of the symptoms. This is especially useful when images from the CT scan demonstrate lesions at two levels.

THE TECHNIQUE

For the L4 nerve at the L4–5 level, the skin is anesthetized under fluoroscopic control opposite the spinous process of L4, 5 to 6 cm from the midline, and a thin lumbar puncture needle is passed in the coronal plane angled at 45° toward the midline until contact is made with the transverse process of L4. The needle is withdrawn, reintroduced 1 cm caudal to the transverse process, and advanced toward the L4–5 foramen. When the needle reaches the L4 nerve, the patient experiences pain in the leg. It is important to ascertain if this is the pain that the patient has complained of. Injection of 1 to 2 ml of renographin demonstrates the tunnel of soft tissue in which the nerve runs laterally and caudally. At this point injecting 2 to 3 ml of 0.25% bupivacaine will abolish the pain. For the L5 nerve at the L5–S1 level the skin is anesthetized in the same way opposite the spinous process of L5 and the needle is advanced in the coronal plane and at 45° toward the midline. It is withdrawn slightly when it hits the transverse process of L5, introduced again to pass caudal to the process, and advanced until it contacts the L5 nerve at the L5–S1 foramen. To block the S1 nerve the needle is introduced posteriorly through the first sacral foramen and advanced to contact the anterior ramus. The remainder of the procedure is as described above.

Electromyography

Dr. J. R. Donat, neurologist at the University Hospital in Saskatoon, writes as follows:

Electromyography is probably not necessary in patients with definite and well localized findings of radiculopathy on physical examination. It may occasionally confirm or help localize radiculopathy in patients with minimal findings or normal examination.

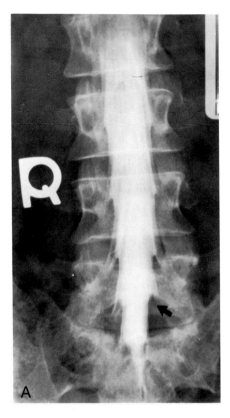

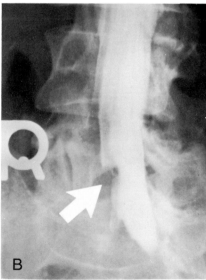

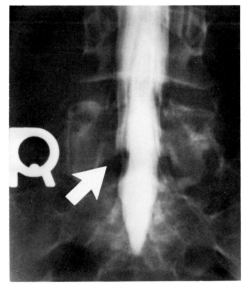

Fig. 11-1 (A) AP myelogram L5–S1 disc herniation on left. The S1 nerve sheath on the left is cut off (arrow). **(B)** AP and oblique myelograms showing L5–S1 disc herniation on right. There is a defect in the contrast column (arrows). **(C)** AP myelogram showing one-level central degenerative stenosis at L4–5. The contrast column is almost completely blocked at this level. **(D)** Lateral myelogram of the same patient. At the L4–5 level the contrast column is indented anteriorly by a bulging disc (not a herniation) and posteriorly by the enlarged articular process. **(E)** AP myelogram. The column is almost completely interrupted at the L4–5 level because of marked one-level central stenosis, degenerative in type. **(F)** Lateral view of the same patient. The block at L4–5 is again seen. The AP diameter of the contrast column is reduced in size; mild developmental stenosis is present. (*Figure continues.*)

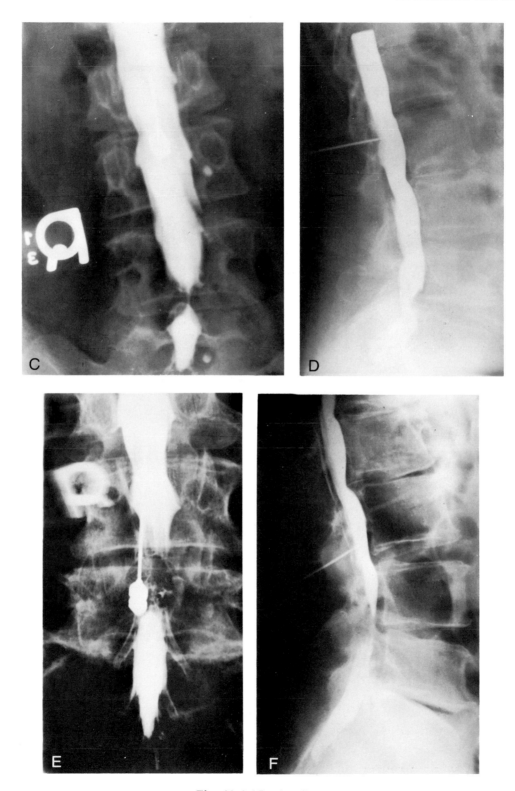

Fig. 11-1 (*Continued*).

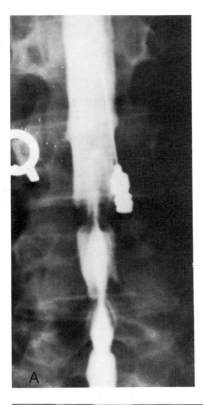

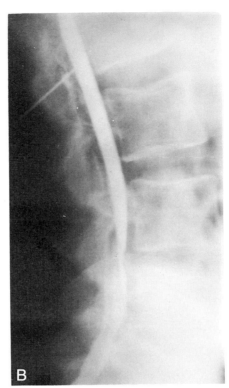

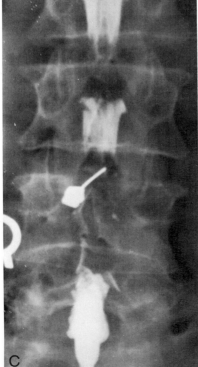

Fig. 11-2 (A) AP myelogram. Defects can be seen in the contrast column at the L4–5 and L5–S1 levels, indicating the presence of degenerative central stenosis at two levels. **(B)** The same patient, lateral view. The AP diameter of the contrast column is reduced. This suggests the presence of mild developmental stenosis. **(C)** AP myelogram. The contrast column is interrupted at the L3–4, L4–5, and L5–S1 levels, indicating that very marked central degenerative stenosis is present at these three levels. (*Figure continues.*)

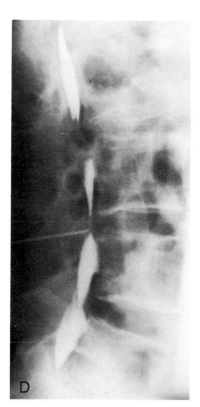

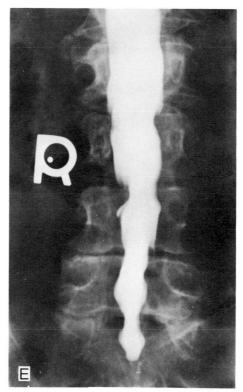

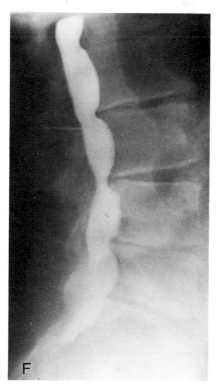

Fig. 11-2 (*Continued*). **(D)** The same patient, lateral view. The AP diameter of the contrast column is markedly reduced. Developmental stenosis is complicated by degenerative stenosis. **(E)** AP myelogram. Marked irregularity of the contrast column, which is narrow from L3–4 to the sacrum. **(F)** The same patient, lateral view. The contrast column is indented anteriorly at every level by bulging of degenerated discs. At the lower levels the column is also indented posteriorly by enlarged articular processes. Multilevel degenerative central stenosis is present.

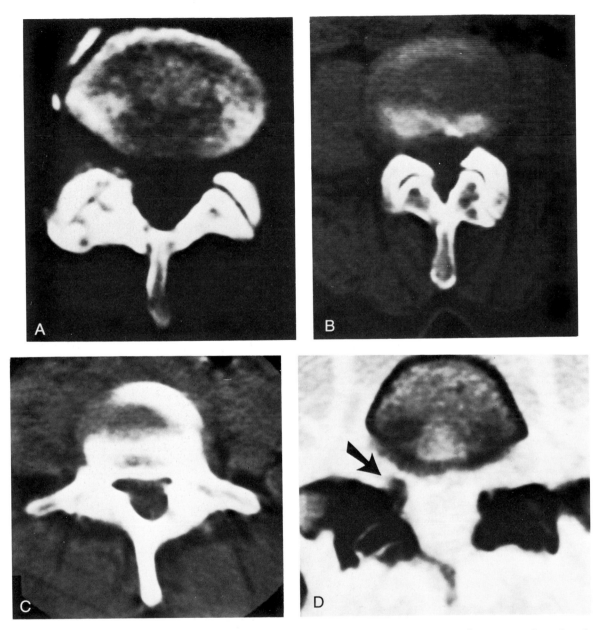

Fig. 11-3 (A) CT scan at the L4–5 level. On the right (viewer's left) the posterior facets are enlarged and fragmented. Marked posterior facet degeneration is present. **(B)** CT scan at the L4–5 level. Tropism of the facets is present. On the right (viewer's left) the facets are oblique. On the left they are more in the sagittal plane. **(C)** CT scan at the L4–5 level. The laminae are asymmetrical. The lamina on the right (viewer's left) is displaced forward releative to that on the left. The central canal is displaced to the left. **(D)** CT scan at the L5–S1 level. A large osteophyte arising from the anterior surface of the superior facet (arrow) has narrowed the right lateral canal. (*Figure continues*.)

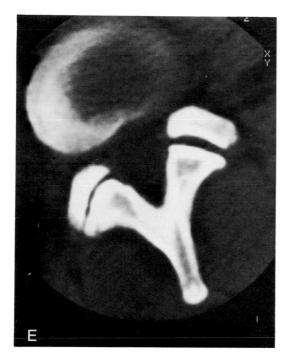 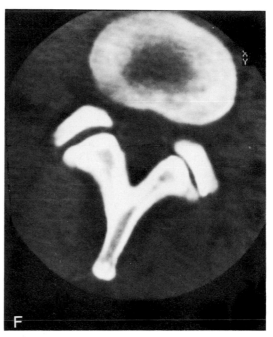

Fig. 11-3 *(Continued).* **(E)** CT scan at L4–5 with rotation. The posterior joint on the left (viewer's right) is open because of capsular laxity and the superior facet has moved forward to narrow the left lateral canal. **(F)** The same patient. Rotation in the opposite direction has opened the posterior joint on the right (viewer's left) and the right lateral canal is narrow. Instability at L4–5 with increased abnormal movement is present.

Routine nerve conduction studies are normal or show only non-specific findings in patients with radiculopathy. However, they help exclude other conditions such as a neuropathy which may confuse the diagnosis.

Electromyography per se may show fibrillation potentials and motor unit changes in denervated muscles. The distribution of abnormalities may help localize the lesion to a particular root. Denervation of para-spinal muscles confirms that the lesion involves nerve roots, but has little localizing value. Unfortunately, the EMG is negative in patients whose symptoms are due to irritation of dorsal roots.

Several new techniques for detecting lesions at sites proximal to those usually studied by routine nerve conduction methods are currently under investigation. These include the F-wave, H-reflex, and spinal evoked potentials.

The F-wave is a late response due to recurrent discharge of motor neurons following stimulation of their peripheral branches. Delay of F-waves evoked by stimulation of peroneal or posterior tibial nerves may suggest lesions of the L5 or S1 ventral roots. The H-reflex is the electrophysiological equivalent of the tendon reflex. Delay of the H-reflex recorded from the soleus muscle following stimulation of the tibial nerve at the knee may suggest a lesion of the S1 dorsal or ventral roots. Both these late responses are easily recorded with equipment generally available in EMG laboratoes.

Spinal evoked potentials are recorded over the cauda equina or spinal cord following stimulation of peripheral nerves. This technique may be useful in detecting lesions of the L5 dorsal root which are not accompanied by weakness, reflex changes or EMG abnormalities. However, it requires computerized averaging of very large numbers of responses.

Clinical electromyography requires a great deal of skill and judgment. Undue confidence in equivocal or non-diagnostic abnormalities leads to frequent false positive diagnosis. The results of electromyography should always be considered in relation to the history, physical examination, and results of other investigations.

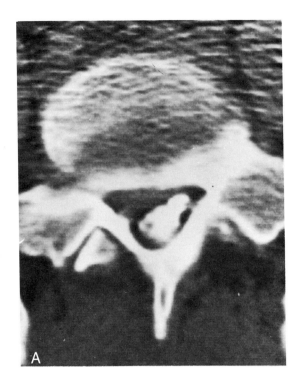

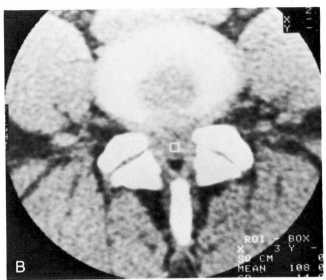

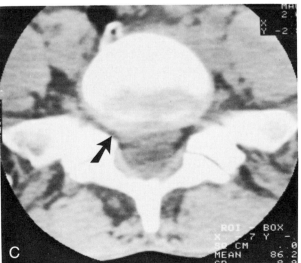

Fig. 11-4 (A) Disc herniation. Metrizamide myelogram followed by CT scan. At the L5–S1 level the contrast is displaced posteriorly on the right by a disc herniation. **(B)** Disc herniation. Scan at L4–5. A large central disc herniation fills the central canal. The mean density of the shadow, as indicated by the white rectangle (the cursor), is 108, the density of a herniation. The mean density of the cauda equina would be much lower. **(C)** Disc herniation. CT scan at L5–S1. The soft tissue shadow of a disc herniation is seen on the right (arrow). The mean density is 86.2. (*Figure continues.*)

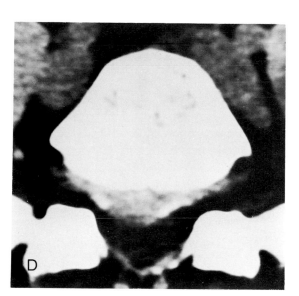

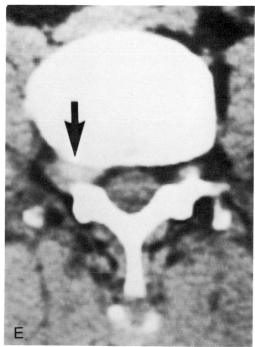

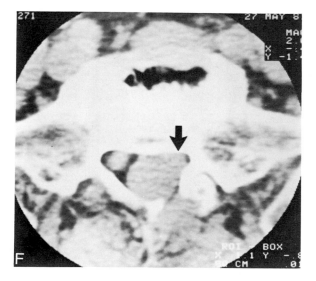

Fig. 11-4 (*Continued*). **(D)** Central disc herniation. CT scan at L5–S1. The soft tissue shadow of the central disc herniation is clearly seen. **(E)** Lateral disc herniation. CT scan at L4–5. The arrow points to a large soft tissue shadow on the right. This herniation would not be demonstrated in a myelogram. **(F)** Fibrosis. CT scan at L5–S1. The arrow points to a poorly defined soft tissue shadow. The mean density of this is 44.2, too low for a herniation, correct for scar tissue.

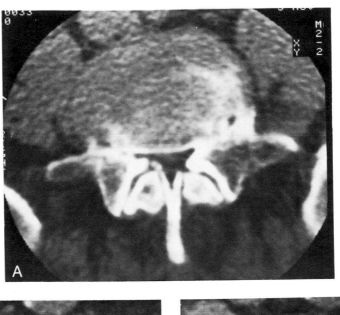

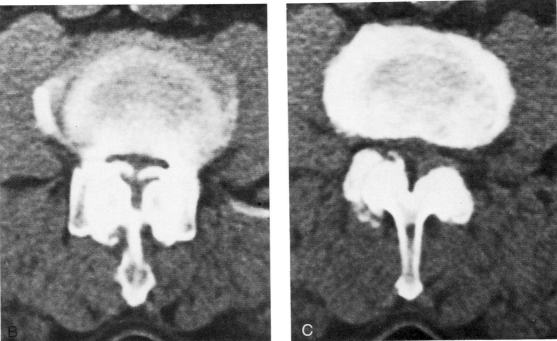

Fig. 11-5 (A) Central stenosis. CT scan at L5–S1. Enlargement of posterior facets on both sides has markedly narrowed the central canal. **(B)** Central stenosis. CT scan at L5–S1. Enlargement of posterior facets on both sides towards the midline has markedly narrowed the central canal. The presence of large osteophytes on the anterior surface of the superior facets has produced even further narrowing. **(C)** Unilateral central and lateral stenosis. Same patient as in (B). CT scan at L3–4. Enlargement of the posterior facets on the righ has produced central and lateral stenosis. (*Figure continues.*)

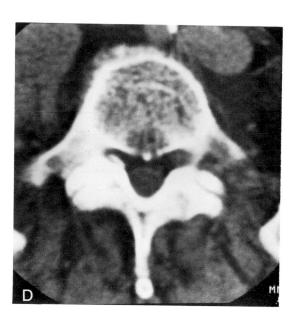

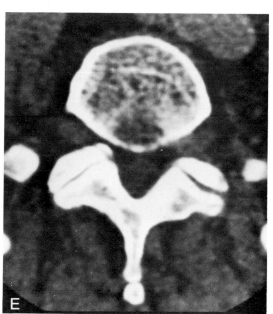

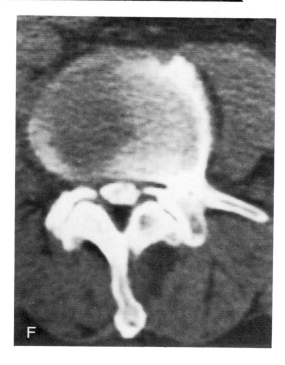

Fig. 11-5 (*Continued*). **(D)** Lateral stenosis. CT scan at the level of the pedicles of L4. The right lateral canal is slightly narrowed just above the point at which the L4 nerve exits. **(E)** Lateral stenosis. The same patient as in (D). CT scan 5 mm below the L4 pedicles. The right lateral canal is very narrow. The shadow of the L4 nerve can be seen lateral to the canal. This stenosis has entrapped the L4 nerve on the right. **(F)** Lateral stenosis. CT scan at L4–5. A large osteophyte is protruding medially from the left superior facet, the subarticular gutter is very narrow and the L5 nerve is entrapped between the superior facet and the back of the vertebral body.

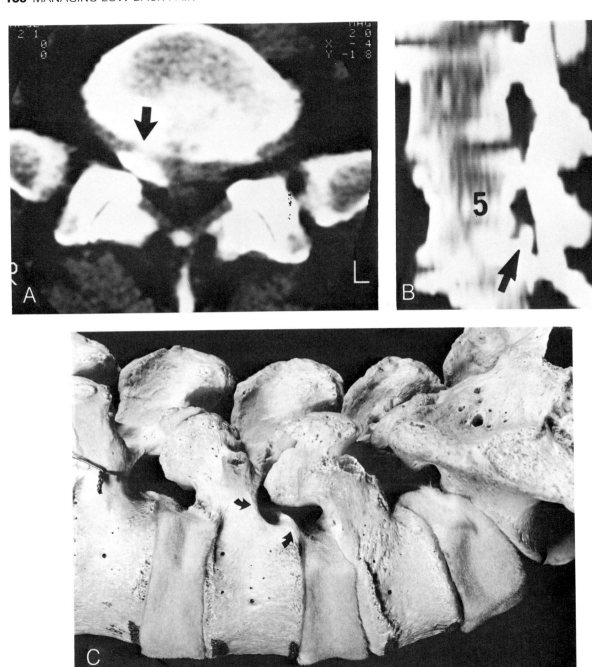

Fig. 11-6 Sagittal reconstructions give useful added information to that obtained from axial images. **(A)** The axial image at L5–S1 demonstrates on the right the presence of a large osteophytic spur arising from the posterolateral aspect of the lower part of the body of L5 (arrow), narrowing the L5–S1 lateral canal and entrapping the L5 nerve. **(B)** The sagittal reconstruction shows the same spur (arrow), which has narrowed the recess anterior to the superior articular process of the sacrum. The L5 nerve passes between the front of the articular process and the back of the spur. **(C)** Lumbar spine showing two sites of nerve entrapment at the L4–5 level.

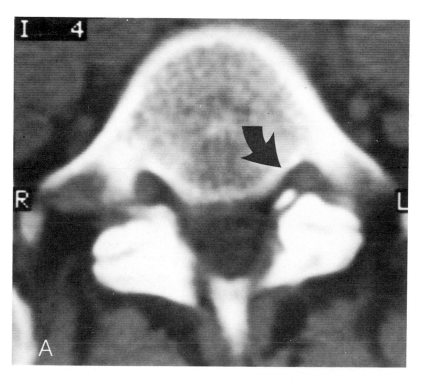

Fig. 11-7 Further demonstration of use of sagittal reconstruction. **(A)** Axial image at the L5–S1 level: On the left is a spur between the back of the body of the sacrum and front of the superior articular process (arrow); the lateral canal is markedly narrowed. **(B)** The sagittal view clearly shows this spur coming from the superior articular process of S1.

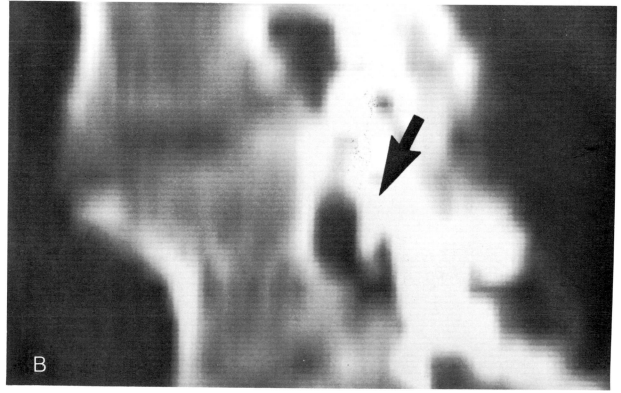

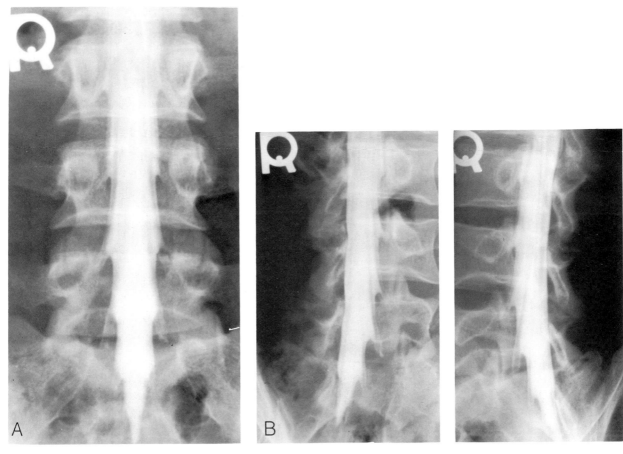

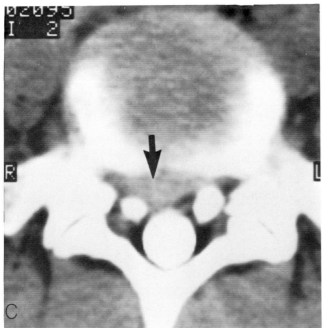

Fig. 11-8 Myelography followed by CT scanning. **(A)** AP view: no abnormality of contrast column or of nerve sheaths. **(B)** Oblique views: no abnormality detected. **(C)** CT following myelogram, three hours later: On the right the S1 nerve is displaced posteriorly by a disc herniation at the L5–S1 level (arrow).

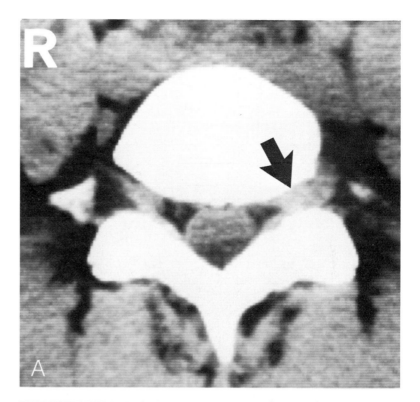

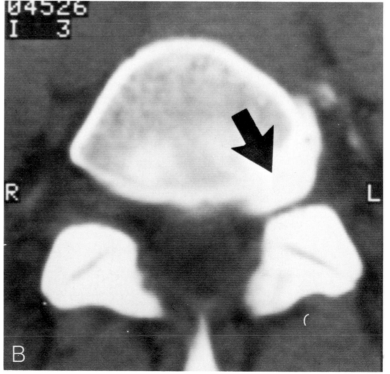

Fig. 11-9 Discogram followed by CT scan. **(A)** At the L5–S1 level on the left the CT image demonstrates the presence of a shadow considered to be due to a disc herniation (arrow). **(B)** The CT image at the same level following discography shows that the contrast injected into the disc has filled the lateral herniation, thus confirming the diagnosis (arrow).

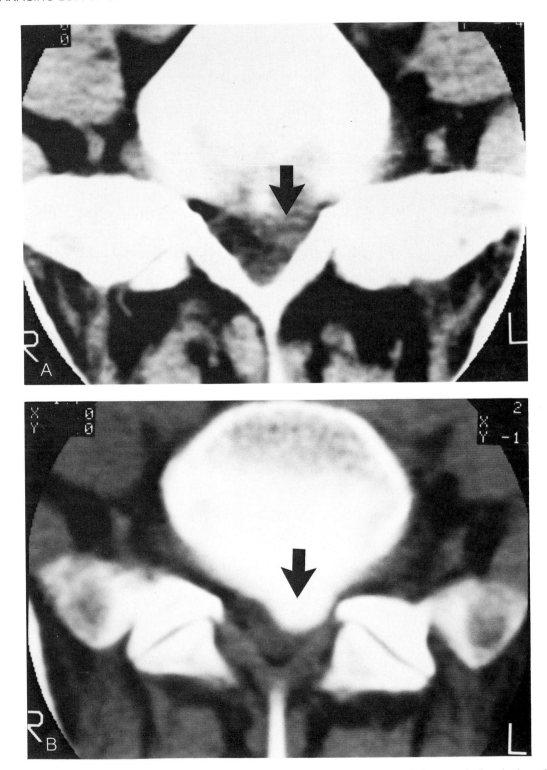

Fig. 11-10 Discogram followed by CT scan. **(A)** At the L5–S1 level on the left (arrow) the shadow from the CT scan suggests the presence of a disc herniation though the mean density of this is low (8.5 H.U.) **(B)** A further CT scan following a discogram shows the presence of contrast in the area under review. This confirms the diagnosis of disc herniation.

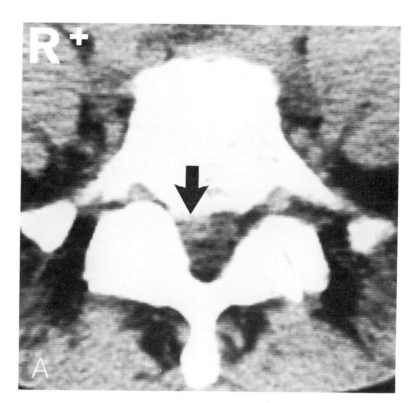

Fig. 11-11 CT scan alone followed some days later by myelogram and CT scan. **(A)** Scan at L5–S1 showing the shadow of a suspected disc herniation on the right (arrow). The density was 75 Housfield units. **(B)** Scan at adjacent L5–S1 level demonstrating a narrow right lateral canal (arrow). (*Figure continues.*)

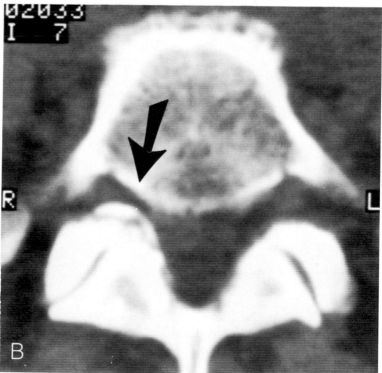

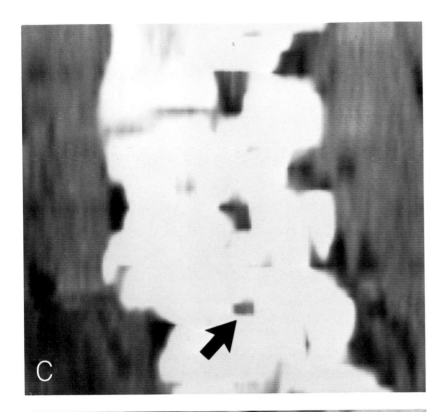

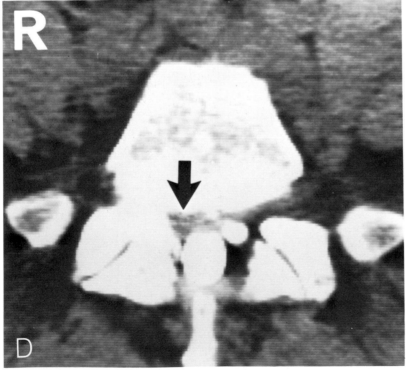

Fig. 11-11 (*Continued*). **(C)** Sagittal reconstruction showing marked stenosis of the L5–S1 lateral canal (arrow). **(D)** Myelogram and CT scan at the same level: The S1 nerve sheath on the right does not fill with contrast (arrow). Disc herniation and right lateral stenosis.

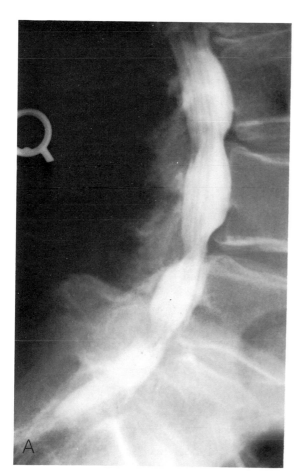

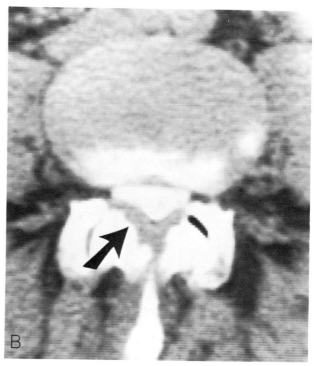

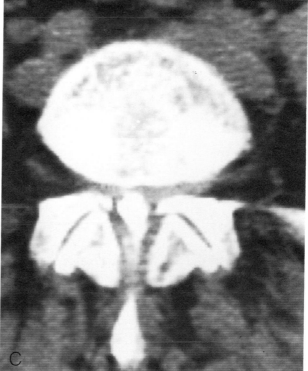

Fig. 11-12 Myelogram followed by CT scan in a patient with degenerative lumbar spinal stenosis. **(A)** Lateral view of contrast column: There is narrowing of the column at the L3–4, L4–5, and L5–S1 levels. **(B)** CT scan: axial image at L3–4 marked thickening of the ligamentum flavum (arrow). **(C)** CT axial image at L4–5: marked central stenosis.

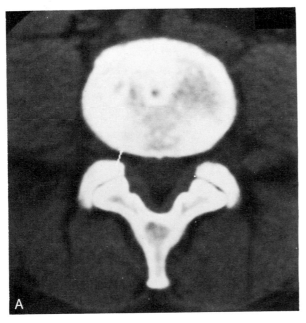
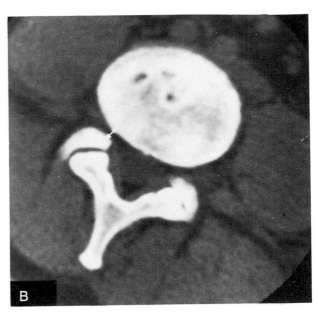

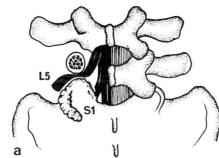

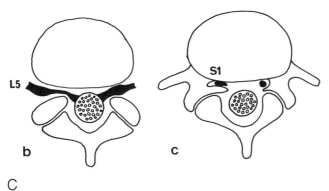

Fig. 11-13 (A) Dynamic lateral stenosis. CT scan at L4–5. Both lateral canals are slightly narrow. Note the diamteter of the right canal (viewer's left). **(B)** The same patient as in (A). With rotation the posterior joint on the right moves forward and the lateral canal becomes narrower than in (A). **(C)** Diagram to demonstrate how two nerves can be entrapped at one level (a) On the viewer's left at the L5–S1 level, the L5 nerve can be entrapped between the pedicle of L5 and the superior facet of the sacrum, and the S1 nerve can be entrapped by an osteophyte that narrows the subarticular gutter deep to the superior facet. (b) The L5 nerve can be entrapped between the superior facet of the sacrum and the pedicle of L5. (c) The S1 nerve can be entrapped between the superior facet of the sacrum and the back of the body of the sacrum or of L5.

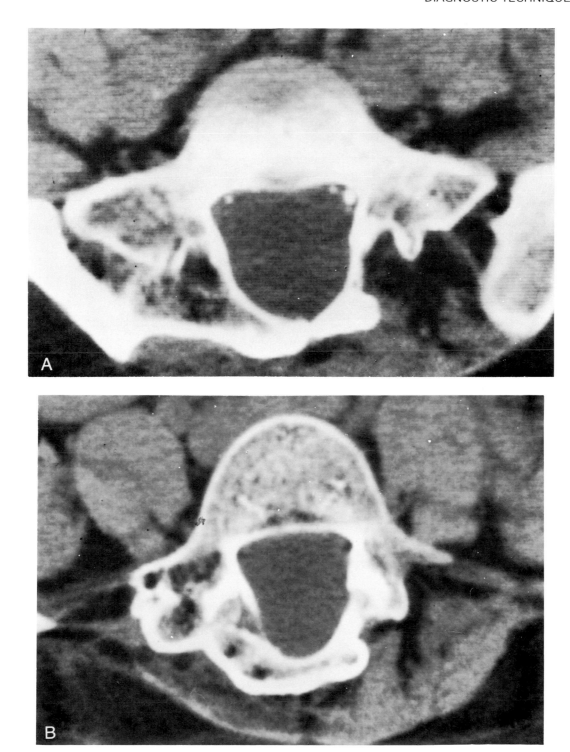

Fig. 11-14 (A) Successful fusion. CT scan at L5–S1. The facet joints are fused. An uninterrupted bar of bone is present posteriorly. **(B)** The same patient. At the L5 level the fusion is equally complete. (*Figure continues.*)

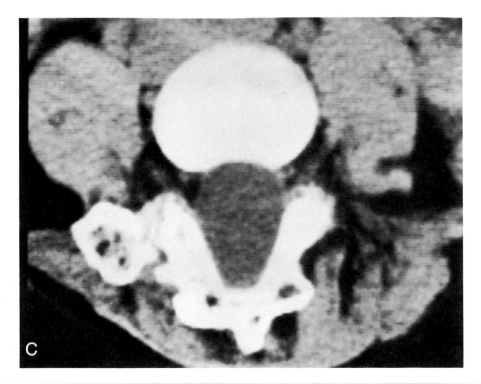

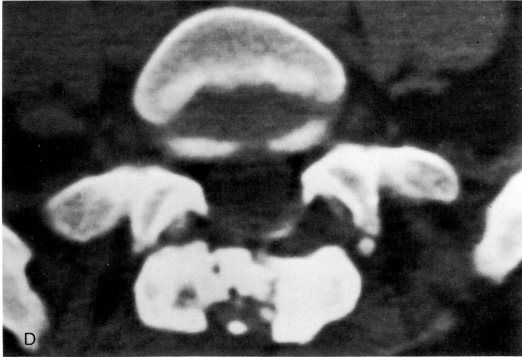

Fig. 11-14 (*Continued*). **(C)** The same patient. At the L4–5 level the fusion is equally solid. Fusion is complete from L4 to the sacrum. **(D)** Another patient. Failed fusion. CT scan at level of upper sacrum. The posterior fusion mass is fragmented. (*Figure continues.*)

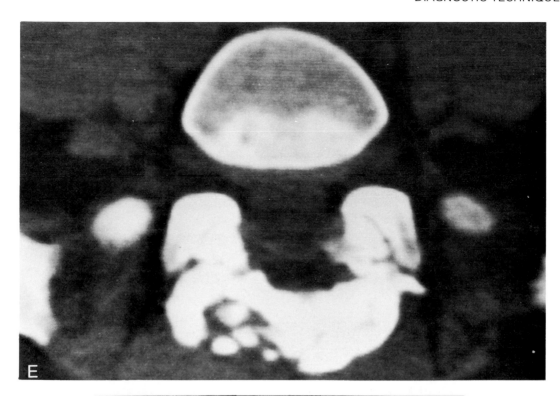

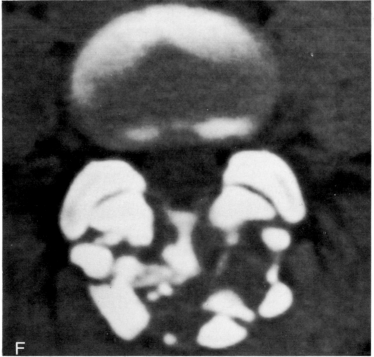

Fig. 11-14 (*Continued*). **(E)** The same patient. At the L4–S1 level the posterior joints are not fused. The posterior bar of bone is fragmented. **(F)** The same patient. At the L4–5 level the posterior joints are not fused. The posterior mass of bone is grossly fragmented.

Psychological Assessment

The value of psychological testing and of an interview with a psychologist interested in the psychological aspects of musculoskeletal lesions has been discussed in Chapter 8. Before any decision is made to advise the patient to consider operative intervention, and in many other cases as well, it is essential that the physician and the psychologist sit down together to discuss the patient's problem in the framework of his or her personality. In some patients the problem is mainly a surgical one; in others mainly a psychological one, and in others it is mixed in nature. In the last group the risks involved in obtaining a good result must be carefully weighed. Often, even when the problem is mainly surgical, knowledge and understanding of the patient's personality and of minor psychological problems helps the surgeon to obtain a better result. Patients with a difficult personality and with major psychological problems often have a serious lesion that requires treatment and they should not be barred from this, provided that future expectations are carefully assessed and the patient informed of them. Many patients who have suffered back and leg pain for several years, especially those who have had several previous operations, are naturally depressed and have suffered a change in personality.

It is surprising how often the opinion of the surgeon and the considered assessment of the psychologist agree. When, on rare occasions, the latter advises strongly against further operative intervention, the wise surgeon heeds this advice.

SYNTHESIS OF CLINICAL EXAMINATION AND DIAGNOSTIC TESTS

The final step in the assessment is to synthesize all that has been done. The reader is again referred to Figure 7-1, in which the various aspects of the problem are set out in tabular form. Some examples serve to make this clear. This assessment gives a concise indication of the treatment required.

Matching the Phase and the Lesion

The patient in Phase I with posterior facet dysfunction is likely to respond to a course of manipulations or a facet injection. The patient in the early stage of Phase II may respond to rest and immobilization. Later in this phase fusion may be required to treat joint instability. In addition, decompression and fusion may be indicated when instability is complicated by a disc herniation or lateral stenosis. The patient in Phase III does not require fusion but may need a decompression for central and/or lateral stenosis.

The Type of Lesion

It is important to define the type of lesion accurately and fully. For example, the symptoms in a patient with central stenosis may be caused largely by interference with the blood supply to the cauda equina and spinal nerves; a decompression should be large enough to relieve this. The patient with several previous operations may be suffering from irritation and stimulation of the sympathetic nervous system. Further operative intervention may make the patient worse. What is required is an epidural steroid injection, a caudal block, or selective nerve block with bupivacaine.

Differential Diagnosis

It is clearly important to consider other conditions that mimic degenerative lesions. We recall the patient with symptoms and signs of an L5–S1 disc herniation who in fact had an abscess in the L5–S1 disc space caused by vertebral osteomyelitis. It may be difficult to differentiate neurogenic and vascular claudication. A neuropathy due to diabetes may mimic a disc herniation or spinal stenosis.

Psychological Assessment

Enough has been said in Chapter 8 for us to appreciate the importance of such evaluation before deciding to carry out any operative procedure and in other cases as well.

SUGGESTED READINGS

Burton CV, Heithoff KB, Kirkaldy-Willis WH, Ray CD: Computed tomographic scanning and the lumbar spine. Spine 4: 356, 1979

Kirkaldy-Willis WH: Five common back disorders: how to diagnose and treat them. Geriatrics 33: 32, 1978

Kirkaldy-Willis WH, Hill RI: A more precise diagnosis for low back pain. Spine 4: 102, 1979

Kirkaldy-Willis WH, Heithoff KB, Bowen CVA, Shannon R: Pathological anatomy of lumbar spondylosis correlated with the CT scan. In Post MJD (ed): Radiographic Evaluation of the Spine. Masson, New York, 1980

Kirkaldy-Willis WH, Farfan HF: Instability of the lumbar spine. Clin Orthop 165: 110, 1982

Mooney V, Robertson J: The facet syndrome. Clin Orthop 115: 149, 1976

Tajima T, Furukawa K, Kuramochi E: Selective lumbosacral radiculography and block. Spine 5: 69, 1980

12

Magnetic Resonance Imaging of the Lumbar Spine

Kenneth B. Heithoff

Magnetic resonance imaging (MRI) has proven to be a valuable adjunct to computed tomography (CT) and other diagnostic radiographic tests of the lumbar spine. Its great usefulness as an adjunct to CT is related to its ability to provide markedly improved soft tissue contrast resolution of lumbar discs and neural elements, as well as the capability of imaging directly in multiple planes (Fig. 12-1). The improved soft tissue resolution allows clear differentiation between soft tissue structures which are often isodense on CT such as disc material, neural elements, intraspinal hematoma, spinal tumors, postoperative recurrent disc herniation versus fibrosis. Spatial resolution is also nearly equal to that of CT.

Unlike CT whose images reflect only attentuation values, MRI images are a composite of T_1 and T_2 proton density, and vascular flow information. Since one can vary the parameters of MR imaging (TE and TR) with resultant different T_1- and T_2- weighting, one can produce widely varying appearances of signal intensity and depiction of normal and pathological anatomy. The selection of the appropriate parameters to best depict the pathology present is essential. No attempt to describe the physics of MRI will be provided in this chapter. Current spine imaging techniques include imaging with partial saturation, T_1-weighted images, and dual-echo spin-echo techniques, which consist of proton density and T_2-weighted images. Variation of these parameters allows a multitude of imaging techniques that provide a unique means of displaying differing parameters of normal spinal anatomy and pathology of the lumbar spine.

TECHNIQUE AND NORMAL ANATOMY

Images with short repetition times (TR) and echo times (TE) produce T_1-weighted images that provide excellent anatomical detail. On T_1-weighted images, the CSF is of low signal intensity (dark) and fat is of high signal intensity (bright or white). Since on T_1-weighted images fat has a very bright signal intensity and neural tissues, CSF, and vascular structures are of low signal intensity (dark), T_1-weighted images produce excellent anatomical detail and high spatial resolution. T_2-weighted images with prolonged TR and TE parameters provide high contrast resolution

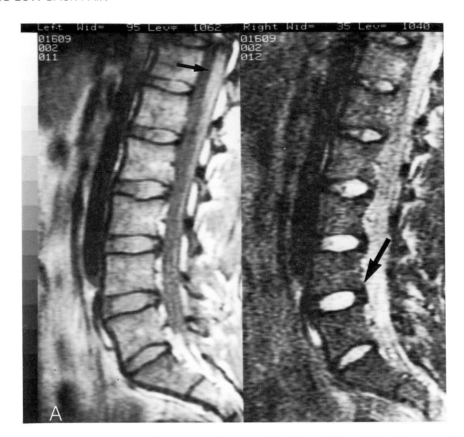

Fig. 12-1 (A) Normal spin-echo sagittal images with proton density and T_2-weighted images. Left, a proton density image depicts the discs as rather homogeneous intermediate signal gray structures. Vertebral bodies are relatively high signal intensity when compared to the T_2-weighted images because of the fat content within the medullary space. Fat is depicted as bright on T_1 and proton density images and becomes low signal intensity on T_2-weighted images as shown on the right. Note visualization of the entire lumbosacral spine from T12–S3 with excellent visualization of the conus (small arrow). CSF is relatively dark on T_1 and proton density images with respect to T_2-weighted images, which show the fluid to become high signal intensity with production of a myelographic effect. Note that on the right hand T_2-weighted images, the normal nuclei are of very high signal intensity due to the well hydrated nature of the normal discs. The annulus is presented as low signal intensity (large arrow). Note that on the left relatively T_1-weighted image, the distinction bewteen the annulus and the nucleus is poor. There is sharp delineation between the hydrated nucleus and the annulus on T_2-weighted images (large arrow). (*Figure continues.*)

between structures containing high contents of "free water" hydrogen ions such as normal disc nuclei, which appear bright, and structures with lesser concentration of "free water" hydrogen, which appear dark. However, because of loss of signal resulting from the prolonged imaging times (TR and TE), the images show poor anatomical detail and spatial resolution. This causes the images to appear "grainy" (Fig. 12-2).

After considerable experimentation, our standard protocol consists of spin-echo, 3 mm contiguous sagittal images, and 5 mm axial images with 1 mm gap. Both the sagittal and axial images are obtained with asymmetric echos (VEMP) with a TR of 1800 and TEs of 20/70; a matrix of 256×128 and 4 excitations. These parameters are continually being reevaluated, however, and are expected to change with new software adaptations and imaging techniques. All scans have been performed on a GE Signa 1.5 Tesla unit (T). Thin section 3-mm sagittal images are felt to be essential to obtain adequate evaluation of the intervertebral nerve root canals in the evaluation of lateral

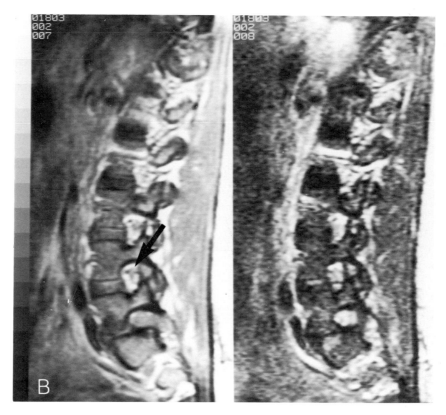

Fig. 12-1 (*Continued*). **(B)** Normal intervertebral nerve root canals: 3-mm sagittal spin-echo images with proton density image on the left and T_2-image on the right; TE/TR 20–70/1500. Note excellent delineation of the exiting nerve root ganglia within the intervertebral nerve root canals (arrow). The ganglion is depicted as a rounded gray structure of intermediate signal intensity. The fat within the intervertebral nerve root canal is bright on both T_1- and T_2-weighted images. The cortical margins of the pedicles and superior and inferior articular processes are of low signal intensity (black) and produce a sharp demarcation of the margins of the intervertebral nerve root canals. Posterior margins of the discs are well visualized and have a straight linear configuration at all levels (small arrow).

spinal stenosis. Spin-echo sagittal technique has been selected since this technique allows a better evaluation of varying degrees of dehydration of the disc than partial saturation technique. In our experience, spin-echo axial images also provide better contrast resolution between herniated disc material and normal neural elements and the CSF. On partial saturation (T_1-weighted) images, herniated disc material, neural elements, and CSF are of similar low signal intensity, causing difficulty in differentiating these structures. Also, we found it difficult or impossible to distinguish between recurrent and residual disc herniation and postoperative fibrosis with partial saturation imaging, whereas recurrent disc herniation can be easily

distinguished from postoperative fibrosis in almost all cases with spin-echo technique (Fig. 12-3).

In the normal patient, lumbar discs are well hydrated and show uniform high signal intensity of the nuclei when visualized in the sagittal plane. The nuclei appear gray on images with short TR and TE and become progressively brighter with increasing imaging times (T_2-weighted images). Degeneration of the disc is associated with loss of water content; thus, the disc becomes darker with the progressive dehydration associated with progressive degeneration of the disc. In the sagittal plane, the normal lumbar disc shows an oval appearance of the nucleus. This is probably not a clear distinction between hydrated

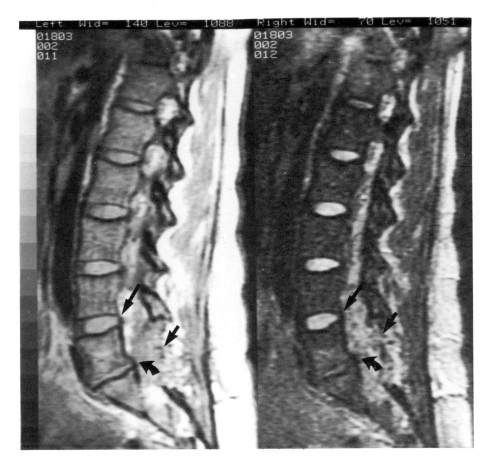

Fig. 12-2 Sagittal T$_1$- and T$_2$-weighted images. TE/TR 20–70/1500. Note: On the left relatively T$_1$-weighted image, the disc is gray and of intermediate signal intensity; on the right, the T$_2$-weighted image shows very bright signal intensity of the discs and clear separation between the hydrated nucleus and the annulus (large arrow). Note the loss of anatomical detail on the T$_2$-weighted image. There is postoperative fibrosis dorsally at L5–S1 (small arrow). Note degenerative dehydration of the L5–S1 disc with loss of signal intensity of the disc and disc space narrowing. Note that the posterior margin of the disc underlying the fibrosis is clearly identified, and one can exclude a recurrent disc herniation despite the presence of fibrosis; thus, a recurrent disc herniation is easily excluded in this patient in whom plain CT was inconclusive.

nucleus and the hydrated inner fibers of the annulus. Many normal discs show a small central posterior projection of increased signal intensity, which either represents dorsally situated nuclear material beneath a thinned annulus or a small punctate region of hydrated inner annular fibers that are more hydrated than the annulus lying on either side of the midline. This small posterior projection should not be mistaken for disc herniation. The outer annulus and the posterior longitudinal ligament form a low signal intensity sharp outer boundary of the disc, which is

normally thin and continuous between the adjacent vertebral bodies. There is a clear distinction between nucleus and annulus, and the ability to visualize disruptions of the annulus allow more accurate evaluation and classification of disc disruptions (Figs. 12-4 to 12-6).

The intervertebral nerve root canals and their contents are well delineated on sagittal MRI images. Epidural fat fills the normal intervertebral nerve root canal and is of high signal intensity on T$_1$ and proton density images. The low signal intensity of the exiting

Fig. 12-3 (A) The postoperative recurrent disc herniation. TE/TR 20–70/1500 is depicted only on the T_2-weighted sagittal image shown on the viewer's right; the recurrent disc herniation is isointense with the fibrosis on the relatively T_1-weighted proton density image. Note the lack of a visualizable annulus on the T_1-weighted image, whereas the annulus is well visualized on the T_2-weighted image and is displaced dorsally by the moderately large recurrent disc herniation (arrow). **(B)** Axial spin-echo images showing the dorsally displaced annulus and hydrated nuclear material. Fortunately, the displaced annulus is of lower signal intensity than the overlying fibrosis (which is of surprisingly high signal intensity) and delineates the periphery of the recurrent disc herniation (arrow). This low signal intensity annular margin of recurrent disc herniation is almost invariably present and provides an excellent demarcation between recurrent herniated nuclear material and the overlying postoperative fibrosis.

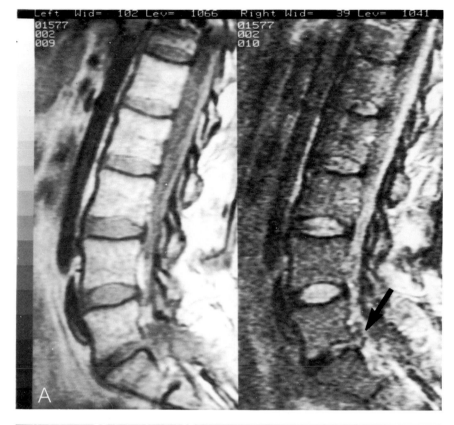

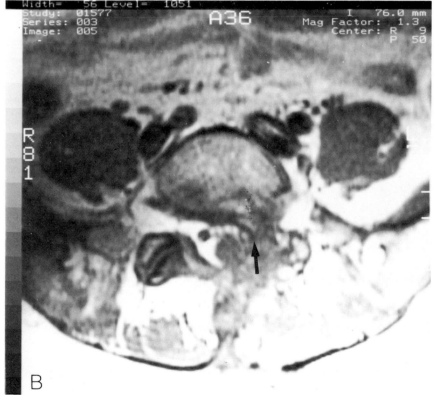

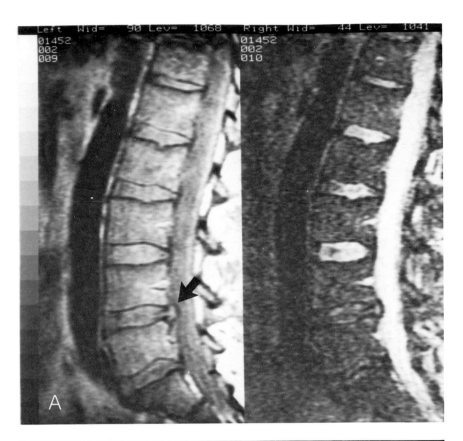

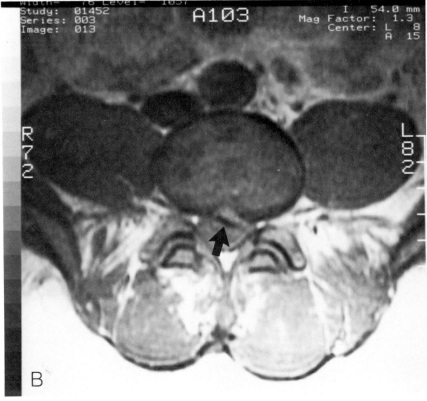

Fig. 12-4 Contained central disc herniation. TE/TR 20–70/1500. **(A)** Sagittal 3-mm images show a moderately large central disc herniation. There is dorsal displacement of hydrated nuclear material with an intact annulus presenting as a linear low density structure separating the herniated nucleus pulposus from the thecal sac (arrow). Note the marked decrease signal intensity on the T_2-weighted images of the degenerated L4–5 and L5–S1 discs when compared with the normal signal intensity of the L3–4 disc (right). The herniated nuclear material is of intermediate signal intensity on the T1-weighted image. Note the bright signal intensity of the CSF on the T_2-weighted image. **(B)** Axial 5-mm images of the same case as Fig. A showing the central and leftsided herniated disc at L4–5 with the low density annulus lying between the thecal sac and the more hydrated dorsally displaced nuclear material (arrow). Note the annular tear on the left.

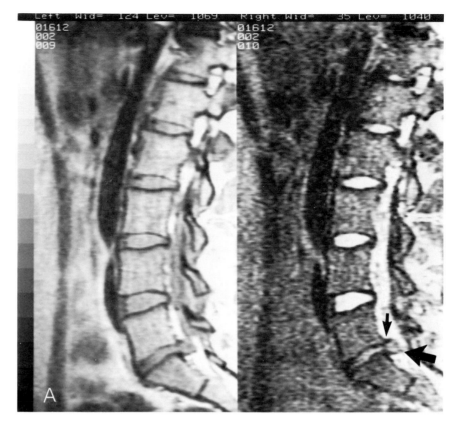

Fig. 12-5 Extruded disc herniations. Technique: spin-echo images TE/TR 20–70/1800. **(A)** Sagittal 3-mm images showing degenerative disc space narrowing and dehydration of the L5–S1 disc with a moderately large extruded disc herniation. Note separation of the annular fibers, which are displaced dorsally to lie at the cephalad and caudal margin of the disc herniation (small arrow) and the intermediate signal intensity herniated nucleus, which projects into the central spinal canal (large arrow). The disc herniations are equally well seen on both proton density images (left) and T₂-weighted images (right). Note the normal signal intensity of the upper lumbar discs from L1–2 through L4–5. **(B)** Axial 5-mm spin-echo images with TR/TE 20–70/1800. Note the dorsally displaced, swollen, edematous left S1 nerve root (large arrow). The left S1 nerve foot is of increased signal intensity compared to the right S1 nerve root secondary to edema (small arrow).

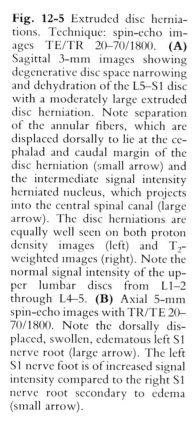

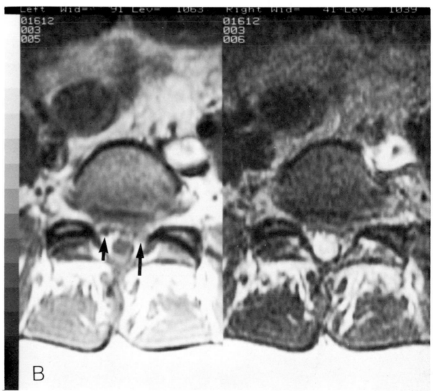

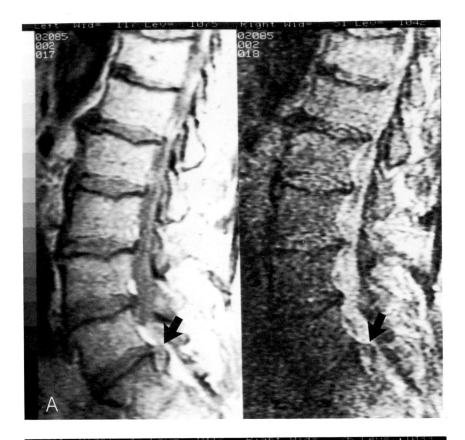

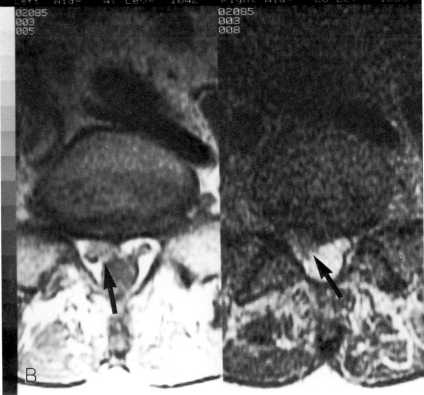

Fig. 12-6 (A) 3-mm sagittal spin-echo images showing large extruded rightsided disc herniation at L5–S1. The image is best seen on the proton density images (left) (arrow). Note the separation of annular fibers and the caudal extension of the large disc herniation. **(B)** Same patient as in Fig. A. Axial spin-echo images show the large extruded disc herniation (right) (arrows). Note the dorsal displacement of the right S1 nerve root on the proton density image (left). (*Figure continues.*)

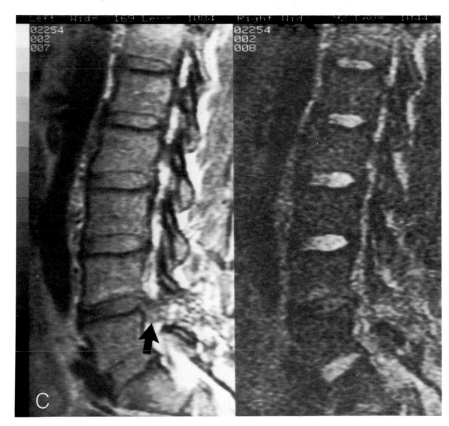

Fig. 12-6 (*Continued*). **(C)** Spin-echo 3-mm sagittal images (TE/TR-20–70/1800) show a large extruded disc herniation. Note the separation of the annular fibers and the large intermediate signal intensity disc herniation on the proton density image (left) (arrow). Note the virtual disappearance of the disc herniation on the T_2-weighted image (right) as the degenerated herniated material is essentially isointense with the adjacent epidural fat. Note the low signal intensity of the involved L4–5 disc on the T_2-weighted images representing dehydration.

nerve root ganglia and epidural veins are well visualized within the epidural fat. The bony cortical margins of the nerve root canals are also of low signal intensity and are sharply demarcated by the high signal intensity of the fat within the nerve root canal. The improved soft tissue contrast resolution of MR is able to resolve differences in signal intensity of the soft tissue structure contents of the intervertebral nerve root canal such as the annulus of the disc, nerve root ganglia, and ligamentum flavum. Thus, a very accurate depiction and diagnosis of soft tissue abnormalities and impingement on the nerve root ganglia and spinal nerve within the intervertebral nerve root canal is now possible with sagittal MR images. These structures are isodense on CT images and pathology within the intervertebral nerve root canals is depicted as homogenous opacification of the canal. This improved soft tissue contrast resolution of MR has proven to be a very valuable adjunct to CT in the evaluation of lateral nerve root entrapment in complicated preoperative cases with suspected concomitant entities such as stenosis, lateral disc herniation, and conjoined

nerve roots, as well as the evaluation of lateral disease in the postoperative patient with fibrosis and/or hemorrhage (Figs. 12-7B and 12-9B).

DISC PATHOLOGY

The ability to dielineate the disc annulus from the nucleus on sagittal images allows very accurate determination and classification of disc protrusion. True annular bulges can be differentiated from contained central disc herniations, and both can be distinguished from extruded and free-fragment herniations (Fig. 12-4). Nuclear material may be either high signal intensity or, when degenerated and dehydrated, of intermediate or low signal intensity and can be differentiated from the low signal intensity of the annulus. Spin-echo images with proton density and T_2-weighted images in both sagittal and axial planes are felt to be necessary for complete evaluation of degenerative disc disease and lumbar spondylosis. Partial saturation, single-echo sagittal imaging does not al-

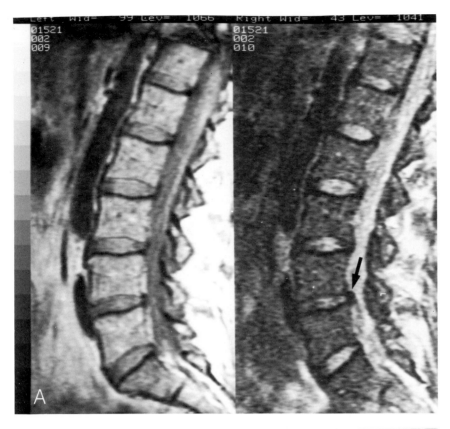

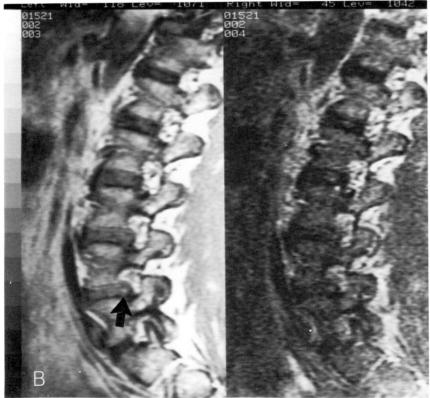

Fig. 12-7 Leftsided L4–5 annular disc herniation. Spin-echo 3-mm sagittal and 5-mm axial images. TE/TR 20–70/1500. **(A)** Sagittal proton density and T₂-weighted images showing a low density disc herniation projecting into the left L4–5 subarticular recess (arrow). Note that the disc herniation is well visualized on the T₂-weighted image (right) and poorly visualized on the proton density image (left). The low signal intensity of this lesion on both the sagittal and axial T₂-weighted images correctly identified this lesion as an annular fragment which projected into the subarticular recess and compressed the traversing left L5 nerve root. This lesion was surgically confirmed. **(B)** Note lateral extension of the disc herniation of Fig. 12-7A into the intervertebral nerve root canal with mild impingement upon the caudal surface of the exiting left L4 nerve root ganglia (arrow). (*Figure continues.*)

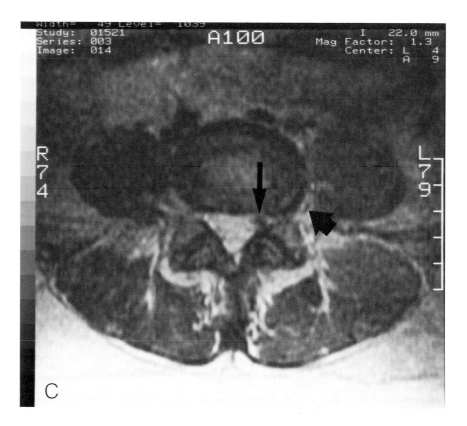

Fig. 12-7 (*Continued*). **(C)** Axial T_2-weighted MRI image showing the left-sided low density L4–5 annular fragment lying within the subarticular recess (large arrow) with impingement upon the left L5 nerve root. Note the generalized posterolateral protrusion of the annulus into the caudal aspect of the intervertebral nerve root canal, which is producing slight lateral displacement of the postgangliotic L4 nerve (large arrowhead).

low accurate evaluation of degenerative disc disease since subtle dehydration and the associated mild decreased signal intensity of the involved disc can be easily missed with this technique (Figs. 12-2, 12-3A and 12-6C). Annular disruption is easily identifiable on the sagittal images. This may be present with or without protrusion of nuclear material (Fig. 12-5). The annulus is best studied on T_1-weighted images because of the more clearly defined anatomical imaging. Disruption of the annulus presents as a separation of the linear low signal intensity structure defining the normal margins of the disc. Extension of nuclear material beyond the disrupted annulus is visualization as a continuation of the high signal intensity nuclear material of the involved disc (Figs. 12-5 and 12-6).

It is well established that dehydration of the nucleus of the lumbar disc is associated with decreased signal intensity. The signal intensity of the herniated nuclear material varies from high to low signal intensity but is most commonly intermediate signal intensity. Herniated annular fragments are of low signal intensity (Fig. 12-7). MRI sagittal images best depict annular

disruption and disc herniation. However, axial images are necessary to evaluate properly the degree of nerve root impingement caused by the disc herniation. Currently, one can clearly identify the position of the overlying nerve root with respect to the disc herniation on many sagittal MR images, however, the degree of nerve root compression is poorly depicted. As previously mentioned, we have found spin-echo images to provide the most useful information and resolution of herniated nuclear material in both preoperative and postoperative patients. Partial saturation images often provide poor delination of the herniated disc since the disc herniation and annulus too often tend to be isointense with respect to the adjacent nerve roots, CSF, epidural veins, and fibrosis, if present. Since we rely heavily on an accurate depiction of the morphology of the posterior margin of the disc in the evaluation of nerve root compression and/ or displacement in our correlation of disc protrusion and its significance with respect to the patient's symptoms, routine spin-echo axial and sagittal spin-echo images are performed. (Fig. 12-8). Free fragment disc

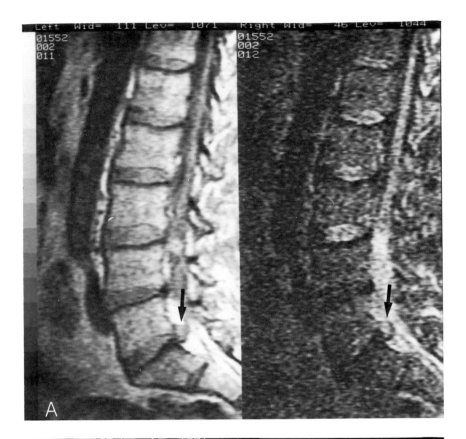

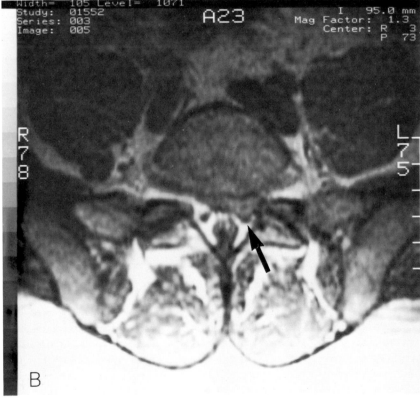

Fig. 12-8 Large extruded left-sided L5–S1 disc herniation. Spin-echo 3-mm sagittal and 5-mm axial images; TE/TR 20–70/1500. **(A)** Proton density and T$_2$-weighted images clearly show a large leftsided L5–S1 disc herniation. However, the position of the S1 nerve root with respect to the disc herniation is not well visualized in the sagittal plane (arrow). **(B)** Axial proton density MRI clearly shows dorsal displacement and compression of the left S1 nerve root by the large central and leftsided disc herniation (arrow). The axial images are essential to delineate the presence and severity of nerve root impingement caused by disc herniations.

herniations are clearly defined in the sagittal plane as elongated protrusions of nuclear material extending well beyond the confines of the disc annulus (Fig. 12-9).

Epidural Hematoma

Intraspinal hematomas can be easily confused with a free fragment disc herniation when evaluated by CT, and serial examinations are required to document resolution. However, acute hemorrhage has a characteristic MR appearance and is easily distinguished from herniated nuclear material (Fig. 12-9C). Therefore, when the appearance of an intraspinal mass suggests the possibility of an intraspinal hematoma, MRI is the diagnostic procedure of choice. The distinction is clinically important since the treatment of choice for epidural hematoma is conservative management. Eventual resolution of the hematoma occurs without surgical intervention in most cases. This lesion is not rare (we have studied approximately 40 cases), and is most often associated with either degenerative disc disease (21 of 25), or significant facet degeneration (3 of 25). Only one of the first 25 cases studied was truly "spontaneous." We have seen two cases associated with lytic spondylolisthesis. Given these associated lesions, we believe that these lumbar epidural hematomas result from a tear of a fragile epidural vein in patients suffering a disc herniation or with underlying instability and torsional injury.

Discitis and Osteomyelitis

MRI is more sensitive in depicting changes within the vertebra resulting from infection and neoplasm than CT, and MRI has become the procedure of choice in the study of discitis and osteomyelitis (Fig. 12-10), as well as metastatic disease and myeloma of the spine. Inflammation presents as increased signal intensity of the disc and vertebral body on T_2-weighted images and decreased signal intensity of the vertebral body on T_1-weighted images. MRI detects these abnormalities very early in the disease process and is a very sensitive modality for following the resolution of discitis and osteomyelitis during antibiotic therapy. With healing, the abnormal increased signal intensity of the disc and vertebra on T_2-weighted images reverts to normal. We have followed three patients with severe discitis and osteomyelitis to complete healing with serial MRI scans

at 1-month intervals. They all showed an increased signal intensity of the vertebral bodies and increased signal intensity of the disc in the acute inflammatory phase; whereas the involved disc was dehydrated and of low signal intensity on preoperative MRI images. There was a gradual decrease in the high signal intensity of the involved vertebral bodies and discs on T_2-weighted images during healing. All involved discs showed a degenerated, low signal intensity appearance after complete healing. Persistent abnormal increased signal intensity of the disc or vertebra on T_2 MRI images indicates residual inflammation.

Stenosis

MRI has proven to be a very valuable adjunct to CT in the evaluation of spinal stenosis. High field strength magnets (1.5 T) allow thin 3-mm sections to be obtained in the sagittal plane. This allows multiple sections to be obtained through each intervertebral nerve root canal with excellent depiction of focal lateral spinal stenosis and nerve root impingement. Although the lack of signal from cortical bone was initially thought to preclude adequate bony imaging, cancellous bone contains fat that produces excellent signal on T_1-weighted images. Thus, MRI imaging of the bony spine is excellent.

In our experience, lateral spinal stenosis is most common at L5–S1. Our initial concept of lateral spinal stenosis based on Kirkaldy-Willis' teaching was that loss of disc height and subsequent cephalad and forward subluxation of the superior articular processes (SA) of S1 produced bony impingement of the exiting L5 nerve root ganglia (L5–S1) between the superior articular process of S1 below and the pedicle of L5 above.

More recently, we have identified a more common type of lateral spinal stenosis at the L5–S1 level. Dr. Charles Ray, of the Institute for Low Back Care in Minneapolis, was the first to call attention to an up/down (cephalocaudad) component of bony lateral spinal stenosis he had observed at surgery. A review of our experience revealed that the majority of patients with lateral spinal stenosis at L5–S1 had an up/down type of nerve root impingement that was, in most cases, due to uncinate spurring. These uncinate spurs are focal dorsolateral bony osteophytes that arise from the posterolateral margin of the L5 vertebral body and project into the caudal and ventral aspect of the intervertebral nerve root canals, resulting in varying

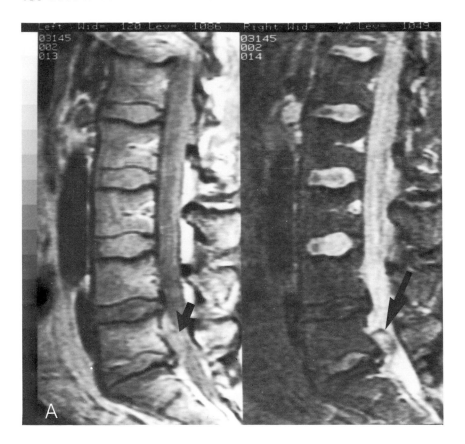

Fig. 12-9 Spin-echo images TE/TR 20–70/1500. **(A)** Large free fragment L5–S1 disc herniation with cephalad migration to the midbody of L5 (arrows). Note that the free fragment herniation is much better visualized on the T_2-weighted images since the intermediate signal intensity of the large free fragment disc lying dorsal to the L5 vertebral body is nearly isointense with the CSF on the proton density image (left). Note the severe dehydration of the L4–5 and L5–S1 discs on the T_2-weighted images (right) as opposed to the more normal hydration of the upper lumbar discs from T12–L1 through L3–4. This degree of dehydration of the L4–5 and L5–S1 disc is difficult to appreciate on the proton density image and even more difficult on T_1-weighted images. (*Figure continues.*)

degrees of cephalocaudad compression of the exiting L5 nerve roots ganglia (Fig. 12-11).

The etiology of these spurs is degenerative overgrowth and spurring of vestigial uncinate processes similar to those present in the cervical spine. The spurs are felt to be traction spurs due to attachment of Sharpey's fibers. They are quite uniform in their appearance from patient to patient, oval in configuration, and lie in the medial half of the nerve root canal.

It is theorized that these spurs cause nerve root compression because as the lumbosacral nerve roots become extradural, the nerve root ganglia (L5) are held in place within the ventral half of the intervertebral nerve root canal by ligamentous attachments (Hoffman's ligaments). Therefore, the ganglion is not free to migrate dorsally into the dorsal half of the intervertebral nerve root canal away from the compressive spur and is vulnerable to compression. The dorsal portion of the canal contains only fat and the ligamentum flavum, which extends over the superior

articular process of S1 and attaches to the undersurface of the pedicle of L5. The trochlear effect of the exiting L5 nerve root also maintains the position of the L5 nerve root ganglion within the ventral half of the intervertebral nerve root canal. This characteristic may mislead the surgeon during probe exploration of the canal, i.e., the probe may pass through the dorsal half of the canal without obstruction. This could cause the surgeon to assume incorrectly that no stenosis exists, when in fact the ganglion is severely compressed within the ventral half of the canal.

On axial images, the typical uncinate spur appears as a rounded, oval, bony overgrowth projecting into the middle one third of the intervertebral nerve root canal. The uncinate spur lies directly caudal to the exiting L5 nerve root ganglion within the ventral one half of the nerve root canal. Axial images may be difficult to interpret with respect to compression of the ganglion since the thin slices obtained at the L5–S1 level often show the ganglion on one image and the uncinate spur on the image immediately

Fig. 12-9 (*Continued*). **(B)** The same patient as Fig. A. Note the severe up/down lateral spinal stenosis at L5–S1 on the right (arrows). Proton density and T_2-weighted images clearly demonstrate that the lateral stenosis is due to both posterolateral bulging of the L5–S1 disc (arrow) on the proton density images (left), as well as cephalocaudad constriction of the intervertebral nerve root canal due to the severe loss of disc height at the L5–S1 level. **(C)** Sagittal 3-mm images in a patient with a small L4–5 disc herniation (small arrow) and an associated moderately large epidural hematoma lying caudal to the degenerated L4–5 disc and dorsal to the L5 vertebral body. Note that the lesion extends to the basivertebral plexus at the level of the mid vertebral body. Note also the moderate decreased signal intensity of the L5–S1 disc and the small to moderate size contained central disc herniation at the L5–S1 level. Note the disruption of the annulus at the L4–5 level with failure of visualization of this low density structure dorsal to the narrowed L4–5 disc on the proton density image (small arrows). The characteristic appearance of the epidural hematoma is of high signal intensity on both T_1-weight T_2-weighted images. Note that on the T_2-weighted image (right), the signal intensity of the hemorrhage is considerably greater than either the hydrated disc or the adjacent CSF. This is also true on the proton density image but less apparent (left).

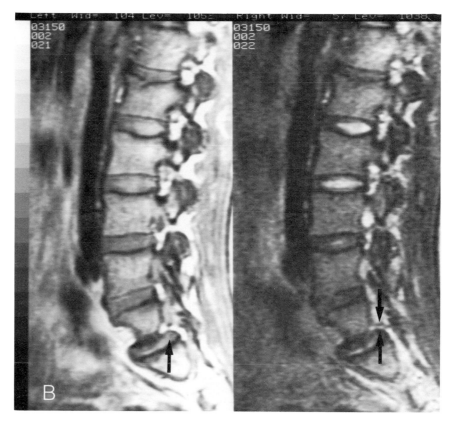

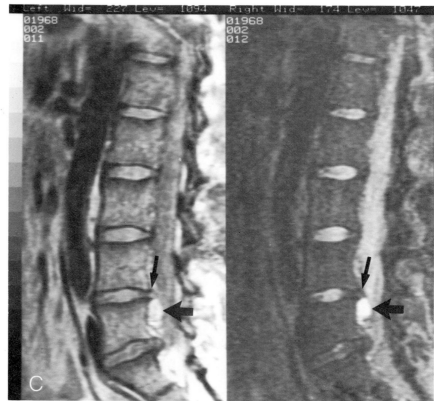

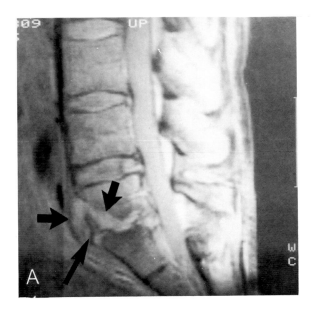 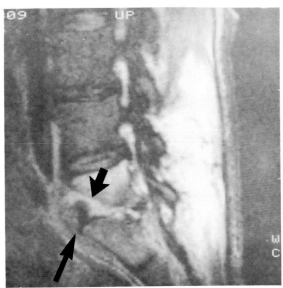

Fig. 12-10 Discitis and osteomyelitis. **(A)** Sagittal spin-echo MRI TE 30–90/TR 2.5; Siemens 1 T magnetom. The proton density images on the left show the large purulent fluid collection within the involved L5–S1 disc and the associated perivertebral mass (short arrows). Note severe destruction of the anteroinferior aspect of the L5 vertebral body with formation of a sequestrum (long arrow). The affected L5 and S1 vertebral bodies show increased signal intensity on the T_2-weighted images secondary to the inflammatory involvement of both L5 and S1 vertebrae on either side of the infected L5–S1 disc. (*Figure continues.*)

caudal, without showing the nerve root compression. However, a ganglion compressed in the cephalocaudad direction appears enlarged in the axial plane. When uncinate spurring is noted, this asymmetry of the affected ganglion should be looked for on the axial images. Confirmation of the presence and quantification of the degree of nerve root compression by uncinate spurring, however, is best visualized on sagittal images. For these reasons, we find that sagittal reformatted CT images and sagittal MRI images are critically important in the evaluation of lateral spinal stenosis (Fig. 12-11).

Nerve root compression within the intervertebral nerve root canals by either bony lateral spinal stenosis or encroachment by pathological soft tissue is visualized both as a decrease in the fat content of the intervertebral nerve root canal as well as a decrease in the overall cross-sectional area of the canal on the sagittal images. Since the lateral disc margin is distinguishable from the ganglia on direct sagittal MR images of the intervertebral nerve root canals, the exact

cause of nerve root compression within the canal can be delineated. Lateral disc herniations can be differentiated from fibrosis in the postoperative patient and from thickening of the ligamentum flavum and bony lateral spinal stenosis in the preoperative or postoperative patient (see Fig. 12-12).

Complex Spine Problems

MRI is most useful as an adjunct to CT in complicated spine cases either postoperatively or when multiple concomitant pathological entities are present or suspected. Nerve root impingement by bony stenosis (both front/back and up/down), lateral disc herniation, enlargement of the ganglia due to conjoined nerve root, and postoperative fibrosis and/or focal thickening of the ligamentum flavum can all be differentiated (Fig. 12-12). This is in contradistinction to CT in which these pathological lesions, when present singly or in conjunction with each other, show similar attenuation values. Therefore, when CT was

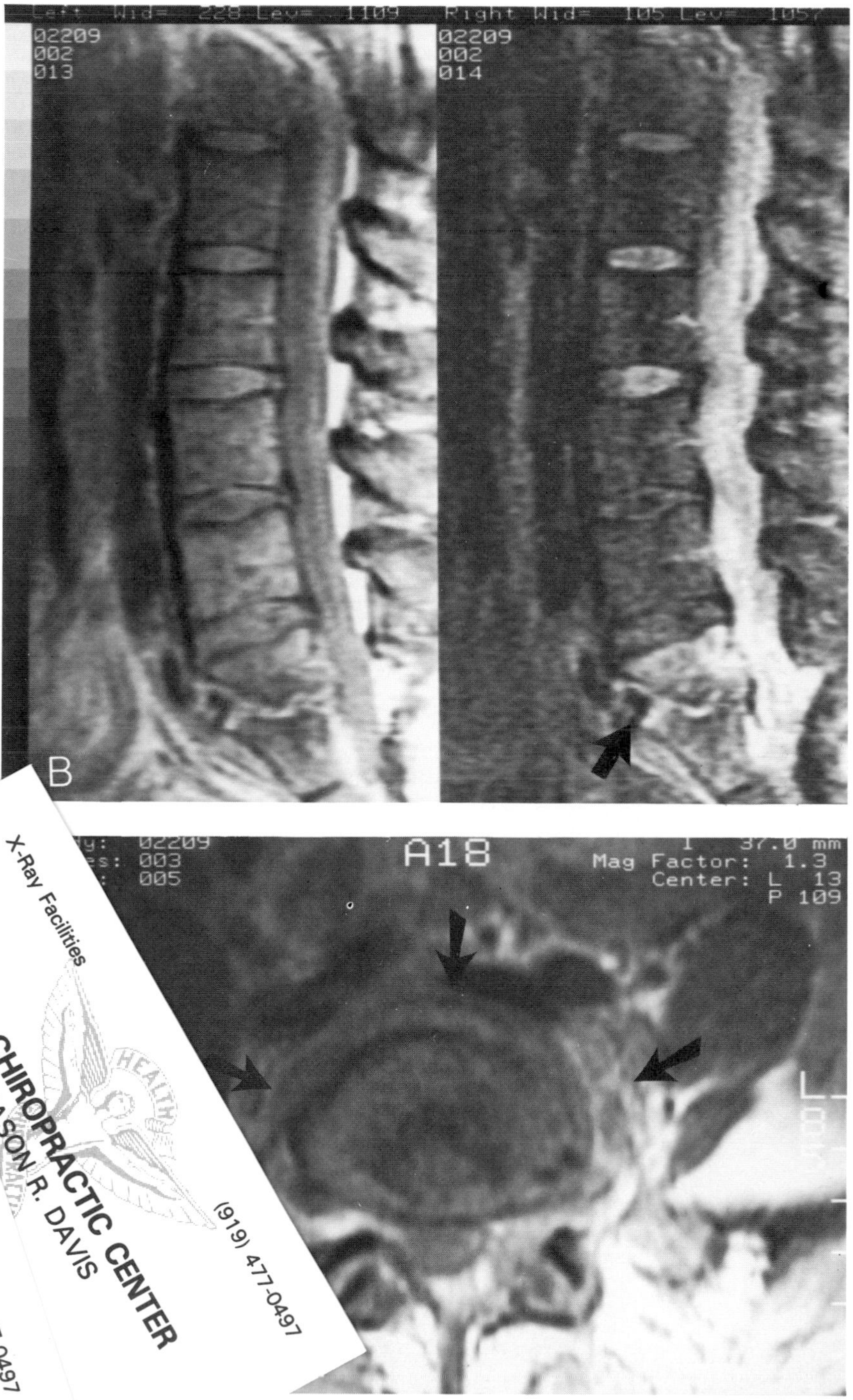

Figure 12-10 (*Continued*). **(B)** Spin-echo sagittal proton density and T$_2$-weighted images of the patient in Fig. A obtained 1 month after the initial study shows a decrease in the soft tissue inflammatory mass involving the disc space and a decrease in the paraspinous soft tissue mass. The sequestrum of the L5 vertebral body is still visualized (arrow). Both the L5 and S1 vertebral bodies show persistent increased signal intensity on T$_2$weighted images but are less signal intense than on the initial study. **(C)** Proton density axial images of the examination of patient in Fig. B shows persistence of the perivertebral soft tissue abnormality as well as the evidence

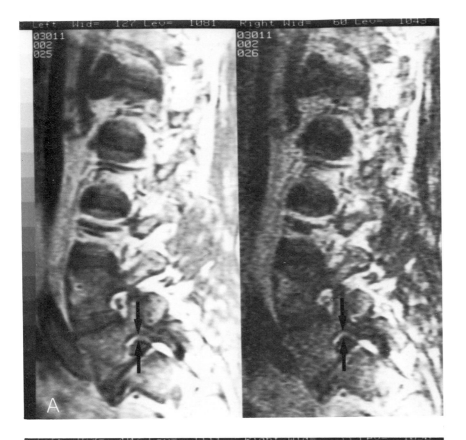

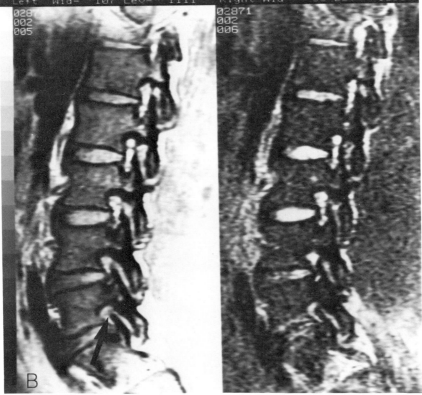

Fig. 12-11 Lateral spinal stenosis and lateral disc herniation. **(A)** Sagittal spin-echo 3-mm MRI images TE/TR 20–70/1500. Note the severe up/down bony lateral spinal stenosis at L5–S1 on the right secondary to a large focal osteophyte projecting from the dorsilateral aspect of the L5 vertebral body (arrows). This uncinate spur is the most common cause of lateral spinal stenosis in our practice and up/down stenosis is much more common than front/back stenosis at L5–S1. **(B)** Sagittal MRI images in this patient show moderate bony lateral spinal stenosis due to hypertrophic overgrowth of the superior articular process. Note that the superior articular process underrides the pedicle and impinges on the exiting left L5 nerve root ganglia (arrow). This is the classic lateral spinal stenosis described by Kirkaldy-Willis. This "front/back" stenosis is less common than the cephalocaudad spinal stenosis at the L5–S1 level. (*Figure continues.*)

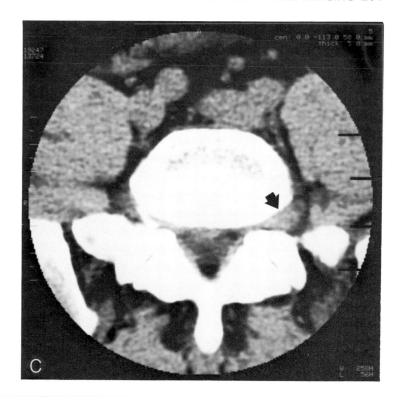

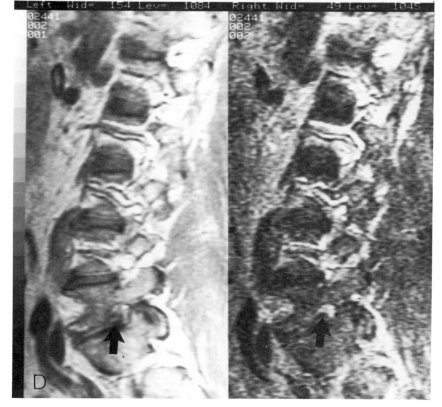

Fig. 12-11 (*Continued*). **(C)** Axial CT scan showing apparent enlarged left L5 nerve root ganglia. From this image, one cannot differentiate between simple enlargement of the ganglia, up/down stenosis, or a superimposed lateral disc herniation (arrow). **(D)** Sagittal MRI of the pateint in Fig. C shows that the abnormality within the left L5–S1 intervertebral nerve root is a laterally herniated disc occupying the caudal and ventral one-half of the intervertebral nerve root canal which causes caphalo-caudad compression of the exiting left L5 nerve root ganglia (arrows). Note that the improved soft tissue resolution of MRI is able to clearly delineate the disc herniation, which is of low signal intensity, from the intermediate signal intensity nerve root ganglia lying cephalad to it.

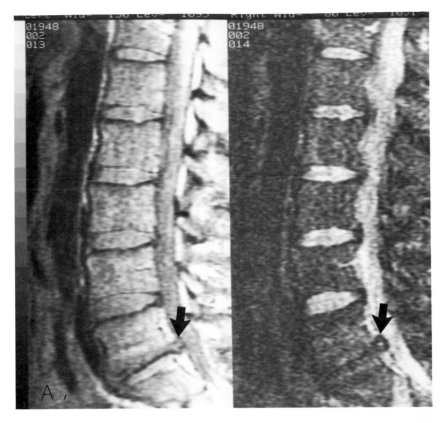

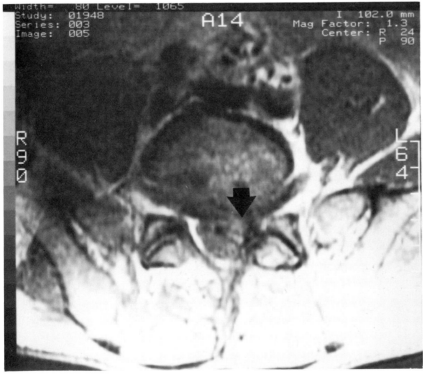

Fig. 12-12 Postoperative fibrosis and recurrent disc herniation. **(A)** Sagittal proton density (left) and T_2-weighted images (right). Note the moderately large recurrent disc herniation at L5–S1 on the left. This is more easily identified on the T_2-weighted images as a low signal intensity degenerated disc herniation (arrow). **(B)** Axial proton density image TE=20, TR=1500. Note the difficulty in distinguishing between the large recurrent disc herniation (arrow) and the overlying fibrosis on the axial image alone. T_2-weighted sagittal and axial images are very useful in the evaluation of the postoperative patient for recurrent disc herniation versus fibrosis. (*Figure continues.*)

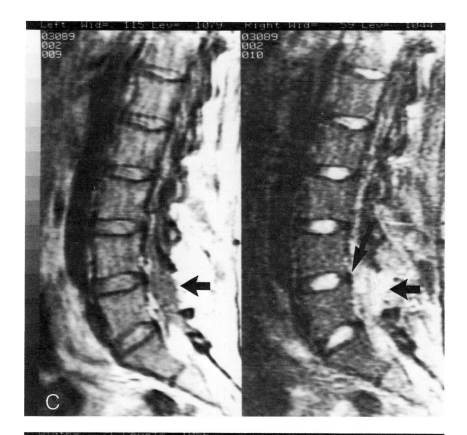

Fig. 12-12 (*Continued*). **(C)** Note the absence of recurrent disc herniation in this patient. The annulus of the disc is intact and well visualized as a low signal intensity structure (large arrow). Postoperative fibrosis lies dorsal to the L4–5 disc and L5 vertebral body (arrow). **(D)** Axial MRI of the patient in Fig. C. Note the high signal intensity of the postoperative fibrosis surrounding the left L5 nerve root (arrow). On the CT examination, the fibrosis surrounding the nerve root did not allow exclusion of recurrent disc herniation. The high signal intensity of the postoperative fibrosis studied on MRI permitted definite exclusion of a recurrent disc herniation.

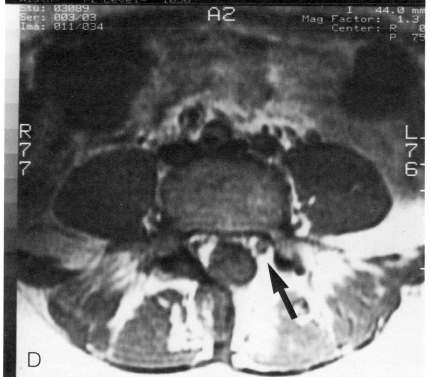

previously the only modality available to study the intervertebral nerve root canal, one could not clearly delineate for the clinician and surgeon whether the abnormal soft tissue within the nerve root canal was merely a compressed ganglia in a patient with lateral spinal stenosis, or represented concomitant soft tissue disease such as lateral disc herniation, conjoined nerve root, or postoperative fibrosis which was isodense with the compressed nerve root ganglia. Therefore, we routinely use MRI when faced with a complicated postoperative patient with disease within the central spinal canal or intervertebral nerve root canals, and preoperative cases in which there is a question of concomitant lateral disc herniation and bony lateral spinal stenosis and/or a nerve root variant such as a conjoined nerve root.

Currently, the GE Signa system is capable of providing routine images in the orthogonal planes (sagittal, coronal, and axial) as well as nonorthogonal planes (oblique). Primary imaging in the sagittal plane with MRI represents a significant improvement in spatial resolution of the sagittal images of the spine compared to CT. The spatial resolution of CT in the sagittal reformatted images is equal to the table incrementation (i.e., if the table is moved 3 mm for each image, the spatial resolution of the reformatted images is 3 mm). The spatial resolution of high field strength MRI is now less than 1 mm.

Improved axial imaging now allows visualization of individual nerve roots in most cases and, consequently, clumped nerve roots in patients with adhesive arachnoiditis. In some complicated postoperative cases, MRI is the only modality capable of clearly differentiating between the various soft tissue structures within the central spinal canal and intervertebral nerve root canals.

Synovial Cysts and Chondromata

MRI is useful in the evaluation of central and subarticular recess stenosis; however, CT is equally useful in most cases. Degenerative spondylolisthesis, a relatively common cause of central and subarticular recess stenosis, may be complicated by synovial cyst formation. In fact, most patients with synovial cysts have underlying degenerative spondylolisthesis. Contrary to previous reports in the literature, synovial cysts and chondromas are often associated with clinical symptoms resulting from nerve root compression.

MRI can clearly visualize the fluid within the synovial cysts on T_2 weighted images and, therefore, differentiates synovial cysts from synovial chondromas. This distinction is important in light of recent clinical research, which has shown that injection of steroids into the zygapophyseal joint which communicates with the synovial cyst may dramatically decrease or completely relieve the symptoms related to nerve root compression and seems to be an alternative to surgery. On the other hand, symptomatic synovial chondromas or noncystic masses of the ligamentum flavum that produce nerve root compression do not respond to this treatment. Synovial cysts most commonly arise at the medial margin of the degenerated facet joints. The synovial cyst has a characteristic appearance with its flat base paralleling the ligamentum flavum at the medial margin of the zygapophyseal joint. The rounded medial aspect of the cyst projects in a anteromedial direction rather than dorsally as would be expected with disc herniation (Fig. 12-13). In some patients, the ligamentum flavum and posterior margin of the disc are characterized by such extensive soft tissue prominence and fibrocartilaginous reaction at the margin of the disc that the cyst margins are not clearly defined. Very occasionally, they can vary in position and may occur within the lateral aspect of the nerve root canal beneath the lateral attachment of the ligamentum flavum to the base of the superior articular facet. A recent case proven by MRI presented as a mass in the posterolateral aspect of the intervertebral nerve root canal. The cyst was dorsal in position and isodense with respect to the ganglia and ligamentum flavum on CT. Because of its unusual location, the etiology of the mass was indeterminate; MRI showed the mass to be clearly cystic and contained by the ligamentum flavum. The association of these lesions with degenerative spondylolisthesis is so strong that any rounded soft tissue mass projecting into the central spinal canal from the medial margin of the facet joint in patients with degenerative spondylolisthesis at that segment should be considered to be a synovial cyst and/or chondroma until proven otherwise.

Isthmic Spondylolisthesis

The most common cause of nerve root compression and sciatica in lytic spondylolisthesis is a cephalocaudad compression of the exiting L5 nerve root ganglia

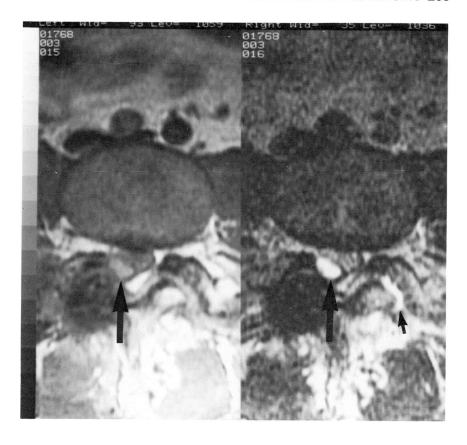

Fig. 12-13 Spin-echo axial images. TE/TR 20–70/1500. The spin-echo images show a large synovial cyst, which is of high signal intensity on the rightsided T_2-weighted images (large arrow). Note severe degenerative overgrowth of the facet joints at L4–5, as well as the increased fluid within the degenerated left L4–5 facet joint (small arrow). The cyst is of intermediate signal intensity and nearly isointense with the CSF on the proton density images (large arrow, leftsided image).

between the pedicle of L5 cranially and the L5–S1 disc plate and S1 vertebra caudally. MRI is a very useful adjunct to CT in delineating the exact pathology occurring within the intervertebral nerve root canal in these patients. Since the L5 Ganglia is very compressed and flattened and fills the entire nerve root canal in patients with severe up/down spinal stenosis, CT cannot differentiate the disc margin from the ganglia. When disc asymmetry is present (which is often the case because of fibrocartilaginous build up at the margin of the L5–S1 disc), one cannot determine on CT examination whether a concomitant lateral disc herniation is present. Sagittal MRI does allow an excellent visualization of the soft tissue of the nerve root canal and discrimination of herniated disc material from ganglia. T_2-weighted images distinguish between thickened, redundant, low signal intensity annulus and lateral herniated nuclear material (Fig. 12-14).

MRI appears to show less severe constriction of the intervertebral nerve root canal and contents than reformatted CT images of the same patient. This apparent discrepancy may be due to a combination of improved spatial resolution of sagittal MRI and/or an underestimation of the degree of compression of the ganglia on MRI. The latter results because of the low signal intensity of the adjacent bone as the increasingly stenotic canal obscures the margins of the adjacent ganglia, which is of intermediate signal intensity.

Axial MRI images are not as useful as axial CT images when studying the intervertebral nerve root canals because of this indistinct differentiation of low signal intensity structures and the relatively thick 5 mm MR images that result in significant partial volume imaging. Recent improvements in software have improved the axial images, and additional improvements may be expected.

Postoperative Spine

For reasons previously described in this chapter, MRI has become our procedure of choice in the postoperative patient. In our experience, it is more accurate than metrizamide-enhanced CT imaging and

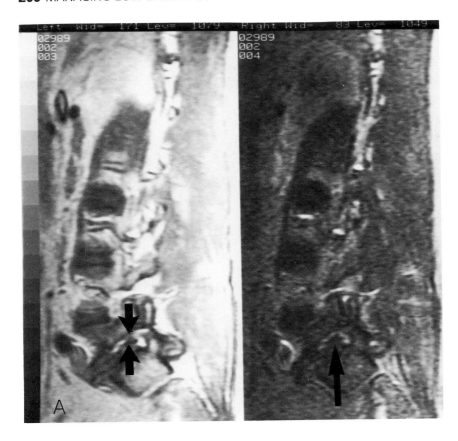

Fig. 12-14 Lytic spondylolisthesis. **(A)** Spin-echo sagittal 3-mm images TE/TR 20–70/1500. Sagittal images show very severe cephalocaudad bony lateral spinal stenosis in a patient with lytic spondylolisthesis. There was marked disc space collapse in this patient and the nerve root ganglion is severely compressed between the pedicle of L5 cranially and the S1 vertebra and L5–S1 disc plate caudally (arrows). (*Figure continues.*)

is less invasive. If adequate fat grafting has been performed and no appreciable postoperative perineural fibrosis is present, the diagnosis of recurrent disc herniation with plain CT in a postoperative patient is no more difficult than in a nonoperated patient nonenhanced CT. In these patients nonenhanced CT remains the procedure of choice in our practice since it is considerably less expensive than MRI and better evaluates the bony spine.

However, since a considerable number of patients have some degree of postoperative fibrosis and a recurrent isodense disc herniation underlying the fibrosis cannot be entirely excluded, an omnipaque-enhanced CT and/or MRI is necessary to exclude a recurrent disc herniation in those patients with recurrent postoperative symptoms. Since one cannot accurately predict in advance which patients will have postoperative fibrosis, many of our postoperative patients studied prior to the advent of MRI received both a plain CT and an enhanced CT when fibrosis

was present. Although a contrast-enhanced CT is a very accurate means of delineating a recurrent disc herniation, it is invasive; and the cost of performing both a plain and intrathecal enhanced CT is equal to or greater than that of MRI.

We recently performed a prospective double-blind study comparing the accuracy of metrizamide enhanced CT and MRI in the evaluation of postoperative recurrent disc herniation versus fibrosis. Fifty patients were studied with both metrizamide enhanced CT and MRI. Surgery was performed in 27 patients. There was correlation of CT and surgical findings in 20 patients (74%) and MRI surgical correlation in 23 patients (85%). There were three false-positive CT studies (11%), no false-negative studies and four indeterminate examinations (15%). There was one false-positive MRI examination (4%), two false-negative examinations (7%), and one indeterminate study (4%). Therefore, in this small series, MRI is more accurate than metrizamide-enhanced CT in the differ-

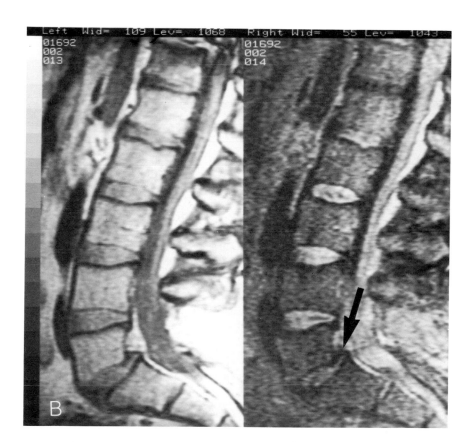

Fig. 12-14 (*Continued*). **(B)** Midline sagittal MRI of another patient showing 15% lytic spondylolisthesis, redundancy of the annulus, and degenerative thickening and dehydration of the dorsal aspect of the disc (arrow). **(C)** Sagittal images of the patient in Fig. B show an associated lateral disc herniation at L5–S1 on the right, which projects into the intervertebral nerve root canal and produces moderately severe cephalocaudad compression of the exiting left L5 nerve root ganglia (arrow).

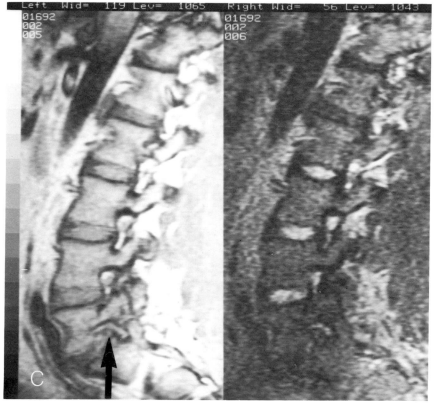

entiation of postoperative disc herniation from fibrosis and is less invasive. Thus in the postoperative patient presenting with symptoms of a recurrent disc herniation, we feel MRI is the procedure of choice.

SUMMARY

MRI has become an invaluable diagnostic adjunct to CT in the study of the lumbar spine. MRI provides improved resolution of soft tissue structures, which leads to more accurate diagnosis of degenerative disc disease and lateral nerve root entrapment as well as spinal neoplasm, infection, and hematoma. MRI is the procedure of choice in the study of complicated spine pathology in postoperative patients. CT currently remains the procedure of choice in the study of degenerative disease of the lumbar spine in the nonoperated patient because of its superb bone and soft tissue imaging and its inexpensiveness when compared to MRI. MRI imaging can be expected to improve with software modifications and new imaging techniques. MRI will play an increasingly prominent role in lumbar spine imaging.

SUGGESTED READINGS

Abdullah AF, Chambers RW, Daut DP: Lumbarnerve root compression by synovial cysts of the ligamentum flavum. Report of four cases. Radiology 153: 855, 1984

Berger PE, Atkinson D, et al: High resolution surface coil magnetic resonance imaging of the spine: normal and pathologic anatomy. Radiographics 6: 573, 1986

Burton CV, Heithoff KB, Kirkaldy-Willis W, Ray CD: Computed tomographic scanning and the lumbar spine. II. Clinical considerations. Spine 4:356, 1979

Burton CV, Kirkaldy-Willis WH, Yong-Hing K, Heithoff KB: Causes of failure of surgery on the lumbar spine. Clin Orthop 157: 191, 1981

Carrera GF, Williams AL, Haughton VM: Computed tomography in sciatica. Radiology 137: 433, 1980

Chafetz NI, Genant HK, Moon K, et al: NMR in the diagnosis of a lumbar disc rupture. Presented at the 2nd Annual Meeting of the Society of Magnetic Resonance in Medicine. San Francisco, California, August 16–19, 1983 Crenshaw C, Kean DM, Mulholland RC, et al: The use of nuclear magnetic resonance in the diagnosis of lateral canal entrapment. J Bone Joint Surg 66B: 711, 1984

Edelman RR, Shoukimau GM, Stark DD, et al: High resolution surface coil imaging of lumbar disc disease. AJR 144: 1123, 1986

Franklin EA, Jr, Berbaum KS, Dunn V, et al: Impact of MR imaging on clinical diagnosis and management: Prospective study. Radiology 161: 377, 1986

Johansen JG, Barthelemy CR, Haughton VM, et al: Arachnoiditis from myelography and laminectomy in experimental animals. AJNR 5: 97, 1984

Lipson SJ, Muir H: Experimental intervertebral disc degeneration morphologic and proteoglycan changes over time. Arthritis Rheum 24: 12, 1981

Maravilla KR, Lesh P, Weinreb JC, et al: Magnetic resonance imaging of the lumbar spine with CT correlation. AJNR 6: 237, 1985

Modic MT, Feiglin DH, et al: Vertebral osteomyelitis: assessment using MR. Radiology 157: 157, 1985

Modic MT, Masaryk TJ, Paushter DM: Magnetic resonance imaging of the spine. Radiol Clin North Am 24: 229, 1986

Modic MT, Weinstein MA, Pavlicek W, et al: Nuclear magnetic resonance imaging of the spine. Radiology 148: 747, 1983

Modic MT, Pavlicek W, Weinstein MA, et al: Magnetic resonance imaging of intervertebral disc disease. Clinical pulse and sequence considerations. Radiology 152: 103, 1984

Moon KL, Jr, Genant HK, Helms CA, et al: Musculoskeletal applications of nuclear magnetic resonance. Radiology 147: 161–171, 1983

Nelson MA: Lumbar spinal stenosis. J Bone Joint Surg 55A: 596, 1973

Paine KWE: Clinical features of lumbar spinal stenosis. Clin Orthop 115: 77, 1976

Paushter DM, Modic MT, Masaryk TJ: Magnetic resonance imaging of the spine: applications and limitations. Radiol Clin North Am 23: 551, 1985

Paushter DM, Dengel FH, Modic MT, et al: Clinical applications of nuclear magnetic resonance: central nervous system—brainstem and cord. Radiographics 4: 97, 1984

Pech P, Haughton VM: Lumbar intervertebral disc: correlative MR and anatomic study. Radiology 156: 699, 1985

Sherman JL, Citrin CM, Gangarosa RE: MR appearance of CSF pulsations in the spinal canal. AJNR 7: 879, 1986

Williams AL: CT Diagnosis of degenerative disc disease. The bulging annulus. Radiol Clin North Am 21: 289, 1983

Van Zanten TEG, Teule GJJ, Golding RP, et al: CT and nuclear medicine imaging in vertebral metastases. Clin Nucl Med 11: 334, 1986

Yong-Hing K, Kirkaldy-Willis WH: the pathophysiology of Degenerative disease of the lumbar spine. Orthop Clin North Am 14: 491, 1983

13

Making a Specific Diagnosis

Thomas N. Bernard, Jr.
William H. Kirkaldy-Willis

Making a specific diagnosis is the logical prerequisite to initiating effective therapy for low back pain. The knowledge gained from the preceding chapters serves as the foundation for achieving this goal.

A thorough clinical history and physical examination combined with certain diagnostic radiographic investigations facilitates localization of the anatomical source of pain. In some instances, the response to treatment confirms the diagnosis. The basic foundation of knowledge is then combined with information from all sources and pieced together much like a jigsaw puzzle to arrive at the precise diagnosis (Fig. 13-1).

The following discussion will describe the process involved in making a specific diagnosis when confronted with referred pain syndromes, radicular pain syndromes, and in complex situations.

REFERRED PAIN SYNDROMES

Referred pain syndromes predominently cause low back pain with variable radiation of referred pain into an extremity. Included in this category are posterior joint syndrome, Maigne's syndrome, sacroiliac joint syndrome, muscle (myofascial) syndromes, spondylolisthesis, and segmental instability. In general, these are less well known causes of low back pain and the signs, symptoms, and pattern of referred pain in this group may mimic nerve root compression lesions.

Posterior Joint Syndrome

This commonly occurring condition usually arises in the dysfunctional or unstable phase of spondylosis, causing an ill-defined (sclerotomal) type of pain. Referred pain to the buttocks, posterior thigh, and below the knee mimic radicular pain. The absence of nerve root tension signs helps distinguish a posterior joint syndrome from nerve root entrapment lesions.

Abnormal coupled motion may be detected with anteroposterior and lateral dynamic bending radiographs during the dysfunctional or unstable phase of spondylosis.

When familiar pain is reproduced and then abolished by injection to the suspected posterior joint, then the diagnosis is confirmed. Successful manipulative treatment to the symptomatic posterior joint also confirms the anatomical source of pain and the contribution of that structure to the patient's current pain complex.

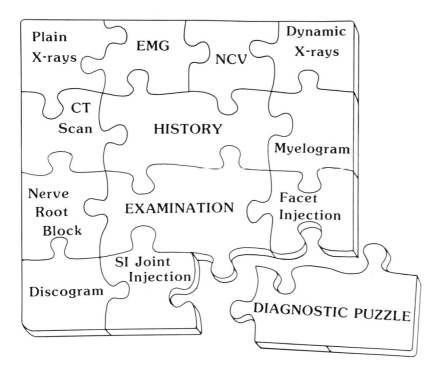

Fig. 13-1 The diagnostic puzzle. Although each piece of the puzzle has relative importance, the composite picture is needed for an accurate diagnosis.

Maigne's Syndrome

Dysfunction of the thoracolumbar posterior joints may lead to referred pain to the iliac crests on the symptomatic side. Since attention is usually directed to the referral site of pain, the source is frequently overlooked.

When Maigne's syndrome is suspected, the diagnosis is confirmed by alleviation of pain following injection or manipulation to the symptomatic posterior joints.

Sacroiliac Joint Syndrome

Referred pain from the sacroiliac joint may radiate to the buttocks, posterior thigh, groin, and occasionally to the lateral calf and ankle. This pain pattern is similar to posterior joint syndrome and may mimic radicular pain from a herniated nucleus pulposus or lateral spinal stenosis. The lack of nerve root tension signs and absence of motor, reflex, or sensory deficits helps to distinguish sacroiliac joint syndrome from nerve root compression lesions (Table 13-1).

When manipulation or injection to the sacroiliac joint effectively breaks the cycle of pain, the diagnosis is confirmed.

Muscle (Myofascial) Syndromes

These soft tissue lesions may be easily confused with other more common causes of low back pain since the reference zone or referral pattern of pain is similar to posterior joint syndrome, sacroiliac joint syndrome, herniated nucleus pulposus, and lateral spinal stenosis.[1–3]

Palpation of the trigger point in the symptomatic muscle usually reproduces familiar pain and frequently stimulates referred pain. The increased muscle tone produces a ropy consistency to palpation when compared to the unaffected contralateral muscle.

The diagnosis is confirmed by the physical findings and response to treatment by either passive stretching or injection of a local anesthetic into the trigger point.

Spondylolisthesis

Degenerative and isthmic spondylolisthesis are easily recognized by conventional radiography. Frequently, it is difficult to determine which component of the motion segment is the anatomical source of pain. Referred pain from the posterior joints, lytic

Table 13-1 Distinguishing Referred and Radicular Pain

Characteristic	Referred Pain	Radicular Pain
Symptoms	Deep, boring, ill-defined, poorly localized	Sharp, well localized, electric-like
Radiation	Posterior joint, sacroiliac joint, and muscle syndromes may radiate to the postero-lateral thigh, calf, rarely to the foot	Follows the sciatic nerve distribution to the buttocks, posterior thigh, and calf to the foot; or femoral nerve distribution to the anterior thigh.
Sensory alteration	Rare	Frequently follows a dermatomal distribution
Motor weakness	May have subjective weakness, but objective weakness or atrophy is rare	Frequent objective weakness and atrophy with prolonged duration of symptoms
Reflex deficit	Rare	Frequent
Nerve root tension signs	Absent; sciatic stretch testing may cause back pain or reveal hamstring tightness	Frequent sciatic notch tenderness and popliteal and peroneal nerve tenderness

defect, or lumbar disc or radicular pain from the nerve root may explain the clinical syndrome. To confirm the spondylolisthesis as the source of pain, the entire motion segment must be studied by dynamic radiographs, provocative and analgesic injections to the posterior joints, lytic defect, and lumbar discs. When radicular symptoms exist, selective nerve root sheath infiltrations are often diagnostic and therapeutic.

Sacroiliac joint syndrome frequently coexists with spondylolisthesis and when present must be considered as the primary or coexisting source of pain.

Segmental Instability

This condition is usually manifested in the late dysfunctional or early unstable phase of spondylosis. A reliable symptom is the history of a "catch" in the back when moving from forward flexion to the erect standing position.

Radiographically, with minimal instability, there are exaggerated changes in the anterior or posterior disc height on dynamic flexion and extension lateral radiographs (Fig. 13-2). As instability progresses, excessive translation may occur between motion segments producing spondylolisthesis or retrospondylolisthesis.

In spite of radiographic instability, the entire three joint complex must be evaluated to confirm the anatomical source of pain. Provocative and analgesic injections to the posterior joints and lumbar discs determine the contribution of each structure to the overall pain complex.

RADICULAR PAIN SYNDROME

These nerve root entrapment lesions usually cause low back pain and leg pain. They are clinically distinguished from referred pain syndromes by the presence of nerve root tension signs and motor, reflex, or sensory deficits (Table 13-1). These syndromes include herniated nucleus pulposus, lateral spinal stenosis, and central spinal stenosis.

Herniated Nucleus Pulposus

The symptoms and signs of a classic herniated nucleus pulposus are well known and usually may be easily distinguished from referred pain syndromes. Myelography has been the "gold standard" by which other techniques are judged for radiographic confirmation of a herniated nucleus pulposus. However, myelography has an unacceptibly high false-negative rate for small central disc herniations, lateral herniations, and 25% of all herniations at the lumbosacral junction.[4,5]

Nonenhanced high resolution computerized tomography starting at the midbody of L3 scanning to the sacrum with 3- to 5-mm overlapping sections with bone and soft tissue window axial and sagittal reformations is adequate for the diagnosis of most lumbar disc herniations.

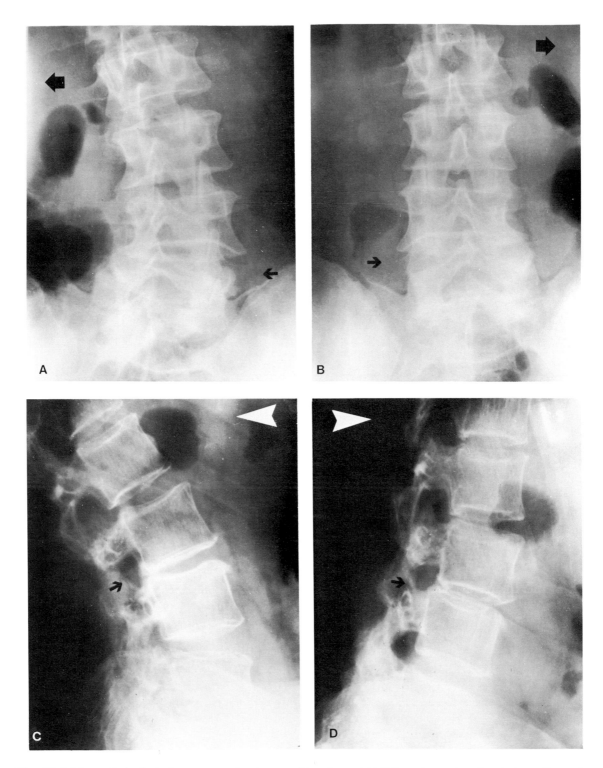

Fig. 13-2 The radiological changes seen in the unstable phase. **(A)** When the patient bends laterally to the right (viewer's left), the body of L4 moves laterally to the left relative to the body of L5 (arrow). **(B)** The same patient as in (A). On attempted lateral bending to the left (viewer's right), the spine remains erect. The body of L4 shifts to the right (arrow). Instability is seen at L4–5. **(C)** In this lateral view in extension the body of L3 is displaced slightly forward on that of L4 (arrow). **(D)** The same patient as in (C). In flexion the body of L3 is further displaced forward on that of L4 (arrow). Instability is due to degenerative spondylolisthesis. (*Figure continues.*)

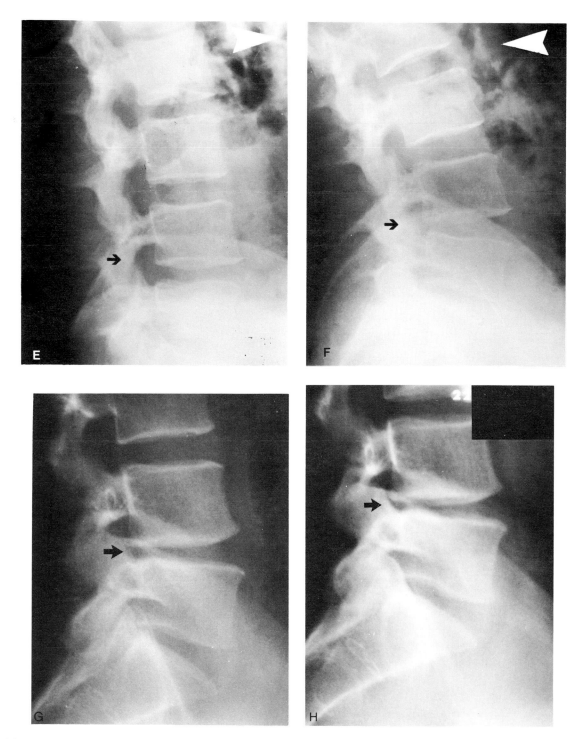

Fig. 13-2 (*Continued*). **(E)** Lateral view in flexion. Posterior aspects of the vertebral bodies (arrow) are aligned normally. **(F)** The same patient as in (E). In extension the body of L4 is displaced posteriorly on that of L5 (arrow). Retrospondylolisthesis is indicative of instability of minor degree. **(G)** Lateral view in flexion. The vertebral body of L4 is displaced posteriorly on that of L5 (arrow). **(H)** The same patient as in (G). In extension the body of L5 is further displaced posteriorly on that of L5. The anterior aspect of the L4–5 disc has opened. Marked retrospondylolisthesis indicates gross instability. (*Figure continues.*)

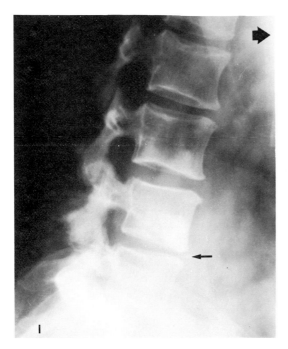

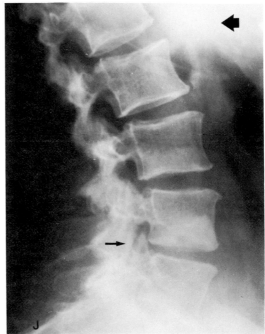

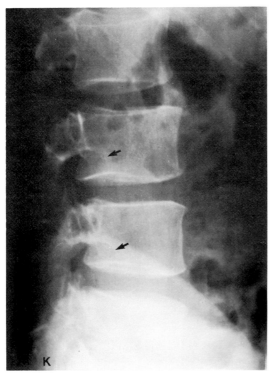

Fig. 13-2 (*Continued*). **(I)** Lateral view in flexion. Loss of disc height at L4–5 (arrow). On either side of the disc the anterior aspects of the bodies are closely approximated (instability). **(J)** The same patient as in (I). In extension retrospondylolisthesis of L4 on L5 (arrow) is present. Thus signs of instability in both flexion and extension are present in this patient. **(K)** At the L3 and L4 levels abrupt loss of pedicle height (arrow) is apparent compared with that at L2 (above the arrow). At L3 and L4 the base of the pedicles lies over and not behind the vertebral bodies. This change is caused by rotation of L3 on L2 and indicates instability in this case. (*Figure continues.*)

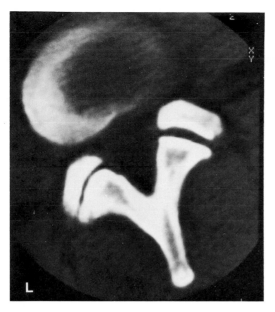 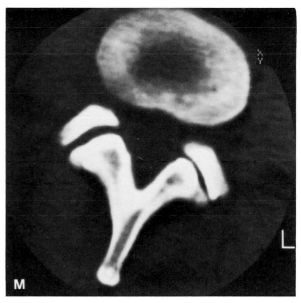

Fig. 13-2 (*Continued*). **(L)** CT scan at L4–5. When the spinous process rotates to the left, the left posterior joint opens widely. **(M)** CT scan of the same patient at L4–5. When the spinous process rotates to the right, the right posterior joint opens. Instability is seen at L4–5.

Central Spinal Stenosis

Central spinal stenosis may be suspected when there is a history of exertional paresthesias, dysesthesias, and weakness involving both lower extremities relieved by rest. Unlike vascular claudications, neurogenic claudications take longer to abate after a period of rest.

The diagnosis is confirmed by water soluble myelography, which reveals the "global extent" of the lesion. Enhanced computerized tomography allows assessment of the reduction of the sagittal diameter of the spinal canal and demonstrates the presence of lateral spinal stenosis that frequently coexists with central spinal stenosis.

Lateral Spinal Stenosis

Buttock and lower extremity pain occur more often than back pain, and exertional claudications usually involve only one extremity in lateral stenosis.

Computerized tomography with sagittal reformations allows assessment of the patency of the radicular canals. Clinical and radiographic lateral stenosis is confirmed by a selective nerve root sheath infiltration, which is diagnostic and frequently therapeutic.

COEXISTING LESIONS

Table 13-2 lists the specific diagnoses of 1,293 patients treated at the University Hospital Low Back Pain Clinic over a 12-year period. The less well-known causes deserve recognition since they occur nearly as often as the well-known causes.

In one third of patients more than one anatomical source of pain from a coexisting lesion was found. The most commonly occurring coexisting lesions are posterior joint and sacroiliac joint syndromes, lateral and central spinal stenosis, herniated nucleus pulposus and lateral spinal stenosis, multiple muscle syndromes, and spondylolisthesis and sacroiliac joint syndrome.

Failure to recognize these coexisting lesions may lead to a less specific diagnosis and a poorer response to treatment.

Solving Complex Problems with Special Techniques

In most cases, the pieces of the diagnostic jigsaw puzzle fit, and the diagnosis is confirmed by a specific test or response to treatment. (Table 13-3). Yet, some-

Table 13-2 Specific Diagnoses of 1,293 Patients

Diagnosis	% of Total Cases
Well-known causes	
Herniated nucleus pulposus	14
Lateral spinal stenosis	13
Central spinal stenosis	5
Spondylolisthesis	9
Segmental instability	4
Less well-known causes	
Sacroiliac joint syndrome	23
Posterior joint syndrome	22
Maigne's syndrome	Less than 1
Muscle syndromes	6
Remaining causes	3
Pseudarthrosis	
Postfusion stenosis	
Inflammatory	
Infection	
Neoplasm	
Arachnoiditis	
Lateral femoral nerve entrapment	
NonSpecific	

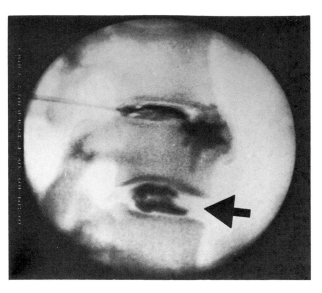

Fig. 13–3 Normal lumbar discogram (arrow). This disc accepted 0.8 cc of saline and 0.6 cc of contrast with a firm end point and produced no pain. The needle in the L2–3 disc demonstrates an abnormal nucleogram of a limbus vertebra. Familiar pain was reproduced during injection of both saline and contrast.

times the diagnosis remains obscure and conventional testing fails to localize accurately the anatomical source of pain. Under these circumstances, special radiographic techniques are useful to refine the diagnosis.

Some of these special techniques are based on provocative and analgesic testing. When familiar pain is reproduced by injection of saline or radiographic contrast and then abolished by injection of a local anesthetic, then that structure contributes to the pa-

Table 13-3 Most Reliable Means to Make a Specific Diagnosis

Syndrome	Diagnostic Indicator
Posterior joint syndrome	Response to manipulation or injection
Sacroiliac joint syndrome	Response to manipulation or injection
Maigne's syndrome	Response to manipulation or injection
Muscle (myofascial) syndromes	Response to injection or stretching
Herniated nucleus pulposus	Physiologic lumbar disc evaluation with postdiscography computerized tomography
Lateral spinal stenosis	Computerized tomography with sagittal reformations followed by selective nerve root sheath infiltrations
Central spinal stenosis	Myelography followed by computerized tomography
Spondylolisthesis	Plain radiographs
Segmental instability	Dynamic lateral bending radiographs
Discogenic syndrome	Physiological lumbar disc evaluation

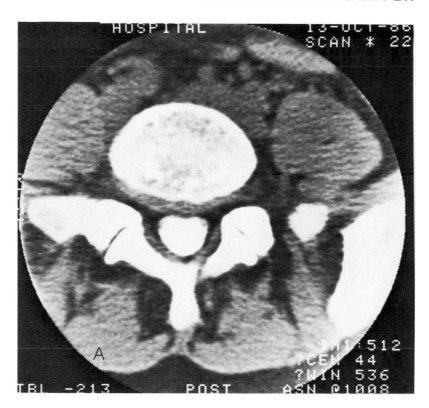

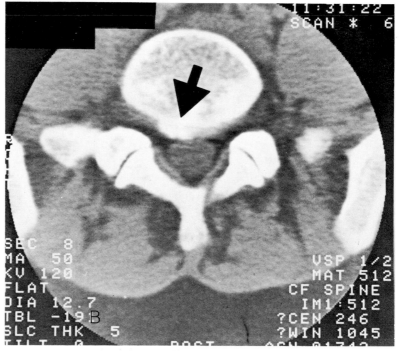

Fig. 13-4 (A) "Bulging disc" at L5–S1. During physiological lumbar disc evaluation, familiar back and right leg pain were reproduced. **(B)** Postdiscography CT scan shows a small central disc protrusion central to right at L5–S1 (arrow).

tient's overall pain complex. This hypothesis is the basis for provocative and analgesic injections to the posterior joints, sacroiliac joints, lumbar discs, and selective nerve root sheath injections.

Physiological Lumbar Disc Evaluation (Discography)

The radiographic appearance of a contrast-enhanced lumbar disc, by itself, has little diagnostic value. This observation has been the basis for condemnation of the diagnostic merit of this procedure.[6-10] Others have recognized the usefulness of discography in selecting fusion levels and localizing the anatomical source of low back pain.[11-16]

The nucleogram is only one component of the physiological lumbar disc evaluation, which is a volumetric, manometric, provocative, and analgesic challenge to the lumbar disc. The normal lumbar disc accepts 0.5 to 1.5 cc of saline or contrast with a firm end point during injection and a predictable nucleographic pattern. A normal disc produces no pain during injection.

Myelography, computerized tomography, and magnetic resonance imaging only provide a static assessment of a disc. The physiological disc evaluation is a dynamic assessment of a lumbar disc and provides information not available by any other means. The most important determination is confirmation of the disc as the anatomical source of pain.

This procedure is also useful to (1) determine the significance of a "bulging" disc, or small protrusion (2) determine the symptomatic levels in multiple disc herniations, (3) evaluate lateral disc herniations, and (4) evaluate the status of lumbar discs at adjacent levels of a known abnormal motion segment.

Contained discogenic disease is usually manifested by a normal myelogram and computerized tomogram. Provocative and analgesic challenge of the disc is the only means to establish this diagnosis.[17] (Figs. 13-3 and 13-4).

On the T-$_2$ weighted image of magnetic resonance imaging, normal and degenerative discs may be contrasted (Fig. 13-5). The appearance of a degenerative disc by MRI does not imply that this is the anatomical source of pain. Physiological lumbar disc evaluation is still required to correlate the abnormal appearing discs seen on MRI to the clinical findings.

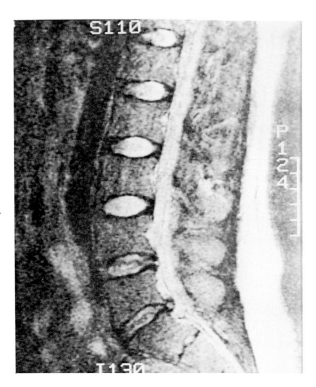

Fig. 13-5 T-$_2$-weighted sagittal image with the proximal discs from L3–4 appearing normal. The L4–5 disc is degenerative and the L5–S1 disc is herniated. The L4–5 disc in this patient was painful during physiological disc evaluation and contributed to familiar back pain. The L3–4 disc was normal by all criteria.

Postdiscography Computerized Tomography

Combining lumbar discography with computerized tomography provides invaluable information not attainable by other means. The nucleographic morphology of the normal, degenerative, and herniated disc may be demonstrated (Figs. 13-6 and 13-7).

Postdiscography computerized tomography allows assessment of the significance of small disc herniations, distinguishes between nerve root anomalies and disc herniations, and delineates the type of disc herniation (protrusion, extrusion, or sequestration) (Figs. 13-6 and 13-7).

Lateral disc herniations, which are usually missed by myelography, may be demonstrated by nonenhanced computerized tomography. Physiological lumbar disc evaluation with postdiscography com-

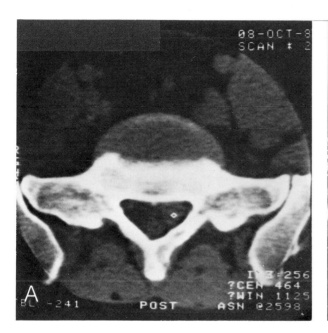

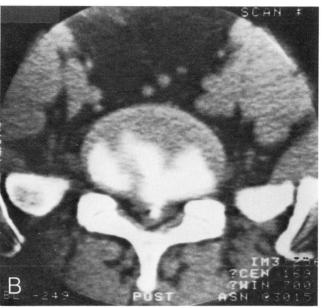

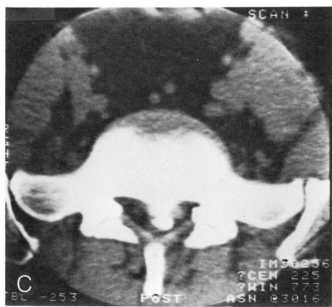

Fig. 13-6 Left-sided herniated nucleus pulposus at L5–S1 on the axial view. The marker is on disc material. **(B)** Physiological lumbar disc evaluation was confirmatory. Postdiscography CT scan shows a grossly degenerative disc with contrast extending into the epidural space. **(C)** Axial image 5 mm distal to Fig. 13-6B reveals distal extension of the herniation. (*Figure continues.*)

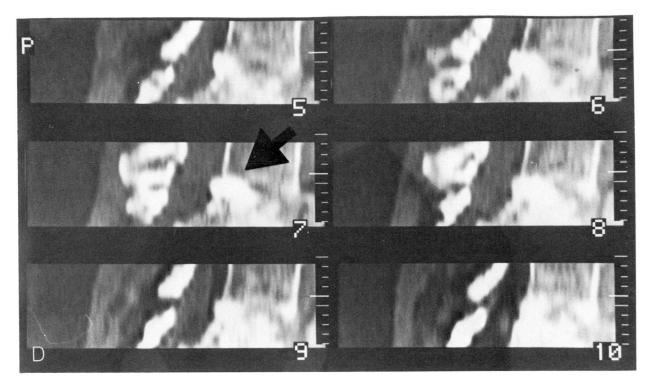

Fig. 13-6 (*Continued*). **(D)** Sagittal reformation shows distal extension of the herniation (arrow). The composite picture gives accurate localization, which facilitates operative treatment.

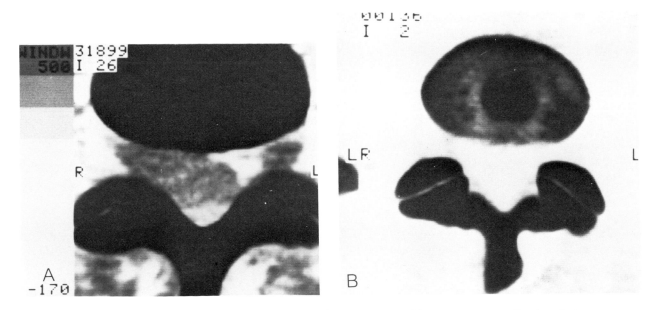

Fig. 13-7 A radiodensity in the right radicular canal at L4–5 was felt to represent a disc herniation on a nonenhanced CT scan. A physiological lumbar disc evaluation did not reproduce the patient's symptoms and was normal by all criteria. **(B)** The postdiscography CT scan reveals a normal nucleogram without communication with the right radicular canal. A lumbar myelogram revealed a composite nerve root sleeve at that level.

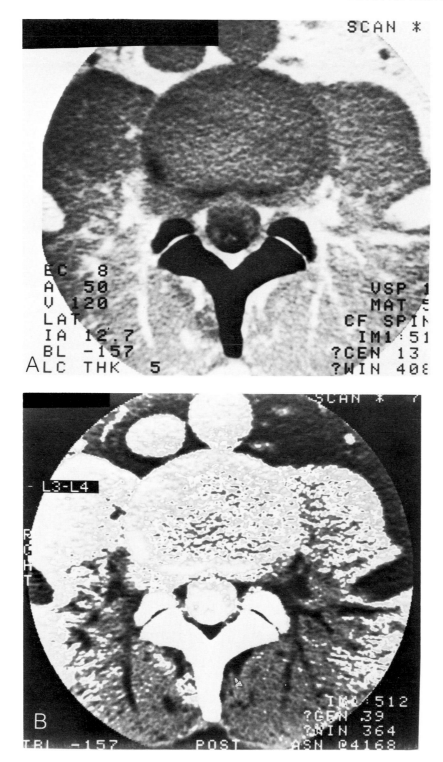

Fig. 13-8 CT and postdiscography CT scanning in various modes to facilitate accurate imaging. This patient experienced recurrence of low back and right leg pain 3 years after an L4–5 laminotomy for a disc herniation. **(A)** A possible lateral disc herniation is seen at L3–4. **(B)** The blinking or identity mode is useful to distinguish disc material from the surrounding soft tissues. (*Figure continues.*)

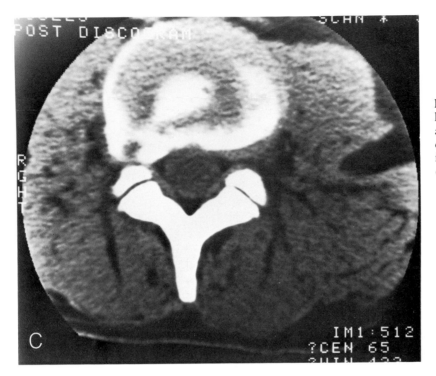

Fig. 13-8 (*Continued*). **(C)** A physiological disc evaluation confirmed the anatomical source of pain, and the postdiscography scan demonstrated a radial fissure communicating with the lateral disc herniation.

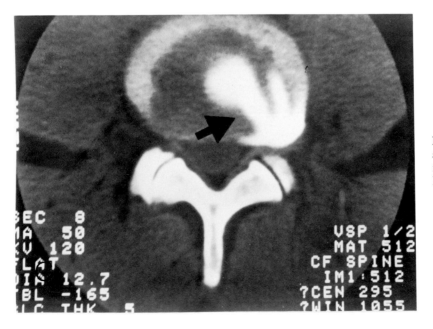

Fig. 13-9 Postdiscography CT scan in another patient demonstrates contrast filling a radial fissure (arrow) and enhancing a lateral disc herniation.

Fig. 13-10 (A) CT. This sagittal reformation demonstrates a normal L3–4 radicular canal. Both the L4–5 and L5–S1 (arrow) radicular canals are abnormal. A selective nerve root sheath infiltration confirmed that the L5 nerve root was symptomatic. **(B)** Magnetic imaging. This new imaging technique has great promise for demonstrating soft tissue tumors and intramedullary brain or spinal cord lesions. Although excellent soft tissue anatomical detail or neural tissue and intervertebral discs are revealed, at present, bone imaging remains inferior to computerized tomography. On this T_1-weighted sagittal image, the exiting nerve roots are clearly seen in the radicular canals.

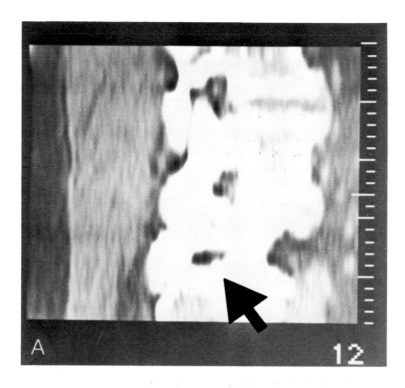

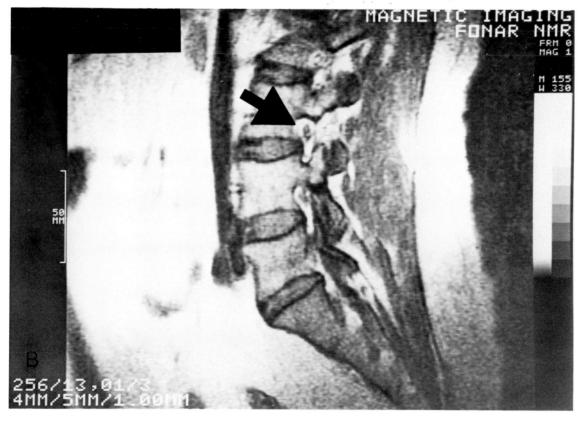

puterized tomography is the most reliable means to confirm a lateral disc herniation as the anatomical source of pain (Figs. 13-8 and 13-9).

Selective Nerve Root Sheath Injection

When the axial and reformatted computerized tomograms suggest lateral stenosis at one or more levels, a selective nerve root sheath injection may confirm whether a given nerve root contributes to the patient's current pain complex (Fig. 13-10). This is a provocative and analgesic test, which may be diagnostic and therapeutic.[18–21]

During radiculography, a normal nerve root sheath is not unduly sensitive to infiltration with contrast medium. A symptomatic nerve root will usually reproduce radicular pain during contrast infiltration and during the initial moment of injection of a local anesthetic and steroid preparation (Figs. 13-11 and 13-12). Reproduction of familiar pain and elimination of nerve root tension signs after nerve root sheath infiltration confirms the role of a particular nerve in the patient's pain complex.

Pain relief from a selective nerve root sheath infiltration should last as long as the local anesthetic acts. When a water soluble steroid is added to the injection, long-standing and occasionally permanent pain relief may be afforded. Complete initial pain relief correctly identifies the symptomatic nerve root. Only temporary pain relief implies that the nerve root is significantly compromised.

The Previously Operated Lumbar Spine

Individuals with continued pain following previous lumbar spine surgery represent one of the most chal-

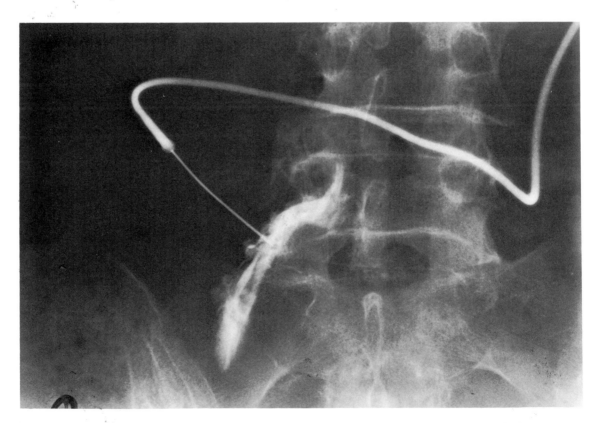

Fig. 13-11 Selective nerve root sheath infiltration. A normal nerve root sheath produces little or no pain during infiltration. A symptomatic nerve root may reproduce familiar pain during infiltration, which may be blocked by a local anesthetic. This illustrates a right L5 selective nerve root sheath infiltration.

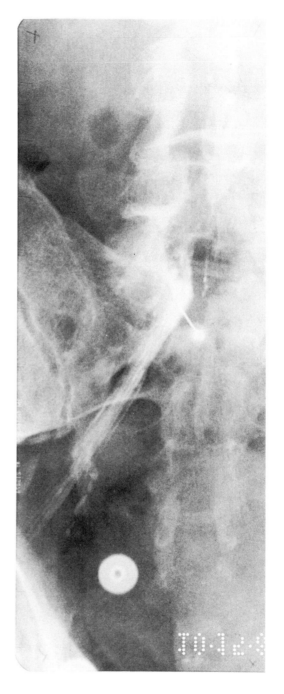

Fig. 13-12 S1 selective nerve root sheath infiltration demonstrates contrast flowing toward the pedicle region of S1 and then toward the sciatic notch.

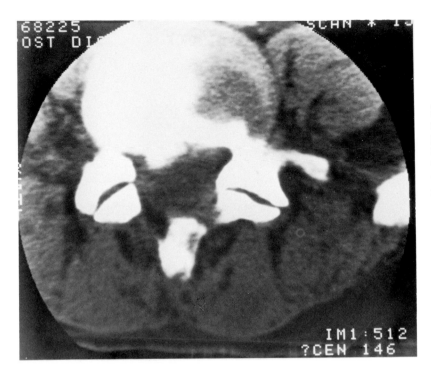

Fig. 13-13 This patient experienced recurrence of right lower extremity pain 3 years following an L4–5 laminotomy and discectomy. The enhanced CT scan did not clearly distinguish between scar tissue or recurrent disc herniation. A physiological lumbar disc evaluation reproduced familiar pain in the right lower extremity. This postdiscography CT scan reveals contrast enhancement of a recurrent disc herniation, which was confirmed operatively.

lenging patient groups. Myelography and intrathecal enhanced computerized tomography frequently reveal postsurgical changes, which are difficult to interpret. Standard diagnostic testing often fails to distinguish clearly between scar tissue and recurrent disc herniation.

These complex cases must be approached by studying the entire motion segments at the operated and adjacent levels. Dynamic bending radiographs will reveal instability or dysfunctional motion. Provocative and analgesic injections to the posterior joints, lumbar discs, and suspected nerve root sheaths are required for a thorough evaluation.

Physiological lumbar disc evaluation with postdiscography computerized tomography clearly distinguishes between scar tissue and recurrent disc herniation (Fig. 13-13).

SUMMARY

A precise diagnosis is the foundation for a rational plan of therapy for low back pain. This requires an understanding of the pain sensitive structures in the axial skeleton and an appreciation of how these structures produce referred and radicular pain.

Combining the information obtained from a careful clinical history and physical examination with the additional knowledge gleaned from certain special radiographic investigations confirms the anatomical source of pain and makes possible a specific diagnosis.

REFERENCES

1. Simons D, Travell J: Myofascial origins of low back pain. Postgrad Med J 73: 81, 1983
2. Simons D, Travell J: Myofascial origins of low back pain. Postgrad Med 73: 99, 1983
3. Simons D: Myofascial pain syndromes due to trigger points: Principles, diagnosis and perpetuating factors. Manual Med 1: 67, 1985
4. Gurdjian E, Webster J, Ostrowski A, et al: Herniated lumbar intervertebral discs—an analysis of 1176 operated cases. J Trauma 1: 158, 1961
5. Macnab, I: Negative disc exploration. J Bone Joint Surg 53A: 891, 1971
6. Bosacco S: Lumbar discography: redefining its role with intradiscal therapy. Orthopedics 9: 399, 1986

7. Fox A: Lumbar discography—a dissenting opinion. J Can Assoc Radiol 34: 88, 1983

8. Holt E: Fallacy of cervical discography. JAMA 188: 799, 1964

9. Holt E: The question of lumbar discography. J Bone Joint Surg 50A: 720, 1968

10. Shapiro R: Current status of lumbar discography. Radiology 159: 815, 1986

11. Brodsky A, Binder W: Lumbar discography. Its value in diagnosis and treatment of lumbar disc lesions. Spine 4: 110, 1979

12. Collins H: An evaluation of cervical and lumbar discography. Clin Orthop 107: 133, 1975

13. Gresham J, Miller R: Evaluation of the lumbar spine by discography and its use in selection of proper treatment of the herniated disk syndrome. Clin Orthop 67: 29, 1969

14. Hartman J, Kendrick J, Lorman P: Discography as an aid in evaluation for lumbar and lumbosacral fusion. Clin Orthop 81: 77, 1971

15. Patrick B: Lumbar discography: a five year study. Surg Neurol 1: 267, 1973

16. Simmons E, Segil C: An evaluation of discography in the localization of symptomatic levels in discogenic disease of the spine. Clin Orthop 108: 57, 1975

17. O'Brien J: The role of fusion for chronic low back pain. Orthop Clin North Am 14: 639, 1983

18. Bundens D, Rechtine, G: Lumbar nerve root injections as an adjunct to sciatica diagnosis. Orthop Rev 14: 45, 1985

19. Krempen J, Smith B: Nerve-root injection. A method for evaluating the etiology of sciatica. J Bone Joint Surg 56A: 1435, 1974

20. Tajima T, Furukawa K, Kuramochi E: Selective lumbosacral radiculography and block. Spine 5: 68, 1980

21. Wippula E, Jussila P: Spinal nerve block. Acta Orthop Scand 48: 458, 1977

14

Differential Diagnosis of Low Back Pain

John H. Wedge
Stanley Tchang

Many different diseases can present as low back pain. The purpose of this chapter is not to classify the numerous different causes of back pain but rather to describe a method of approaching the problem of differential diagnosis. The reader is referred to other sources for an exhaustive encyclopedic classification of the etiology of low back pain.

We find Macnab's classification[1] of back pain simple, concise, and useful. He lists the causes as follows:

1. Viscerogenic
2. Neurogenic
3. Vascular
4. Psychogenic
5. Spondylogenic

As soon as the physician thinks of back pain in this way, the likelihood of mistaking a more serious cause for degenerative disease is reduced. A small number of causes of back pain often lead to diagnostic problems. Failure to do a thorough examination or to order the appropriate investigations at the outset is the usual error. A thorough abdominal examination may direct attention away from the spine to the source of viscerogenic pain, an elevated ESR to an infection, and a bone scan to a tumor.

We will emphasize those conditions that are commonly missed, it is extremely valuable always to remember the lesions listed in Table 14-1. Likewise, Table 14-2 lists investigations to be made for back pain of undetermined origin.

VISCEROGENIC BACK PAIN

In practice, visceral pain is not very often confused with pain originating in the spine. Usually, sufficient specific symptoms and signs are present to localize the problem correctly. For example, carcinoma of the pancreas can cause severe and persistent back pain. However, this lesion causes other problems that turn attention away from the spine. Hollow viscus perforation or colic seldom closely mimics "typical back pain," nor do gynecologic conditions. Low back pain of mechanical spondylotic origin is normally relieved by rest, whereas lesions in solid or hollow viscera are not so relieved.

NEUROGENIC BACK PAIN

Serious delay in diagnosis can result from failure to appreciate the fact that neoplasms of the cord and cauda equina and nerve roots and inflammatory le-

Table 14-1 Important and Often Missed Causes of Back Pain

Vascular
    Abdominal aortic aneurysm
    Peripheral vascular disease

Neurogenic
    Nerve Root Tumors
      Neurofibroma
      Neurilemmoma
    Spinal cord tumors
    Diabetic neuropathy

Spondylogenic
    Multiple myeloma
    Secondary malignancy
    Osteoid osteoma
    Pathologic fracture (osteoporosis)
    Vertebral osteomyelitis
    Ankylosing spondylitis

sions can mimic spondylogenic pain. Neurofibromata and neurilemmomata cause erosion of bone, often at the intervertebral foramina (Fig. 14-1). Spinal cord and cauda equina tumors give characteristic appearances on myelography (Fig. 14-2). Central and lateral spinal stenosis (see Chapter 10 for symptoms and signs) can be diagnosed by myelography and CT scanning.

Diabetic neuropathy can cause nerve root irritation.[2] A clinical picture that is indistinguishable from sciatica can result and this similarity may lead to long and serious delays in diagnosis. One often sees patients with symptoms unrelieved by laminectomy in whom the diagnosis of diabetes has been missed or ignored simply because this condition was not suspected and a fasting blood sugar was not done.

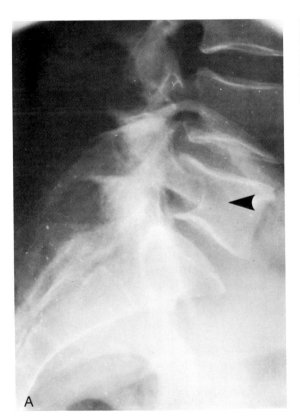 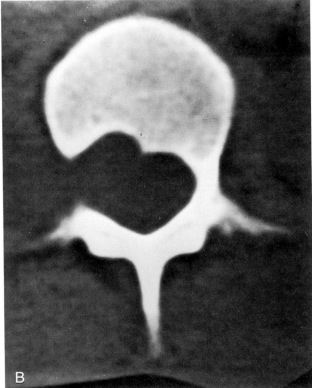

Fig. 14-1 (A) Lateral radiograph of spine shows enlarged intervertebral foramen typical of neurofibroma. **(B)** In another patient CT scan reveals neurofibroma that enlarges the foramen and erodes the posterior aspect of the vertebral body.

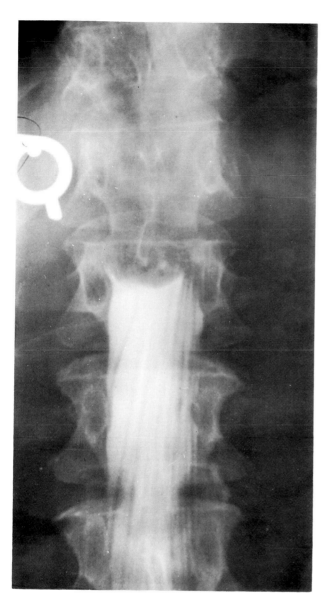

Fig. 14-2 Typical myelogram (water-soluble contrast) of an intrathecal tumor, in this instance a meningioma.

VASCULAR BACK PAIN

Abdominal Aortic Aneurysm

Abdominal aortic aneurysm can produce nagging, chronic back pain. Careful examination of the abdomen including auscultation may reveal the source of the symptoms. The lateral radiograph of the lum-

bar spine may show erosion of the anterior aspect of the vertebral bodies or calcification of an enlarged aorta (Fig. 14-3).

Peripheral Vascular Disease

Peripheral vascular disease with claudication can be confused with spinal stenosis. The major difference in the clinical features is the response of the pain to rest. While pain from both vascular and neurogenic claudication is relieved by rest, neurogenic pain may not be induced as quickly by exercise done with the spine held in flexion (as in bicycling). Vascular pain will be induced more quickly regardless of the position of the spine. Pain from spinal stenosis may actually be temporarily reduced by walking, but not that originating from vascular disease. The pain from stenosis is not usually relieved as promptly by rest as is pain of vascular origin.

PSYCHOGENIC BACK PAIN

Back pain is seldom ever purely psychogenic in origin. It is unwise to assume that the complaint of low back pain is made solely to gain attention or receive compensation, though this does happen occasionally. Outright malingering is rarely seen. This very complex issue is discussed in Chapter 8.

SPONDYLOGENIC BACK PAIN

The symptoms produced by bone lesions are relatively limited in nature and quality: the conditions producing these symptoms are numerous. However, subtle variations in the symptoms together with other clinical findings lead to suspicion of the correct diagnosis. The age of the patient, the character of the pain, weight loss, fever, deformity, and bone tenderness are most helpful in making the correct diagnosis.

Multiple Myeloma

Multiple myeloma is the most common malignant primary bone tumor and early in its course can easily be overlooked as the cause of back pain. The complaints may be nonspecific, but the astute physician senses the general lack of well-being of the pa-

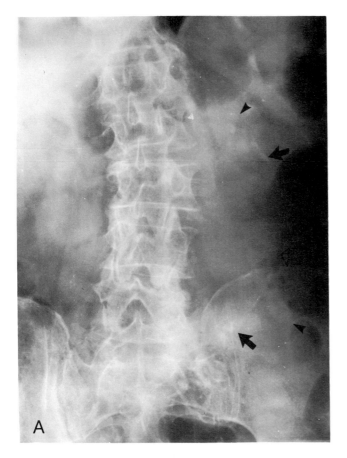

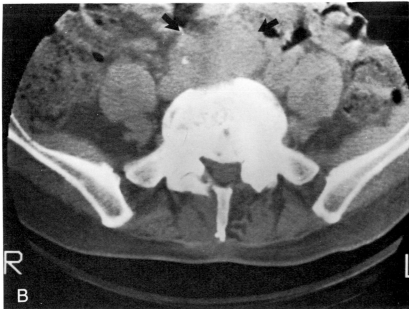

Fig. 14–3 (A) AP radiograph of spine in a patient with a large abdominal aortic aneurysm. Note calcification outlining the aneurysm (arrows). **(B)** In another patient CT scan shows an aneurysm eroding anterior aspect of lumbar vertebral body.

tient. Abnormalities on serum-protein electrophoresis studies and the presence of Bence Jones proteinuria usually clinch the diagnosis. However, at times both findings may be absent. Further difficulty may be encountered because the early radiographic picture is that of diffuse osteoporosis (Figs. 14-4, 14-5). The typical appearance of multiple "punched out" lesions is often absent (Fig. 14-6). Sternal puncture to obtain bone marrow for histology may be necessary.

Metastases

Secondaries from breast, thyroid, lung, kidney, and prostate can present as back pain. The distinguishing feature is the unrelenting, intense, and progressive nature of the pain. The patient looks anxious, fatigued, and often desperate for relief. Back pain due to degenerative disease is seldom if ever unrelenting and, as stated previously, usually responds to bed rest. Removal of a breast primary may be so far remote from the present that the patient does not volunteer the essential information. It is wise to assume that low back pain following a mastectomy is due to secondaries until proof to the contrary is obtained. Once such metastases are suspected, appropriate investigations lead to the correct diagnosis (Figs. 14-7, 14-8). Often a needle biopsy of the spine under fluoroscopic control is the most direct route to the diagnosis (Fig. 14-9). However, it is important to remember that neoplasms that metastasize to bone may lose their characteristic microscopic appearance. Often the pathologist can be confident that malignant tissue is present but may not be able to diagnose the tissue of origin.

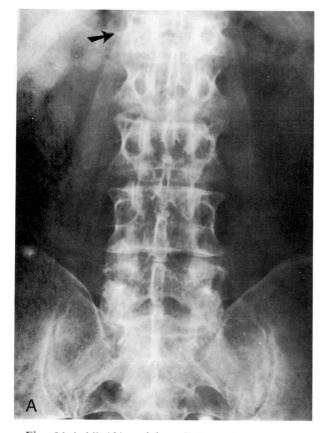 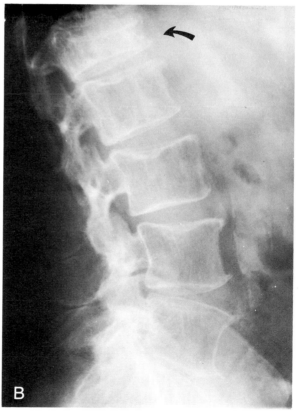

Fig. 14-4 AP **(A)** and lateral **(B)** radiographs showing diffuse osteopenia and fracture of L1 in multiple myeloma. The typical appearance of multiple punched-out lesions is often absent.

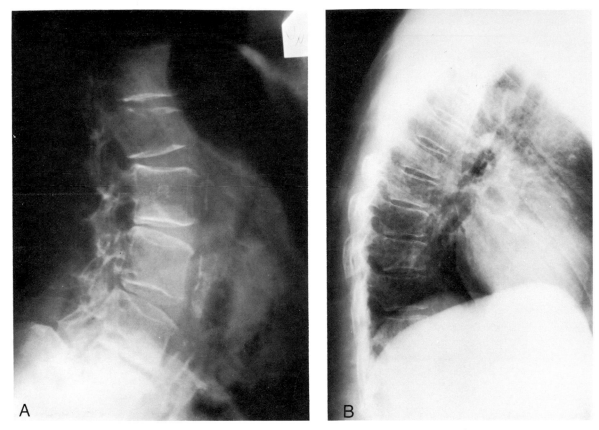

Fig. 14-5 Another patient with diffuse osteopenia and a fracture of L2.

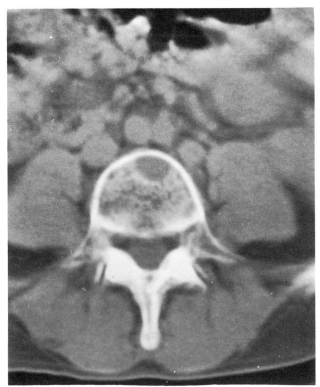

Fig. 14-6 CT scan showing typical lesion of multiple myeloma in the anterior aspect of a vertebral body.

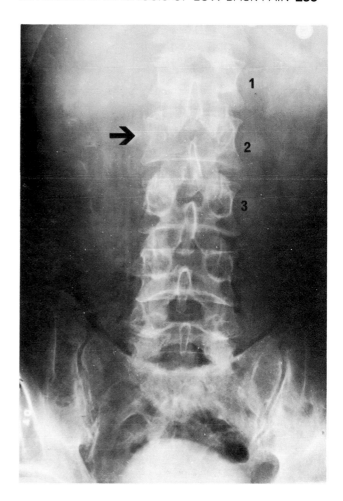

Fig. 14-7 Secondary to the spine from carcinoma of the colon. Note destroyed pedicle of L2 (arrow).

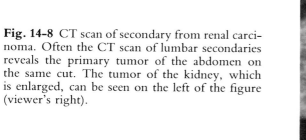

Fig. 14-8 CT scan of secondary from renal carcinoma. Often the CT scan of lumbar secondaries reveals the primary tumor of the abdomen on the same cut. The tumor of the kidney, which is enlarged, can be seen on the left of the figure (viewer's right).

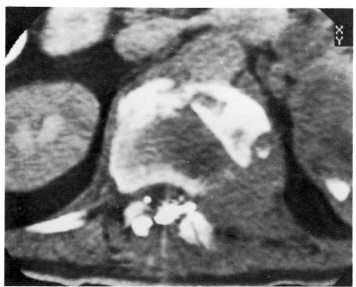

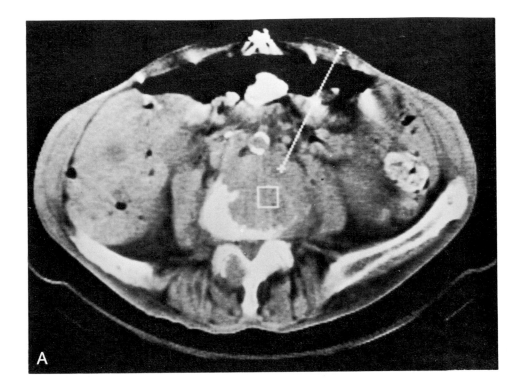

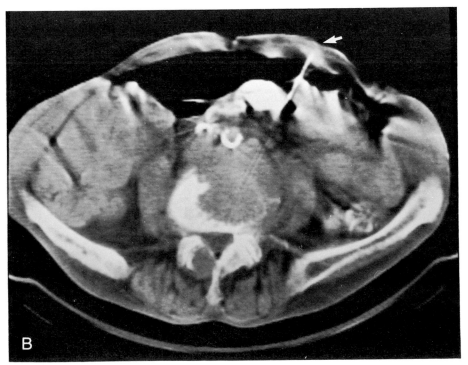

Fig. 14-9 The CT scanner is valuable in selecting the site for introduction of a biopsy needle. **(A)** Secondary in the vertebral body and the safe route from the exterior for the needle are shown. **(B)** Biopsy needle is introduced under CT control.

Osteoid Osteoma

Osteoid osteoma or osteoblastoma of the spine can also present a diagnostic problem. The characteristic history of night pain relieved by mild analgesics may be missing. Hamstring spasm with marked limitation of straight leg raising is often found with osteoid osteomata of the lumbar spine but can lead the physician further away from the correct diagnosis. Persistent back pain in a young adult in the absence of radiographic findings is an indication for a radioisotope bone scan (Fig. 14-10). Tomography of the area of increased isotopic uptake will usually localize the lesion to an articular process, lamina, or pedicle. The CT scan is extremely valuable in localizing the lesion (Figs. 14-11, 14-12).

Osteoporosis

Osteoporosis can result in compression fractures. Acute pain superimposed on chronic discomfort, often in the absence of a history of trauma, may be the presenting symptom. The patient may recall only

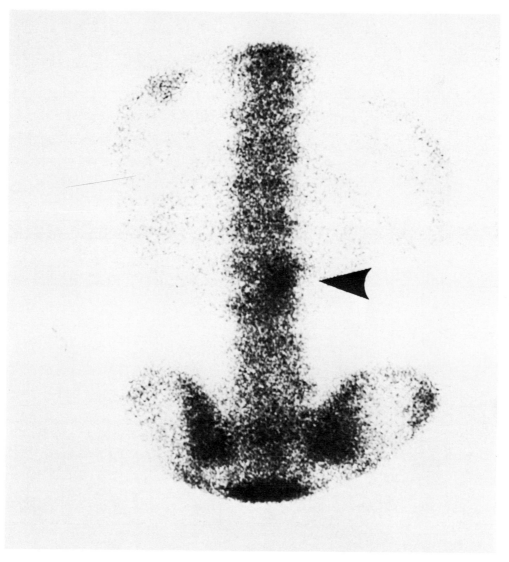

Fig. 14-10 Radioisotope bone scan of an osteoid osteoma in lamina of L2 (arrow).

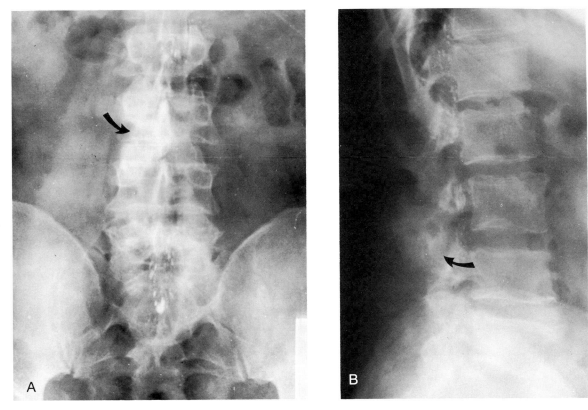

Fig. 14-11 AP **(A)** and lateral **(B)** radiographs of an osteoblastoma in the inferior articular process of L3.

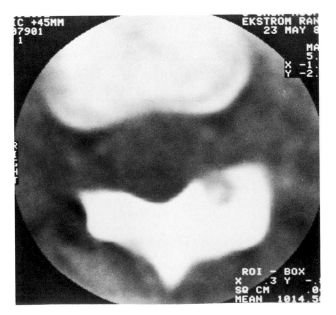

Fig. 14-12 CT scan of osteoid osteoma showing radiolucent nidus and surrounding sclerotic bone.

a "snap" associated with mild back pain that occurred when she simply bent to pick up a small object. More intense pain may not develop for hours or until the next day. A fracture may not be seen on the initial radiographs. Usually, however, osteoporosis and bi-concave vertebral bodies as well as a recent fracture are seen on the radiograph (Fig. 14-13). It is important to think of the possibility of compression fracture in the osteoporotic spine so that the patient is not subjected to the cost and inconvenience of extensive investigations.

Vertebral Osteomyelitis

Vertebral osteomyelitis due either to *Mycobacterium tuberculosis* or pyogenic organisms is perhaps the most frequently missed diagnosis. It is particularly important to remember infection as a cause of low back pain in diabetics, drug addicts, alcoholics, pa-

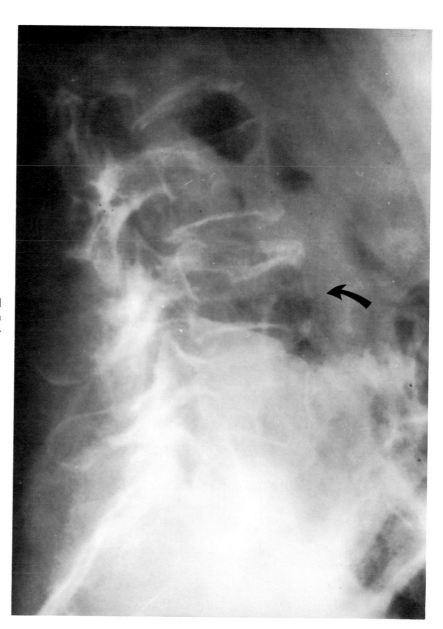

Fig. 14-13 Severe osteopenia and fracture of L3 in a 54-year-old woman who had been on corticosteroid therapy for many years.

tients on corticosteroid drugs, those who have had recent urethral instrumentation, those with disseminated malignancy, and otherwise debilitated patients. No rise in body temperature may be present and the white blood cell count may be normal. In a recent series of cases of osteomyelitis diagnosis was delayed more than 3 months from the appearance of initial symptoms in 50% of patients.[3] The most constant clinical finding is marked tenderness over the spinous process of the involved vertebra and the erythrocyte sedimentation rate is almost invariably elevated. Early in the course slight disc-space narrowing and minimal adjacent vertebral body erosion may be the only radiographic findings (Figs. 14-14, 14-15).

Ankylosing Spondylitis

Ankylosing spondylitis may be another diagnostic enigma. Night pain and morning stiffness may be the major complaints, but asymmetric sacroiliac involvement with radiation into the buttock and thigh is not unusual. In fact, it is not unknown for these patients to come to laminectomy before the correct diagnosis is made. Early in the course of the disease, no obvious radiographic changes in the spine or sacroiliac joints may be present (Figs. 14-16, 14-17). An elevated sedimentation rate, a positive HLA-B27 antigen test, and increased uptake on a radioisotope bone scan strongly suggest the diagnosis.

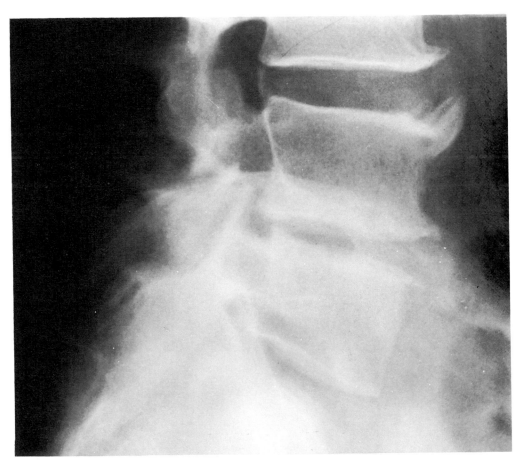

Fig. 14-14 Lateral radiograph showing early osteomyelitis of the inferior aspect of L4 with L4–5 disc-space narrowing. Initially attention was diverted to the obvious degenerative changes at L3–4, which were thought to be the source of the symptoms.

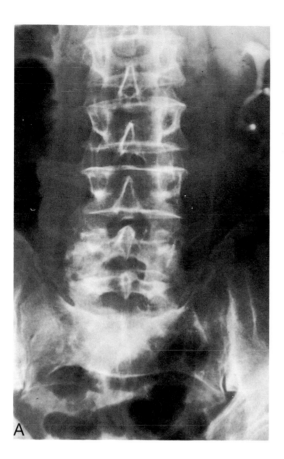

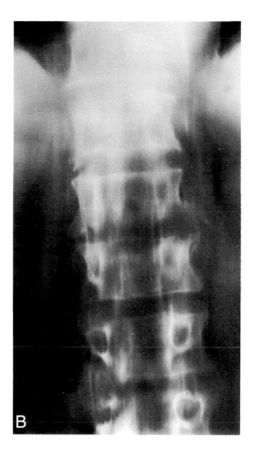

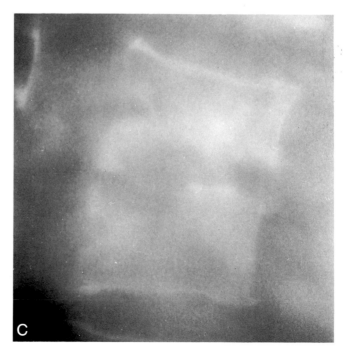

Fig. 14-15 (A) Vertebral infection at L1-L2. This AP radiograph taken 1 week after onset of symptoms does not direct attention to the site of the infection. **(B)** AP and **(C)** lateral tomograms taken 6 weeks later show typical appearance of pyogenic infection of the spine.

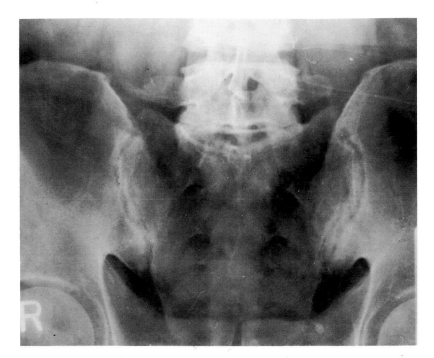

Fig. 14-16 Early ankylosing spondylitis. The sacroiliac joints can be clearly visualized, but note the particular sclerosis.

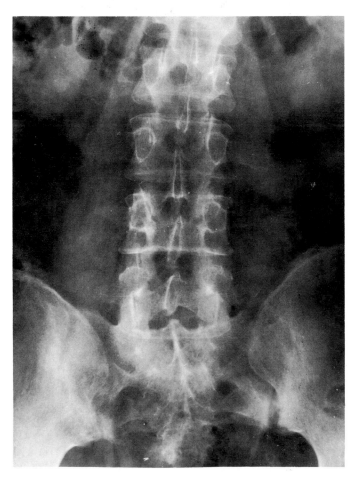

Fig. 14-17 Moderately advanced ankylosing spondylitis. Note obliteration of right sacroiliac joint (viewer's left).

Table 14-2 Investigations for Back Pain of Undetermined Origin

Urine
  Glucose
  Protein
  Uric acid crystals
  Bence Jones protein
  Culture and sensitivity

Blood
  Hemoglobin
  White blood count, differential and smear
  Erythrocyte sedimentation rate
  Fasting blood sugar
  Serum proteins and electrophoresis
  Alkaline and acid phosphatase
  Liver enzymes
  HLA-B27 antigen
  Blood culture

Radiography
  Spinal films, conventional and
    computed tomography (see chapter on investigation)
  Bone scan, gallium scan
  Chest x-ray
  Liver-spleen scan
  Thyroid scan
  Mammography

Biopsy
  Needle biopsy—Gram stain, culture
    and sensitivity, histology
  Open biopsy

SUMMARY

Table 14-1 lists the conditions that are frequently confused with low back pain caused by degenerative lesions in the lumbar spine. The wise physician has this list in mind when examining any patient who presents with the symptoms and signs of low back pain. The diagnosis of the conditions discussed in this chapter will almost always be made by systematically working through the investigations listed in Table 14-2, selecting those tests appropriate to the clinical presentation of the patient. When the problem is approached in this way, particularly if the patient does not respond rapidly to simple conservative measures of treatment, failure to arrive at the correct diagnosis will be a rare occurrence.

REFERENCES

1. Macnab I: Backache. Williams & Wilkins, Baltimore, 1977
2. Tile M: Diabetic neuropathy in orthopaedic practice. J Bone Joint Surg 55B: 662, 1973
3. Wedge JH, Oryschak AF, Robertson DE, Kirkaldy-Willis WH: Atypical manifestations of spinal infections. Clin Orthop 123: 155, 1977

TREATMENT

15

A Comprehensive Outline of Treatment

William H. Kirkaldy-Willis

THE FRAME

In this chapter we consider in broad outline the physical modalities of treatment used in the management of low back pain. Treatment is based on our assumption that frequently the physical problem has mental, emotional, and even spiritual overtones, as shown in Figure 15-1. The importance of the emotions has been stressed by John Sarno.[1] We also think that the individual, made up of these four component parts, must be pictured in the environment composed of home and family, workplace, hobbies and interests, and social activities. This is demonstrated in Figure 15-2.

THE ROLE OF PHYSICIAN AND THERAPIST

It is vitally important that all those physicians and therapists involved in treating low back pain work together as a team, appreciating the fact that at different stages different people have the important role. Volunteers too have much to contribute. Considerable give and take is required all around. It is the task of the leaders to make sure that all concerned feel they are an essential part of the team. In our hospital in Saskatoon many volunteers give a number of services free.

The way in which the treatment of low back pain is organized varies greatly. The patient is often seen first and starts treatment with the family practitioner. Frequently no further treatment is needed. Some patients seek help first from the osteopath or chiropractor.

At this point it is helpful to look at Figure 15-3. This was shown first in Chapter 4 when we were discussing pathophysiology. The chiropractor and the physical therapist have much to offer the patient with muscle dysfunction (2 to 5 o'clock), with a myofascial syndrome (5 o'clock) and in the early stages of pathoanatomy (7 o'clock), though injections of local anesthetic may be required from a physician for these lesions. These two therapists are thus involved in 80% to 90% of treatment in some centers.

The physician and surgeon are more and more involved as the realm of pathoanatomy is approached. Only a small percentage of patients fall into this category but each requires a large amount of work (7 o'clock).

The physical therapist is much involved in the process of functional rehabilitation to treat increasing muscle pathology (8 to 11 o'clock) with other members of the team—physician, osteopath, chiropractor,

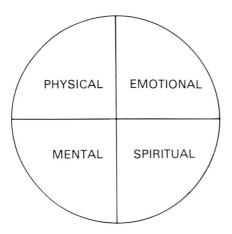

Fig. 15-1 The four aspects in each individual (after Arthur Bell).

Visualization

A number of writers have described the way in which one can form a picture of oneself progressively recovering from illness or injury. The patient is instructed to set aside 10 to 15 minutes at regular intervals three or four times a day. Initially, the patient requires a lot of help from the instructor and is told first in simple terms what is wrong with the back and then is shown how to picture or imagine the process of healing taking place. The patient has to practice and experiment a good deal to acquire this skill. The Simonton method[2] is most effective as it harnesses not only mind and reason but also emotions and subconscious. It can be adapted easily to the field of low back pain.

Supernatural Help

The point of view of the psychiatrist is expressed in Jerome D. Frank's excellent book.[3]

The physician who takes the time and trouble to question and listen to patients will discover that they often have sought the help of a minister, priest, or friends in their church during a serious illness or before a serious operation. This nearly always is a great encouragement to the patient and can bring release from stress, anxiety, fear, and resentment. Often it enables the patient to recover more quickly with less pain. Many physicians encourage their patients as they seek this kind of help. In our modern world the physical and the supernatural are separated into two different compartments. We are suspicious of any kind of supernatural method of treatment for disease. It is most reasonable to protect the patient from "quacks" and from the "occult." Nevertheless, we at least need to keep an open mind about methods of treatment we do not understand.

psychologist, occupational therapist, social worker, industrial advisor, and representative from insurance company or compensation board (Fig. 15-3).

OTHER KINDS OF HELP

Realizing the potential complexity of the problem, even in apparently minor low back injuries, it is good to supplement physical modalities with some of the following. These things are especially important in managing patients with increasing muscle pathology who sometimes present an almost insuperable problem.

Relaxation

Relaxation is described in Chapter 16.

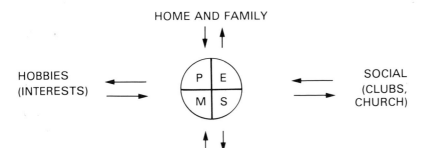

Fig. 15-2 The individual and the environment.

MYOFASCIAL CYCLE

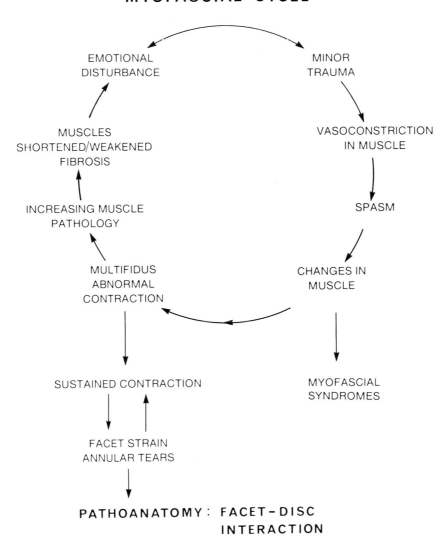

Fig. 15-3 Pathophysiology: overview.

The matter of supernatural healing is dealt with in a simple and convincing way by Agnes Sanford.[4] A Christian herself, she describes how she has helped sick people—both Jews and Christians—with only the vaguest faith in a creator and those with a more definite faith. She recommends that the sick person make contact with the Creator, ask for specific help in healing, imagine this taking place by the process of visualization, and then express thanks before seeing the result.

SURVEY OF MANAGEMENT OF LOW BACK PAIN

An overall view is set out in Table 15-1. Of course, so brief a summary is no more than a guide for the reader. It cannot be applied rigidly in every case. There are many exceptions.

Planning treatment as advocated by the writer is rather complex because of the need to consider two aspects in each instance: the phase and the type of

Table 15-1 Overall View of Scheme of Treatment
(Low back school and elastic back support for most patients)

Phase	Lesion	Treatment
Dysfunction	Facet joints	Manipulation, injection
	Sacroiliac joint	Manipulation, injection
	Muscle syndromes	Stretching, injection
	Piriformis syndrome	Stretching, injection
	Disc herniation	Expectant, discotomy
Unstable Phase	Disc herniation	Expectant, discotomy
	Instability only	Injection, fusion
	Lateral stenosis	Decompression, fusion
	Central stenosis	Decompression, fusion
	Degenerative olisthesis	Decompression, fusion
	Isthmic olisthesis	Decompression, fusion
Stabilization	Disc herniation	Expectant, discotomy
	Lateral stenosis	Decompression
	Central stenosis	Decompression
	Degenerative olisthesis	Decompression, rarely fusion
	Isthmic olisthesis	Decompression, rarely fusion

clinical lesion. If readers bear this in mind, they should not experience much difficulty in following the rationale suggested below. Conservative measures are considered first because they apply to all patients with low back pain. Consideration of the clinical lesions seen in dysfunction (Phase I) comes next. Dysfunction of the intervertebral joints affects both the facet joints and the disc, but the joint symptoms predominate. A discussion of the treatment of instability (Phase II) and stabilization (Phase III) follows because all subsequent lesions may present in either of these phases. Then herniation of the nucleus pulposus is considered because it may occur in any of the three phases, though it is seen most commonly at the end of Phase I or the beginning of Phase II. The other clinical lesions that are discussed subsequently are encountered in both Phases II and III.

CONSERVATIVE TREATMENT

The term conservative treatment is frequently used to describe the measures discussed in this section. However, it is not altogether accurate because more aggressive methods sometimes prove more conservative in the sense of conserving, that is of restoring, normal function quickly. The term "nonoperative measures" has also been used.

Spine Education Program (The Low Back School)

Every patient should attend a class in spine education as early as possible (see Ch. 16 for discussion). Instruction is given by a physiotherapist and an occupational therapist. The structure and function of the lumbar spine are taught in simple terms. The different types of lesion and the way in which these can cause pain are discussed. Instruction is given in low back care, especially as related to the activities of daily living. The class is taught correct posture and pelvic tilting and exercises to be done twice daily to strengthen muscles, especially the abdominal muscles that provide most strength to the back. Weight reduction is often advocated, and the patient may be sent to consult a dietician about this. Individual instruction should be given to each patient at the end of the class, explaining in more detail the nature of the patient's lesion and the way in which the patient can become his or her own doctor to deal with it. A second period of instruction to reinforce what has been taught during the first session is highly desirable.

Manipulation

As discussed in Chapter 17, manipulation is greatly beneficial to many patients in Phase I.

More Intensive Therapy

Many patients benefit greatly from one attendance at the spine education program. Some require further help. For these an intensive course of physiotherapy and occupational therapy is given for several hours a day for 2 to 3 weeks. It is convenient to lodge patients attending from a distance in a hostel adjacent to the hospital. A light elastic garment is often provided for the patient to wear whenever not in bed. It provides support to the back and helps the patient to pull in the abdominal muscles. It permits almost full movement of the spine, and thus does not contribute to muscle atrophy (Ch. 18).

DYSFUNCTION: THE POSTERIOR FACET SYNDROME

As discussed previously, this syndrome is caused by rotational strain to both facet joints and annulus fibrosus. Dysfunction of the facet joints produces most of the symptoms, and treatment is mainly directed there (Table 15-2).

For the acute lesion with severe incapacitating pain, treatment with suitable analgesics and a few days of bedrest is indicated. The value of muscle relaxants and of anti-inflammatory drugs is doubtful.

For less acute and for recurring and chronic lesions

the conservative treatment previously described is prescribed. At this point the physician has a choice between two apparently different forms of treatment.

Manipulation

Undertaken by a practitioner well versed in the art and given daily for 7 to 10 days, manipulation relieves many patients of their symptoms. Few physicians or surgeons have acquired the necessary skill. The physician needs to choose a practitioner whose skill he knows and whose judgment he trusts. The way in which this modality works has long been the subject of controversy. The most reasonable explanation is that manipulation produces a threefold effect: (1) a direct mechanical effect on the facet joints, which may reduce a subluxation of 1 to 2 mm; (2) stretching of hypertonic posterior segmental spinal muscles by the thrust applied by the manipulator with abolition of pain coming from the muscles, ligaments, and tendons because of stretching; (3) increased neural output produced by mechanoreceptor stimulation that may modulate pain perception through the gate control mechanism.

Facet Injection

The technique will be described in detail in a later chapter.[5] After the skin is anesthetized, a lumbar puncture needle is passed under fluoroscopic control to the posterior joint considered to be mainly affected. A 1-ml dose of 0.25% bupivacaine (Marcaine) is injected into the joint. As the needle is withdrawn, 3 to 4 ml are injected into the muscle overlying the

Table 15-2 Plan of Treatment: Phase I: Dysfunction

Lesion	Treatment			
	Conservative	Manipulation	Injection	Operation
Facet joints	Yes	Facets	Facet and muscle	—
Sacroiliac joint	Yes	Sacroiliac and muscle	Joint and muscle	—
Myofascial syndrome	Yes	Stretch muscle	Muscle	—
Piriformis syndrome	Yes	—	Muscle	—
Disc herniation	Yes	Rarely	Epidural steroids	Sometimes

joint. The patient then stands and puts the back through a full range of movement. In many cases injection at one level, usually L4–5, relieves the patient of his pain (Fig. 15-4). If the pain is relieved, no further injection is given, but in some cases it is necessary to repeat the procedure at a second or third level. Facet injections nearly always relieve the patient of pain for several hours. In approximately 50% of cases the patient is free of pain for weeks or months. In some cases relief is permanent. The explanation that best explains the success of injection is (1) that the nerve supply to the joint and capsule is temporarily anesthetized, permitting a minor subluxation to be reduced; (2) that hypertonic contracted ischemic muscle is relaxed when pain coming from it is abolished; (3) that relaxation of the muscle overlying the joint allows the subluxed articular surfaces to move back into correct alignment; (4) that sustained neural activity that summates to produce pain is interrupted and the vicious circle of pain is broken.

Each of the two modalities brings relief to many patients. No guideline can be given as to which should be tried first. If one fails, the other should be tried. Sometimes facet injection followed by manipulation gives good results. In each case the treatment is followed by adherence to the conservative measures previously outlined. In recalcitrant cases, where both manipulation and injection have failed, the application of a "light cast" body jacket to immobilize the spine for 4 to 6 weeks may be very effective. This assists resolution of the inflammatory synovitis in the joint and healing of tears in the capsule and annulus (Table 15-1).

Denervation of posterior joints is occasionally indicated when all other methods have failed to give relief of pain.

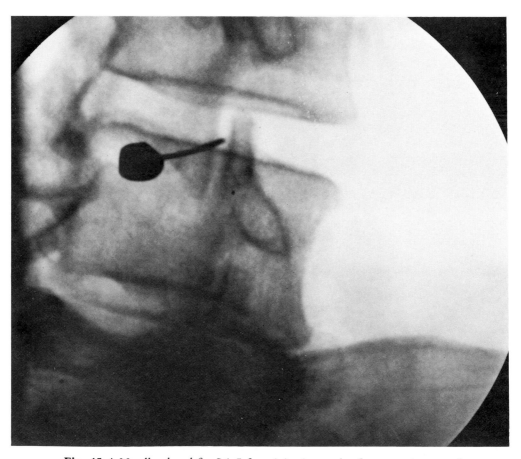

Fig. 15-4 Needle placed for L4–5 facet injection under fluoroscopic control.

DYSFUNCTION: THE SACROILIAC SYNDROME

The presentation is rarely acute and nearly always subacute or chronic. We have seen (Chapter 10) that the symptom complex is well-defined even though the exact pathological nature of the lesion is obscure. The response to treatment is as well defined as the clinical syndrome. Conservative measures are prescribed as previously listed. Definitive treatment is started as soon as the diagnosis is made.

Manipulation

The patient nearly always has reduced movement of the sacroiliac joint as well as pain. Manipulation for 3 to 4 days often relieves the pain and restores the joint movement. Sometimes daily manipulation for 10 days is required. Three types of adjustment are employed: a superior, a direct, and an inferior sacroiliac manipulation. This modality is by far the most certain way of relieving the patient's pain.

Injection

When manipulation fails, injection of 3 to 4 ml of 0.25% bupivacaine into the overlying muscle, the posterior ligaments, and, if possible, the joint sometimes produces marked relief of pain (Fig. 15-5). It is difficult to be certain that the local anesthetic has penetrated into the joint.

Manipulation probably relieves pain by reducing hypertonicity (spasm) in the posterior muscles that maintain the point in a state of fixation; the treatment may also result in restoring movement by shifting the ilium 1 to 2 mm on the sacrum. It is reasonable to assume that injection acts by relieving muscular hypertonicity.

We now think that the most satisfactory procedure is to inject the anesthetic at the upper, middle and lower levels of the joint, 1 ml to the joint and 3 ml to posterior ligament and muscle.

DYSFUNCTION: MAIGNE'S SYNDROME

In this condition there is a facet syndrome, often on both sides, usually at the T12–L1 level but occasionally at the T11–12 or L1–2 level.

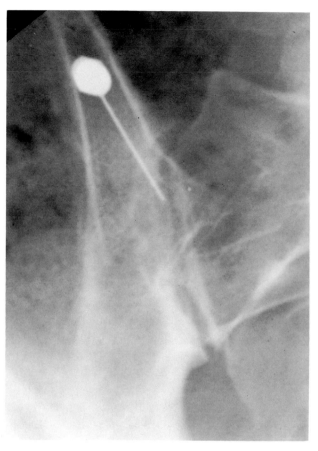

Fig. 15-5 Needle placed for sacroiliac joint injection under fluoroscopic control.

Manipulation

Manipulation is directed to the painful joints and is often effective.

Injection

On occasion it is necessary to inject 0.5 to 1.0 ml of 0.25% bupivacaine to each affected joint and 2 to 3 ml to overlying muscle. One of these methods is nearly always effective in relieving the patient's local and referred pain.

DYSFUNCTION: MYOFASCIAL SYNDROMES

The reader is referred to Chapter 10, in which the clinical presentation of these syndromes is considered.

1. Multifidus syndrome (facet syndrome) (Figs. 10-1 and 10-2)
2. Gluteus medius syndrome (Figs. 10-11 A and B)
3. Gluteus maximus syndrome (Fig. 10-12)
4. Quadratus lumborum syndrome (Fig. 10-13)
5. Piriformis syndrome (Fig. 10-14)
6. Tensor fasciae latae syndrome (Fig. 10-15)

Spraying and Stretching

The first line of attack is to ask the physical therapist or chiropractor to spray the skin over the affected portion of muscle with fluorimethane and then to stretch the segment of muscle manually. Exercises to stretch the muscle further are added to this regimen.

Injection

When the above method fails to relieve the pain and spasm, it is relatively easy under fluoroscopic control to inject the affected segment of muscle with 0.25% bupivacaine. The site for the injection is indicated by the star in each of the illustrations (Fig. 10-1 to Fig. 10-15). The lesion in quadratus lumborum may be higher or lower than shown in Figure 10-14. There are two motor points for gluteus maximus and tensor fasciae latae (Figs. 10-12 and 10-15). After the injection, exercises to stretch the muscle further are recommended. Sometimes it is necessary to repeat the injection.

DYSFUNCTION: THE PIRIFORMIS SYNDROME

Injection

The treatment is to inject 2 to 3 ml of 0.25% bupivacaine into the muscle medial to the spine of the ischium. The injection is made from the buttock with a finger in the rectum or vagina. Details are given in Chapter 20. Almost instantaneous relief of pain is obtained (see Fig. 10-14) (see Fig. 20-58).

THE UNSTABLE PHASE AND STABILIZATION

The Unstable Phase

The clinical diagnosis depends on both the presence of low back pain and radiological evidence of increased abnormal movement. Instability may occur

Table 15-3 Plan of Treatment: Phase II: Unstable Phase

Lesion	Treatment		
	Conservative	Decompression	Fusion
Disk herniation Instab. mild	Yes	Yes	No
Disk herniation Instab. marked	Yes	Yes	Yes
Instability alone Mild	Yes	Cast Immobilization	Denervation
Instability alone Marked	No	No	Yes
Lateral stenosis Instab. mild	Yes	Yes	No
Lateral stenosis Instab. marked	No	Yes	Yes
Central stenosis Instab. mild	Yes	Yes	No
Central stenosis Instab. marked	No	Yes	Yes
Degen. olisthesis	Yes	Yes	Yes
Isthmic olisthesis	Yes	Yes	Yes

alone. In that case only the instability should be treated. Alternatively, it may accompany a disc herniation, spinal stenosis, and other clinical lesions. In this case treatment of the clinical lesion should be followed by treatment of the instability. Patients with mild instability may respond to the conservative measures previously outlined. The application of a "light cast" body jacket may be helpful. Apart from this there are two main methods of treatment of instability: denervation and fusion (Table 15-3).

Denervation of Posterior Joints

The rationale of this procedure is to reduce the number of impulses from pain fibers (S) arising in the posterior joints and thus to prevent summation of impulses from posterior joints and disc and so inhibit pain. Denervation may be carried out percutaneously by creating a thermal lesion that destroys part of the innervation of the posterior joint or by open operation when a more thorough denervation can be performed. It is indicated, occasionally when other modalities fail to relieve pain in dysfunction and, more often, early in the unstable phase in an attempt to obviate the necessity for spinal fusion.[6]

Study of Figure 15-6 shows that each posterior facet joint receives innervation from three levels: at the level concerned, at that above, and at that below. Thus, denervation of three posterior primary rami is required. In our hands, the results of this procedure have not been as good as expected.

Spinal Fusion

There is much confusion over the role of fusion in treating low back pain. Some surgeons advocate fusion of one or two levels when a period of bed rest and wearing a rigid corset or brace or immobilization in a "light cast" jacket have failed to relieve the patient's pain. Others reserve fusion for patients

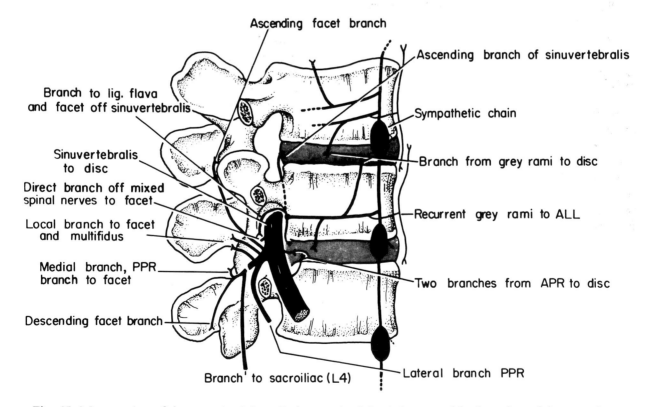

Fig. 15-6 Innervation of the posterior joints. Each posterior joint is innervated by branches of the posterior primary rami from three levels. At each level a small nerve passes directly from the main nerve to the posterior joint. (Figure courtesy of Dr. Stanley Paris.)

who have had prolonged conservative treatment followed by one or more operations for decompression and still have low back pain. In effect they say, "this patient has had every other form of treatment with no relief of pain; a small percentage of patients benefit from fusion; therefore fusion is indicated." Still others choose anterior or posterior interbody fusion for the same reason when a posterior or posterolateral fusion has failed to relieve pain. In the opinion of the writer these approaches are not logical.

The only logical reasons and indications for spinal fusion are, first, that other modalities have been tried and failed; second, that from a psychological viewpoint the operation is reasonable; and, third, that instability is present at one or two levels. The definition of instability (the unstable phase) is pain with increased abnormal movement (as discussed and illustrated by stress radiographs and CT images in Chapter 9). There appears to be no adequate reason for fusion other than radiological demonstration of increased abnormal movement.

At present no consensus as to when posterior and when interbody fusion is the best form of treatment exists. Fusion relieves pain by abolishing movement.[7]

SPINAL FUSION WITH INTERNAL FIXATION

At the present time, there is considerable interest in combining a posterolateral fusion with internal fixation of the affected segments by means of pedicle screws and plates. Pertinent to this is the work of Camille, Steffee and Wiltse. This approach may well prove to be a very satisfactory one. It is still a matter of controversy. The writer is of the opinion that the procedure should only be done by a skilled spine surgeon who is thoroughly conversant with it and aware of the hazards involved.

Stabilization

As seen in Chapter 9, this final phase in the degenerative process can be diagnosed with accuracy by stress radiographs. When this phase is nearly reached, the surgeon can with confidence assure the patient that soon the low back pain will abate. When stabilization has been reached, fusion is seldom if ever indicated though decompression may be required to treat central or lateral spinal stenosis (Table 15-4).

HERNIATION OF THE NUCLEUS PULPOSUS

The pathology, pathogenesis, and clinical picture have been described in previous chapters. To recapitulate briefly, two mechanisms are involved. First, recurrent rotational trauma produces lesions in the facet joints and the annulus fibrosus. In this type circumferential tears coalesce to form radial tears. The posterior annulus thins out at one point. Further minor rotational trauma allows the annulus to bulge locally at that point (a disc protrusion) or to rupture completely (a disc extrusion). Second, a fall onto the buttocks with the lumbar spine in flexion may produce a sudden rupture of the posterior annulus with protrusion or extrusion of the nucleus pulposus.

The Three-Joint Complex

Nearly every case of disc herniation is accompanied by pathology in the facet joints. For this reason the wise physician, confronted by a patient with a disc

Table 15-4 Plan of Treatment: Phase III: Stabilization

Lesion	Treatment		
	Conservative	Decompression	Fusion
Disk herniation	Yes	Yes	No
Lateral stenosis	Yes	Yes	No
Central stenosis	Yes	Yes	No
Combined stenosis	Yes	Yes	No
Degenerative spondylolisthesis	Yes	Yes	Sometimes
Isthmic spondylolisthesis	Yes	Yes	Sometimes

herniation, considers the possibility that this lesion is complicated by facet lesions that may produce pain or instability and by facet subluxation that may result in lateral canal stenosis.

The Phase

Most commonly the herniation occurs at the end of Phase I or early in Phase II. More rarely, it takes place during Phase III, complicating spinal stenosis or degenerative spondylolisthesis.

Expectant Treatment

Resolution of a first disc herniation takes place in approximately 75% of patients over a period of 3 months. With recurrent herniation the chance of spontaneous relief of symptoms is reduced. In a very acute stage the patient is hospitalized and put on bed rest with bathroom privileges. Adequate analgesics relieve the pain, and this helps the hypertonicity and spasm in muscle to subside. Gravity lumbar reduction (see Chapter 19) is of considerable assistance to some patients. The amount of straight leg raising obtained without pain is a useful indication of recovery. At the onset often the leg can be raised no more than 20°. Over 1, 2, or 3 weeks the amount of straight leg raising slowly increases to 30°, 40°, 50°, and 60°. It is unusual to keep the patient in bed for more than 3 weeks. By this time in most cases the acute symptoms have subsided. In a few cases the pain is still severe and the patient is aware that other measures should be begun.

Chemonucleolysis

In several Canadian centers chemonucleolysis is the treatment of choice when expectant measures have failed. In this center it is reserved for patients below the age of 40 with minimal loss of motor power. We manage a large percentage of patients with expectant measures and thus fewer cases by chemonucleolysis. Undoubtedly this latter therapy has a place in treating disc herniations. An immediate complication is anaphylactic shock and a late complication the development of lateral stenosis from loss of disc height and subluxation of posterior facets. Both complications are uncommon. It is essential to order a CT scan before embarking on chemonucleolysis in order to rule out the possibility that lateral stenosis is present along with the herniation.

Fraser, of the Flinders Medical Center, Adelaide, South Australia, reported on a double-blind study on the use of chymopapain at the Toronto meeting of the International Society for the Study of the Lumbar Spine in June 1982. This author recommends the use of chymopapain for the treatment of sciatica due to proven intervertebral disc prolapse when conservative measures have failed before discotomy is considered.

Microsurgery on the Disc

The rightful place of this type of surgery is not yet firmly established. It is reasonable to suppose that the procedure has a role provided that neither central or lateral stenosis, as shown by CT scan, nor marked instability, as shown by stress radiographs, is present.

Discotomy

As previously mentioned it is essential to assess accurately not only the level of the disc herniation but also the presence or absence of instability and of lateral stenosis.

The uncomplicated herniation is approached by either a unilateral or a bilateral minimal partial laminectomy after the level is accurately identified, if necessary by radiography at the time of surgery. The use of magnifying glasses, a headlight, and bipolar cautery minimize the danger of injury to nerves and blood vessels. The operative field should be bloodless throughout the procedure. After retraction of the dura and gentle retraction of the nerve, the disc herniation comes into view. The nerve is retracted medially or laterally as required; the annulus is incised; and the protruded or extruded nuclear material is removed using pituitary forceps. In the case of an extrusion, incising the annulus may not be necessary. It is important to make certain that no loose fragments of material are left within the disc or in the central or lateral spinal canals. Further confirmation of the size of the lateral canals is obtained by measuring them with gauges ranging from 2 to 5 mm in diameter.

In treating a herniation with lateral stenosis, it is necessary to enlarge the lateral canals to 6 mm at this point, using the Quintron sonic tool, Kerrison forceps, or osteotome and mallet.

When the herniation is complicated by marked instability as demonstrated by stress radiographs, it is wise to perform a one-level spinal fusion. At the end of the operation a free fat graft is placed posterior to the dura to prevent adhesions (Fig. 15-7).

The after care is the same whatever the nature of the treatment because a concomitant lesion in the facet joints is virtually always present. The patient receives instruction in low back care and exercises. An elastic support should be worn for 2 to 3 months. The patient should rest at home for 1 month and avoid bending, lifting, twisting, and all heavy work for a further 2 months. It is wise to warn the patient that a disc does not become herniated unless the affected level has been weakened by recurrent injury. This implies that some extra care throughout life is

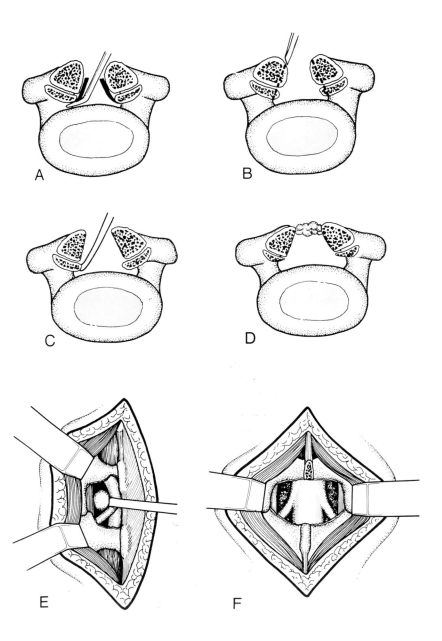

Fig. 15-7 Cross-sectional illustration of the four steps in an operation to treat one-level or multilevel central and lateral stenosis. (**A**) A laminectomy has been performed and a gauge is inserted into the lateral canal to determine its size. (**B**) Removal of the medial third of the inferior articular process with an osteotome. (**C**) Removal of the medial and anterior parts of the superior articular process using the Quintron sonic tool. (**D**) The lateral canals have been enlarged and a free fat graft is placed posterior to the dura. (**E**) Posterior view of a unilateral approach for discotomy. (**F**) Posterior view of a bilateral minimal partial laminectomy for one level central and lateral stenosis.

necessary to avoid becoming overweight, to do exercises daily, and to follow the instructions given in the spine education program.

ONE-LEVEL CENTRAL AND LATERAL STENOSIS

In the early stage, one-level central and lateral stenosis, diagnosed and assessed accurately by the CT scan, may sometimes be managed by the type of conservative measures previously outlined. These are specially indicated when an operation is hazardous because the patient's general condition is poor.[8–11]

Operation

When conservative measures fail, the level of the stenosis is approached through a one-level bilateral minimal partial laminectomy, as described for operation on a disc herniation. After the central portion of the ligamentum flavum is excised on both sides, it may be necessary to remove bone from both the lower edge and the upper lamina and the upper edge of the lower lamina. The inferior articular processes are identified and on each side the medial third of the process is removed using a 1-cm-wide osteotome and mallet until the cartilage of the superior articular process is reached. In doing this, care must be taken not to fracture the base of the inferior process. The medial third of the superior articular process is then removed using the Quintron sonic tool, Kerrison forceps, or osteotome and mallet. Central stenosis is usually relieved by excising the medial third of the inferior and the medial edge of the superior process. In treating lateral stenosis, it is usually necessary to remove more of the superior process until the lateral canal between the anterior surface of the superior process and the back of the vertebral body and disc is at least 6 mm in diameter. Confirmation of canal size is obtained as previously described. Two nerves may be entrapped laterally at any one level. For example at the L4–5 level the L4 nerve may be entrapped just below the pedicle of L4 between the displaced superior process of L5 and the body of L4; the L5 nerve may be entrapped in a narrow subarticular gutter between an enlarged superior articular process of L5 and the back of the L5 vertebral body or the L4–5 disc (Fig. 15-9) (see Chapter 11, Fig. 11-5 to 11-7). In addition, one nerve may be entrapped at either or both of two levels as shown in Figure 15-8. At the end of the procedure a free fat graft, taken subcutaneously, is placed between the dura and the posterior muscles to prevent adhesions.

Instability

When more than a minimal amount of abnormal increased movement is detected by stress radiograms and/or at the time of operation, a one-level fusion should be done at the same operation. Two methods are possible: a posterior facet and intertransverse fusion using iliac crest grafts or a posterior interbody

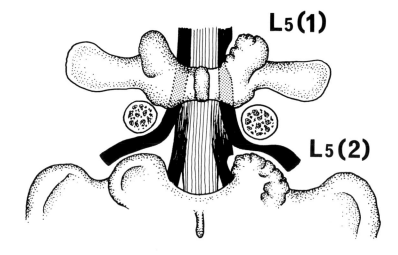

Fig. 15-8 The L5 nerve may be entrapped at one of two different sites: at the L4–5 level, by the medial edge of an enlarged L5 superior facet or between this facet and the back of the L5 vertebral body in the subarticular gutter; and at the L5–S1 level between the superior facet of the sacrum and the pedicle of L5.

fusion. Both of these will be described in detail in Chapter 20.[8,9,12]

CENTRAL AND LATERAL STENOSIS AT SEVERAL LEVELS

Conservative measures are again employed to treat early lesions but are less likely to be effective than in managing one-level stenosis.

Operation

Entry between the laminae is usually made at what is considered the upper or lower end of the stenotic segments. This method may be difficult and time consuming. It is often easier to expose the dura just above or just below the area of the lesion through a normal interlaminar space. Often the interlaminar space is much reduced in size. After the dura is exposed, the aperture is widened as described for treating one-level stenosis, and the medial portions of inferior and superior facets are removed in the same way. From then on, the exposure can be lengthened with Kerrison forceps, with care taken not to injure the dura. It may be difficult to determine the length of the laminectomy. To some extent this can be decided before the operation by studying the myelogram or CT scan and by correlating it with clinical findings. Three examples clarify this point. (1) The patient has clinical signs and symptoms of L5 nerve entrapment. The CT scan demonstrates central stenosis at the L3–4, L4–5, and L5–S1 levels. Decompression of the L5 nerve at the L5–S1 level may well be

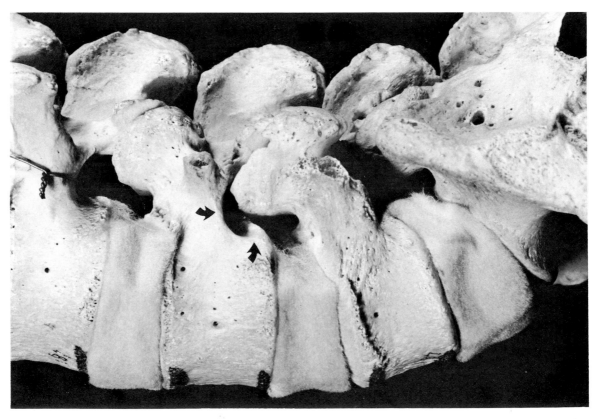

Fig. 15-9 Left lateral view of lumbar spine. At the L4–5 level the L4 nerve may be entrapped between the pedicle of L4 and the tip and anterior aspect of the superior articular process of L5 (arrow on left). The L5 nerve may be entrapped at a slightly lower level and more medially between the anterior aspect of the superior articular process of L5 and a large osteophyte protruding backwards from the posterior surface of the lower part of the body L5–a Heithoff–Dupuis spur (arrow on right).

adequate. (2) The patient has symptoms and signs of entrapment of the L4 and L5 nerves. The CT scan demontrates stenosis at L3–4, L4–5, and L5–S1. Decompression of the L4 and L5 nerves at the L4–5 and L5–S1 levels may well relieve the patient's symptoms. (3) The patient has bizarre symptoms and signs affecting almost the whole of both lower limbs. The CT findings are as described under (2). It is wise to decompress the whole length of the stenotic area.

The presence or absence of pulsation of the dura at operation is another useful guide. When pulsation is absent, the laminectomy should be extended proximally as far as the L2–3 level to restore pulsation. While the laminectomy should be as short as possible, a long laminectomy does not add to the risk of instability, provided that the lateral two thirds of all the facet joints are preserved. At the end of the procedure, a free fat graft is placed posterior to the dura (Fig. 15-10).[10,11,13,14]

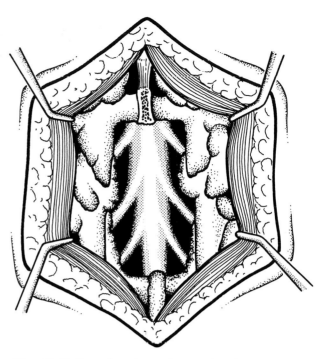

Fig. 15-10 Posterior view of a two-level decompression for central stenosis.

DEGENERATIVE SPONDYLOLISTHESIS

The condition presents either late in Phase II or early in Phase III. Assessment of the phase is most important in deciding what treatment is adequate. Erosion of the articular processes, usually at L4–5, allows the upper vertebra to move anteriorly on the lower as the disc yields. At the L4–5 level, for example, anterior displacement of the inferior process of L4 accompanied by marked erosion of the superior process of L5 entraps the L5 nerve between the processes and the back of the vertebral body of L5.[15]

Conservative Measures

Such measures help some patients. However, it is likely that the patient must put up with back and leg discomfort and pain until the severity of this makes life miserable enough so that the patient requests an operation.

Operation

The approach and the size of the window made by a bilateral minimal partial laminectomy are as described for one-level central or lateral stenosis. The cephalocaudal dimension of the window needs to be slightly greater. Removing the medial part of the inferior articular process is more difficult because it is displaced far forward and because the superior process is eroded. The thin rim of the eroded superior process and the anterior portion of the inferior process are in contact with the nerve. This makes release of the trapped nerve time consuming and difficult.

When marked instability is present, undertaking a one-level fusion—usually a posterolateral fusion—is essential (Fig. 15-11).[15]

ISTHMIC SPONDYLOLISTHESIS

The presentation is most commonly at the L5–S1 level. Posterior joint pain is often at the level above the lesion, at L4–5. Leg pain is due to entrapment of the L5 nerve medial to the L5–S1 foramen. The nerve is compressed or put under tension by the upper part of the pars interarticularis, immediately above the defect.

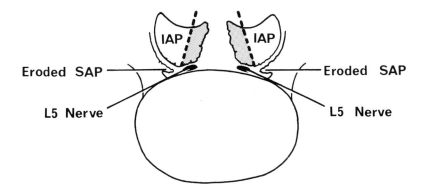

Fig. 15-11 Cross-sectional view illustrating the decompression for degenerative spondylolisthesis at L4–5: IAP, inferior articular process; SAP, eroded superior articular process. Anterior displacement of the inferior process has trapped the L5 nerves on both sides; the amount of the medial portion of the inferior articular processes to be removed is indicated by the dotted lines and shading.

Conservative Measures

Such therapy assists many patients. Pain arising in the posterior joints can be relieved by either manipulation or injection. In some patients the pain experienced arises in the sacroiliac joint. Often a sacroiliac syndrome arises as a complication of spondylolisthesis. The treatment for this has been discussed.

Operation

The plan of treatment propounded by Wiltse[16] and Wiltse et al.[17,18] is a useful guide as to what type of operation should be done. In adolescents with back or leg pain, a fusion (from L5 to the sacrum for a slip at L5–S1 and from L4 to the sacrum for a slip at L4–5) is usually all that is required. In adults with back pain only, a fusion alone usually suffices. In adults with leg pain, decompression alone may be enough. (4) In adults with back and leg pain, the decompression should be followed with a fusion. (5) In patients with spondyloptosis both decompression and fusion should be performed.

Decompression

Removing the loose fragment alone is not enough. It is essential to expose the pars interarticularis just above the defect, identify the nerve and exact site of entrapment, and remove enough of the pars interarticularis at this point to free the nerve (Fig. 15-12). The procedure can be done through a posterior midline incision or through two lateral incisions as described by Wiltse and his group.[18]

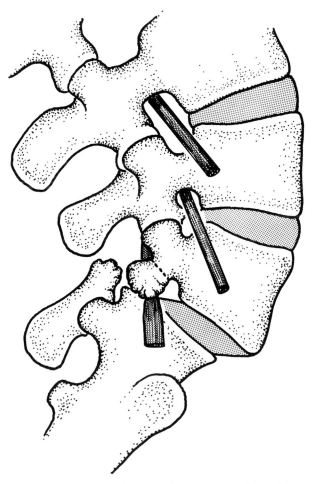

Fig. 15-12 Parasagittal section demonstrating how the L5 nerve is entrapped by the pars interarticularis just above the defect in isthmic spondylolisthesis; the amount of bone to be removed is shown by the dotted line.

Fusion

When fusion alone is to be done, the surgeon can choose either a posterolateral or an anterior-interbody fusion.

When fusion follows decompression, a posterolateral fusion can be undertaken at the same operation. Anterior interbody fusion requires a second operation. Posterior interbody fusion, which theoretically can be done at the same time as the decompression, in the writer's opinion is difficult because of the slip.[16-19]

A Word of Caution

Just as the back pain in spondylolisthesis may arise from a sacroiliac joint, pain after decompression or fusion may have the same origin. Awareness of this possibility and conservative treatment of this separate lesion may save the patient from a second decompression or fusion.

POSTFUSION STENOSIS

Two types are recognized: that due to degenerative changes in the joints just above the fusion—the most common type; and that caused by new bone formation beneath and anterior to the fusion.

Operation

One-level degenerative stenosis above the fusion is relieved by decompression through a bilateral minimal partial laminectomy. Stenosis beneath a fusion presents a more difficult problem. The dura should be exposed just above the top of the fusion and the central portion of the fusion mass removed in a caudal direction. This procedure is time consuming and difficult. Often the dura adheres to the anterior aspect of the fusion.

THE MULTIOPERATED BACK

The first operation should be done with such meticulous attention to detail that it is the last. In practice it is often necessary to consider undertaking a second or third operation. In this situation the personality of the patient, the phase, and the exact site and nature of the lesion should be most carefully assessed.

The most commonly seen lesions, as recorded by Burton et al.[12] are lateral spinal stenosis (58%), central spinal stenosis (7%), arachnoiditis (16%), recurrent disc herniation (12%), and epidural fibrosis (8%). Instability is more common than previously recorded.

Arachnoiditis and epidural adhesions sometimes benefit from epidural steroid injections or from a caudal block. In a few patients, found at reexplora-

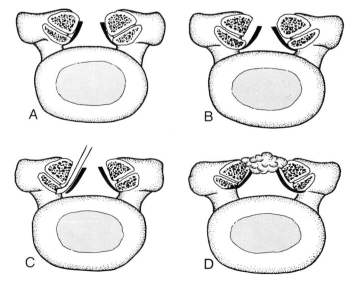

Fig. 15-13 Cross-sectional diagram of the four steps of an operation to decompress the nerves lateral to the dura and in the lateral canal when fibrosis in the multioperated back is present. (**A**) A laminectomy has been performed. (**B**) On the left side the lateral expansion of the ligamentum flavum has been separated from the medial aspect of the inferior articular process and the medial third of this process has been removed. (**C**) the sonic tool is inserted between the ligamentum flavum and the superior articular process to remove its medial and anterior portions. (**D**) The lateral canals have been enlarged and a free fat graft is placed posterior to the dura.

tion to have marked intraspinal fibrosis, repeated epidural steroid administration following the operation has been beneficial.

Operation

The problems encountered are distortion of anatomy because of previous surgery, the presence of adhesions between the dura and the scar tissue posterior to it, and the presence of scar tissue surrounding spinal nerves. The risks encountered during operation are opening of the dura, damage to nerves, and damage to blood vessels leading to hemorrhage, postoperative fibrosis, and nerve ischemia. For these reasons, it is often wise to begin the decompression lateral to the lateral extensions of the ligamentum flavum. These are identified just medial to the inferior articular processes. The plane of cleavage between the ligamentum flavum and the articular processes is developed. The ligament is separated from the superior process anteriorly and laterally. The dura and overlying scar can then be retracted toward the midline, first on one side and then on the other. At this point it is easier to identify the site at which scar adheres to the dura and to excise the scar without opening the dura (Fig. 15-13).

Clearly the advent of magnetic resonance imaging will greatly affect the treatment because it will make the diagnosis much more accurate.

SUMMARY

In this chapter the writer has attempted a brief overall survey of the therapeutic modalities for low back and leg pain. Each of these will be considered in more detail in later chapters in this section.

REFERENCES

1. Sarno J: Mind Over Back Pain. Morrow, New York, 1984
2. Simonton OC, Simonton SM: Getting Well Again. Cancer Control Soc, Azle, TX, 1980
3. Frank JD: Persuasion and Healing. Shocken Books, New York, 1974
4. Sanford A: The Healing Light. Ballentine Books, New York, 1972
5. Mooney V, Robertson J: The facet syndrome. Clin Orthop 115: 149, 1976
6. Edgar MA, Ghadially JA: Innervation of the lumbar spine. Clin Orthop 115: 35, 1976
7. Farfan HF, Kirkaldy-Willis WH: The present status of spinal fusion in the treatment of lumbar intervertebral joint disorders. Clin Orthop 158: 198, 1981
8. Crock HV: Isolated disk resorption. Clin Orthop 115: 109, 1976
9. Crock HV, Venner RM: Clinical Studies of isolated disk resorption in the lumbar spine. J Bone Joint Surg 4B: 491, 1981
10. Getty CJM: Lumbar spinal stenosis. J Bone Joint Surg 62B: 481, 1980
11. Kirkaldy-Willis WH, Paine KWE, Cauchoix J, McIvor GWD: Lumbar spinal stenosis. Clin Orthop 99: 30, 1974
12. Burton CV, Kirkaldy-Willis WH, Yong-Hing K, Heithoff KB: Causes of failure of surgery of the lumbar spine. Clin Orthop 157: 191, 1981
13. Arnoldi CC: Intraosseous hypertension. Clin Orthop 115: 30, 1976
14. Dommisse GF: Arteries and veins of the lumbar nerve roots and cauda equina. Clin Orthop 115: 22, 1976
15. Cauchoix J, Benoist M, Chassaing V: Degenerative spondylolisthesis. Clin Orthop 115: 122, 1976
16. Wiltse LL: The etiology of spondylolisthesis. J Bone Joint Surg 44A: 3539, 1962
17. Wiltse LL, Bateman JG, Hutchinson RH, Nelson WE: The paraspinal sacrospinalis—splitting approach to the lumbar spine. J Bone Joint Surg 50A: 919, 1968
18. Wiltse LL, Widell EH, Jackson DW: Fatigue fracture: the basic lesion in isthmic spondylolisthesis. J Bone Joint Surg 57A: 17, 1975
19. Newman PH: Stenosis of the lumbar spine in spondylolisthesis. Clin Orthop 115: 116, 1976

16

The Back School

Elizabeth S. H. Kirkaldy-Willis

The concept of back school is one of the most important in the management of low back pain. Patients suffering from this condition should attend a back school (spine education program) as early in their treatment as possible. It is as useful in helping the vast majority of patients with minor degrees of pathology as for patients recovering from major surgery. Each patient needs three periods of instruction. The first period of 2 to 2½ hours should be followed 1 to 2 weeks later by a second period of similar duration. In centers where patients attend from a long distance it may be necessary to hold the first instruction period in the morning and the second during the afternoon of the same day. A third period of an additional hour should be held 1 month later to reinforce what has been learned and to test how much of the information given has been retained and is being practiced by the patient.

Many different kinds of programs have been established including (1) the class situation—a therapist instructs six to eight patients; (2) the one-to-one instruction—a doctor or therapist instructs the individual patient; and (3) the industrial back school—a company wants a back school program for their employees. Someone from a back school records on camera employees performing their jobs. A back school program is set up for that specific company including a slide presentation showing how employees can position their backs correctly for the particular job hazards of that company.

The following description is a composite from several different types of programs and is the method we use in Saskatoon.

The instruction should be short, simple, and practical. The patient should participate as fully as possible.

THE SETTING

The setting should be informal. Exercise mats with boxes or chairs are arranged on the floor so that patients can relax lying with hips and knees flexed for at least part of the time spent in the class (Fig. 16-1).

THE OBJECTIVE

The objective of the program is to teach the patient how to help himself or herself. This should be made clear right from the start and repeated two or three times. In our modern society we tend to want everything to be done for us. This attitude leads the patient to expect the physician or therapist to do all the work. For this reason we say, "We understand your trouble. We cannot ourselves do more than a certain amount to help you. However, we can teach you to help and to cure yourself. You will have to work hard to do this. Learn to be good to your back and your back will be good to you." The rest of this chapter is concerned with ways in which the patient can be good to his or her back.

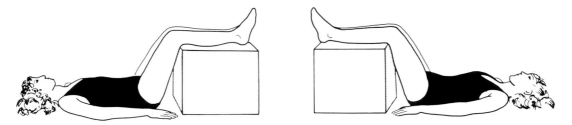

Fig. 16-1 Patients relaxing with hips and knees flexed.

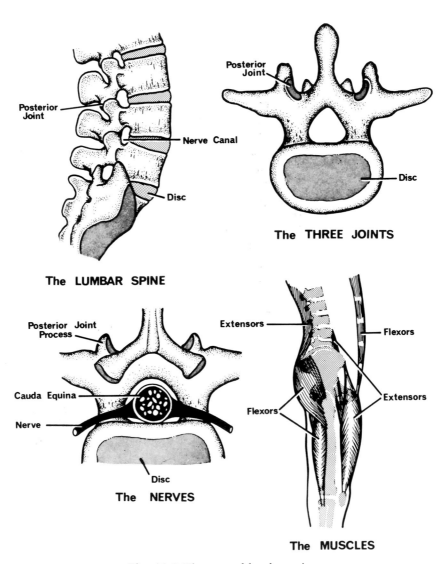

Fig. 16-2 The normal lumbar spine.

THE NORMAL LUMBAR SYSTEM

It is necessary right at the start for the patient to have some knowledge of the way in which the normal lumbar spine functions. Each patient is given a lumbar vertebra to hold while the anatomy is being explained. From top to bottom the lumbar spine has five segments. Each segment has three parts, two small joints at the back and one larger joint in front—the disc. The movement of these three joints is controlled by muscles that bend the spine backward and forward, rotate (twist) it from side to side, and bend it to one side and another. A channel or tube runs down the center of the spine and contains the nerves in a sheath (covering)—the dura. At each level a nerve passes from the sheath to left and right side. It passes along a smaller channel, leaves the spine, and joins other branches to form the nerves that supply the leg (Fig. 16-2).

INJURY TO THE LUMBAR SPINE

The patient who knows something about the normal lumbar spine is better able to understand the reasons for low back and leg pain. Emphasis is placed on simple conditions that are by far the most common causes of pain: poor posture, usually minor and often repeated twisting injuries, and compression resulting from a fall onto the buttocks with the spine flexed (bent forward). The most common type of injury, a posterior joint strain, affects the two small posterior joints at one of the lower two levels. Although this is not serious, it may cause severe pain and spasm (tightness) of the muscles that makes the pain worse. Other, less common conditions that result from these simple posterior joint strains should be mentioned briefly: disc herniation, central stenosis (narrowing of the central tube), lateral stenosis (narrowing of the smaller tubes that contain individual nerves), and instability (weak joints at one level that allow more movement than normal). When the joints do not work normally, muscles also work abnormally. Sometimes they contract (tighten up) and increase the pain. Later on they become weak (flabby) and the spine loses its normal strength (Fig. 16-3). The diagnosis is written on each patient's requisition form. The leader of the class should be aware of all the diagnoses. Patients should be asked if they understand their diagnosis. If a patient is in doubt, it is helpful to explain what is wrong, pointing to the lesion on the diagram on the screen or to the spine model from which the patient is being taught. Again it is very helpful for the patient to handle the vertebrae to see how the spine is constructed.

THE PAIN

As previously stated, pain usually comes from irritation of nerves supplying the posterior joints (Fig. 16-4). This condition may give leg as well as back pain. The common causes of leg pain are a disc herniation and central or lateral stenosis. Irritation of nerves supplying a joint produces electrical impulses that pass along the nerve to the spine and up to the brain where they are recognized as pain.

The Gate

There are two kinds of nerves in the joint—those that are stimulated by movement, rhythm, and activity and those stimulated by injury. The first kind shuts the gate in the spine so that the patient does not feel pain. The second kind results in pain. When the gate is shut (by the first lot of nerves), the painful impulses cannot pass and so the patient feels less pain. It is useful to use the following analogy. Think of a gate on a farm between two fields. Cows (the good impulses that prevent pain) and sheep (the bad painful impulses) are waiting in one field by the gate. If the cows are passing through the gate to the second field, the sheep, because they are smaller, have a difficult time going through; however, if the cows are making no attempt to go through the gate, it is easy for the sheep to do so.

The leader then tells the class how to stimulate the cows (the good impulses) to pass the gate. The following conditions stimulate the cows to go through the gate:

1. Confidence that comes from understanding about one's back problem.
2. Activity (movement), using the back as much as possible without causing pain.
3. Rhythm, learning to move smoothly from one position to another.
4. Avoiding actions that aggravate back pain.

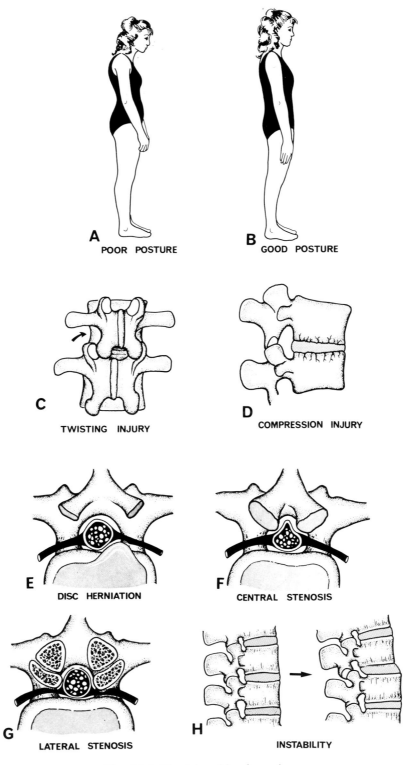

Fig. 16-3 The injured lumbar spine.

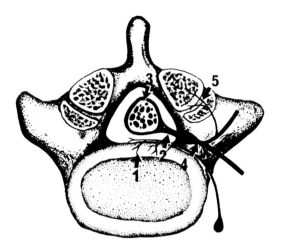

Fig. 16-4 Common sites of nerve irritation. 1. Sinuvertebral nerve from central disc herniation; 2. main spinal nerve from more lateral disc herniation; 3. cauda equina from central stenosis; 4. main spinal nerve and ganglion from lateral canal stenosis; and 5. posterior joint nerves from degeneration of this joint.

The following conditions stimulate the sheep to pass through the gate:

1. Fear: not knowing what is wrong or how serious it is.
2. Holding the back stiffly so that it does not move, or so that it moves in a jerky way.
3. Tenseness and frustration.
4. Not knowing how to avoid actions that increase pain.

In practice all this means that from the start rest and relaxation are important. As the back heals, it is extremely important for the patient to begin to use the muscles to move the back normally and with rhythm. Rhythm can be demonstrated by music—a flowing waltz tune played while the leader moves from place to place around the room demonstrating how to move smoothly while walking, sitting, bending, lifting, and pivoting. The point should be made that the patient is not likely to become pain free until he or she is moving the back almost normally again. Thus, an early return to work (avoiding activities that cause pain) is a most important part of the treatment (Table 16-1).

Table 16-1 Factors that Affect Pain

Decrease pain
Confidence
Movement
Rhythm
Avoidance of painful activity
Increase pain
Fear
Holding back rigid
Tenseness and frustration
Lack of knowledge of how to avoid pain

TREATING BACK STRAINS

Emphasis should be placed on treating back strain, the most common and most easily treated condition. The patient can do a great deal to help himself or herself by following these simple guidelines. As the leader explains the guidelines the patients should be participating (doing the things the leader advises) as far as possible.

Rest and relax for several periods of time each day. (At this point patients should be resting on their backs with hips and knees flexed.)

AIM (Aspirin–Ice–Movement)

Aspirin: one or two tablets three or four times a day helps to relieve pain and counteracts inflammation.

Ice: applied to the back several times a day, reduces muscle spasm (tightness).

Movement: stimulates the good nerves (the cows at the gate) and reduces pain.

Wear a Camp elastic garment or elastic body stocking for both support and help to pull in the tummy muscles, which relieves pain (see Fig. 16-5 B, and Figs. 18-6 and 18-7).

Be aware of posture. Arching the back jams the posterior joints together and increases the pain. Pelvic tilting helps to avoid this by straightening the spine (Fig. 16-5 A). Patients should be taught pelvic tilting first while lying on the floor on the exercise mat (see exercises described below). When they have mastered this, then they should be taught how to pelvic tilt while standing against the wall with their knees slightly flexed (Fig. 16-5 C). They

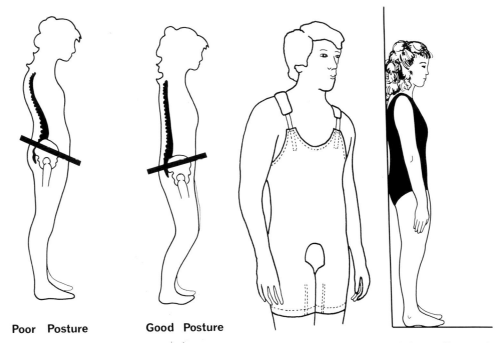

Poor Posture **Good Posture**

Fig. 16-5 (A) Poor and good posture. **(B)** Elasticon support. **(C)** Pelvic tilting while standing against a wall.

should practice pelvic tilting for 5 to 10 minutes several times a day. *Posture Correction:* When patients can pelvic tilt against the wall, attention is directed to the upper spine and the shoulders. The shoulders should not be rounded forward or drawn right back in the military stance, but somewhere in between those two positions, so that the arms fall naturally at the side and the fingers fall along the pants or slacks seam. The neck supports the head, which should be held erect over the shoulders with the chin tucked in gently. At this point the patient should be given some mental images to help "stand tall." The leader can tell the patient to imagine that there is a golden cord attached from the crown of his or her head to a star. Another useful image is to visualize a third eye in between the two bones at the front of the lower neck. The patient should move so that the third eye can have a clear view at all times. To do this, the spine must be straight and the shoulders and neck held erect. Another way to help the patient is to balance a book on his or her head while standing against the wall. Then instruct the patient to walk away

from the wall keeping the book balanced. Good posture is essential for this activity (see Figs. 16-3 A and B, and 16-5 A).

Avoid obesity. The patient should be made aware of the importance of losing weight, of building up abdominal muscles to strengthen the back, and of avoiding stress to the back to obtain a rapid return to normal health. A supervised diet may be suggested as well as regular exercise and the exercise program. Most patients put on weight around the midline, and the leader can point out that when this happens the back is arched to maintain the center of gravity. The obvious example of this is a pregnant woman (Table 16-2).

Table 16-2 Treatment of Back Pain

Rest and relaxation		Elastic support
AIM	Aspirin	Pelvic tilting
	Ice	Reduce obesity
	Movement	

EXERCISE PROGRAM

General Rules

1. Do each exercise slowly. Hold the exercise position for a slow count of five.
2. Start with five repetitions and work up to 10. Relax completely between each repetition.
3. Do the exercises for 10 minutes twice a day.
4. Omit painful exercises from the program.
5. Do the exercises *every day* without fail.

Floor Exercises

PELVIC TILT (Fig. 16-6A)

Lie on your back with knees bent and feet flat on the floor. Pull stomach muscles in slightly and tighten seat muscles. Press low back firmly against the floor, as far as you can without pain. Relax shoulders and breathe normally throughout the exercise. This exercise corrects arching of the back.

MODIFIED SIT-UPS (Fig. 16-6B)

Begin as in Figure 16-6A. Keep your arms by your side. Lift your head so that your chin almost touches your chest. Lift your shoulders off the floor as you reach with both hands for your knees. Touch the top of your knees with your fingers. Lower your shoulders slowly to the floor. Keep your chin tucked in. Then lower your head slowly to the floor. Relax arms and take a deep breath before repeating exercise. Be sure you do not arch your back during any part of this exercise.

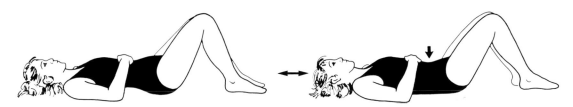

Fig. 16-6A

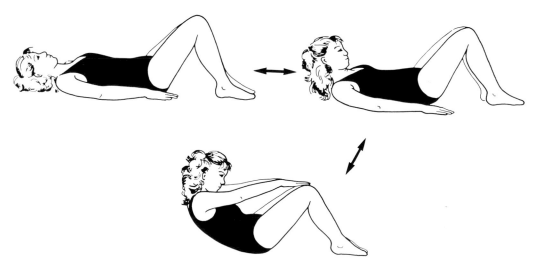

Fig. 16-6B

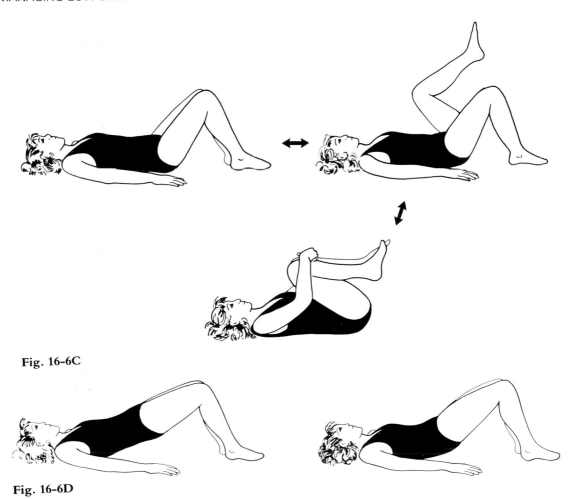

Fig. 16-6C

Fig. 16-6D

DOUBLE KNEE-TO-CHEST OR LOW BACK STRETCH (Fig. 16-6C)

Begin as in Figure 16–6A. Bring both knees to your chest, one at a time. Hug your knees and gently pull them toward you until you feel a mild stretch in your low back. Lower your legs slowly to the starting position, one at a time. Be sure you do not arch your back during any part of this exercise.

SEAT LIFTS (Fig. 16-6D)

Begin as in Figure 16–6A. Lift your seat up off the floor, very slowly, a little at a time. Keep your low back flat. Slowly lower your body, allowing your low back to touch the floor first and then your seat. Be sure you do not arch your back during any part of this exercise.

MOUNTAIN AND SAG. KNEE TO ELBOW (Fig. 16-6E)

Start on hands and knees. Make a mountain out of your back (round your back). Then let your back sag, slowly and carefully like an old horse (arch your back). Repeat 5 to 10 times. Bring your knee to your elbow, then straighten your leg behind you. Watch underneath your body and do not lose sight of your toes; you do not want to arch your back. Then bring your knee back to your elbow and put your knee down. Repeat with the other leg.

HAMSTRING STRETCH (Fig. 16-6F)

This can be done lying, standing or sitting. (1) Begin as in Figure 16–6A. Bring one knee to your chest (Fig. 16–6F). Put both hands around your thigh. Stretch your heel up to the ceiling to extend your

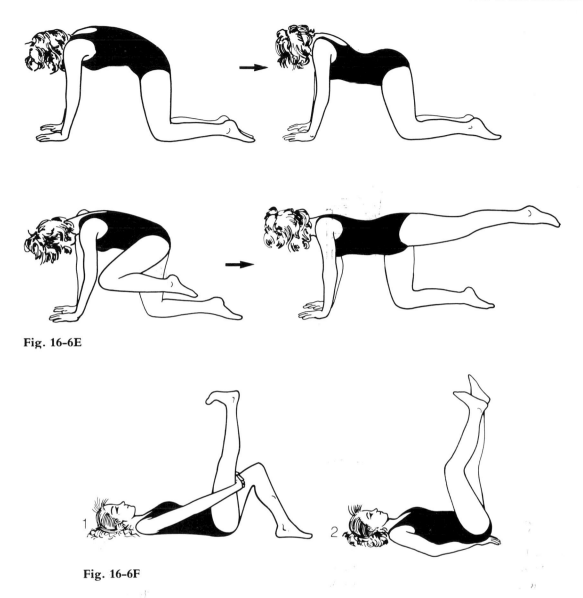

Fig. 16–6E

Fig. 16–6F

knee as far as possible. Gently pull your leg toward you until it is vertical. Dorsiflex your foot at the ankle. Repeat with the other leg. (2) Lying on your back, put your hands under your buttocks. Slowly, lift your legs over your head. *Do not* keep your legs straight when lifting them. Then, flap your feet.

Figure 16–6G shows another exercise for hamstring stretch. (1) Stand with one leg propped on a table or back of a chair. Bend the leg you are standing on until you feel a mild stretch under your thigh. Repeat with the other leg.

(2) Stand with one leg on low platform or stool. Dorsiflex this foot at the ankle. The knee of the leg you are standing on should be slightly bent. Slowly, bend from the hips towards the leg on the stool until you feel a mild stretch under your thigh. Repeat with the other leg.

Figure 16–6H shows a final hamstring stretch exercise. Sit on the floor with one leg bent and the other almost straight. Lean toward the bent leg until you feel a mild stretch under the other thigh. Repeat with the other leg.

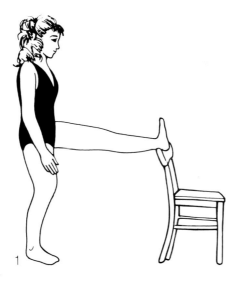

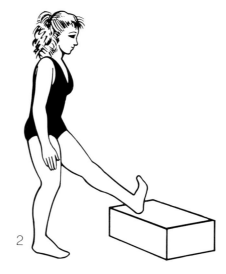

Fig. 16–6G

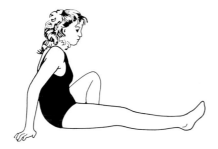

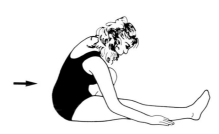

Fig. 16–6H

Swimming Exercises

Swimming in warm water is one of the best activities for patients with low back pain, but diving is inadvisable. Repeat all the exercises 10 times. Omit any that cause pain.

1. With back to the wall, bring knees to chest and rotate to the right and then to the left.
2. Bring knees to chest. Straighten legs, but keep them at a right angle to your body. Spread legs apart, then bring them back together.
3. With legs out in front (as in exercise 2), open legs and then cross them like a pair of scissors.
4. Stand up with back to the wall, raise one leg straight in front, then pull back down. Repeat with other leg.
5. With back to wall, raise knee up to hip level, allowing knee to bend. Straighten and bend knee. Repeat with other leg.
6. Turn with side to wall. Kick outside leg up in front, then behind, then to side and down. Repeat on other side.
7. Face wall and kick one leg out behind, keeping leg straight. Repeat with other leg.
8. Facing bar, put both feet on bar. Bend and straighten knees.
9. With back to the wall, pretend you are riding a bicycle.
10. Back to wall, make a circle with one leg. Be sure foot touches surface of water as well as bottom of pool. Reverse direction. Repeat with other leg.

General Fitness for the Cardiorespiratory System: Aerobic Exercises

Patients with low back pain who have good heart/lung fitness tend to have less frequent and shorter periods of pain. They can accomplish daily tasks or prolonged activity without getting tired so quickly. Because they are fit they have the energy to use their muscles and spine correctly during activity. Patients should choose activities that allow them to exercise long enough for their heart and lungs to work—15 minutes or more if possible without stopping. It is important to increase some activity in the daily schedule gradually. Movement is good for the back. Regular exercise improves the patient's outlook on life a great deal.

RULES FOR SAFE AEROBIC EXERCISES

1. Exercise at least three times a week, on alternate days.
2. Start slowly with a new exercise and progress gradually.
3. Learn the correct technique by having a lesson if necessary. Poor technique can bring on back pain.
4. Avoid the positions that you have been taught are bad for your back.
5. Avoid being competitive. Work at your own speed and ability.
6. A gradual 5 to 10 minutes warm up is invaluable in preventing pain during activity (running on the spot, swinging arms and then stretching slowly). Cool down afterward in the same way.
7. Avoid fatigue. Stop and rest now and then when you start to feel tired.

SOME RECOMMENDED AEROBIC ACTIVITIES

1. Walking—Start slowly and progress to 1 mile in 15 minutes if possible.
2. Swimming—The water supports your body and takes the weight off your low back. Front crawl, back crawl, and side stroke are usually the safest for patients with back pain.
3. Cycling—A stationary bicycle or a regular bicycle. Adjust the seat and the handlebars so that you can sit nearly upright and pelvic tilt. You should be able to reach the lower pedal with leg extended and knee slightly bent.
4. Nonimpact aerobics—Designed for those with back problems. There are low, medium, or high intensity classes. If there is any individual exercise in the class that is done in a position that hurts your back, avoid that exercise (Fig. 16-7).
5. Cross-country skiing—This sport is smooth, rhythmical, and good for your back. Pay attention to your posture and maintain the pelvic tilt.
6. Skating—Skate easily and within your limits to avoid falls. Skate in a smooth rhythmical way. Avoid figure skating and jumps that arch the back.

Relaxation Exercise

Demands and frustrations in daily life cause an increase of tension and stress, which may build up slowly and imperceptibly. By the time it causes pain it is severe. Tension may be felt in different ways—headache, fatigue, or back pain. Tension produces tightness in the muscles of the neck, top of the shoulders, shoulder blades and deep lower back areas. When there is tension in these muscles we cannot move correctly and the muscles can become very painful.

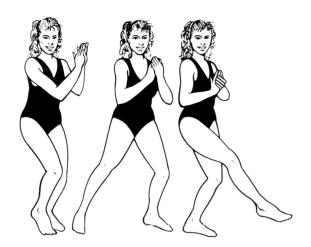

Fig. 16-7 Nonimpact aerobics.

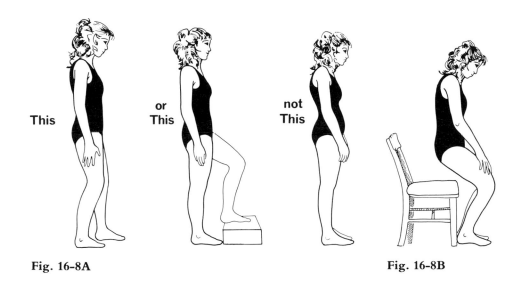

This   **or This**   **not This**

Fig. 16-8A   Fig. 16-8B

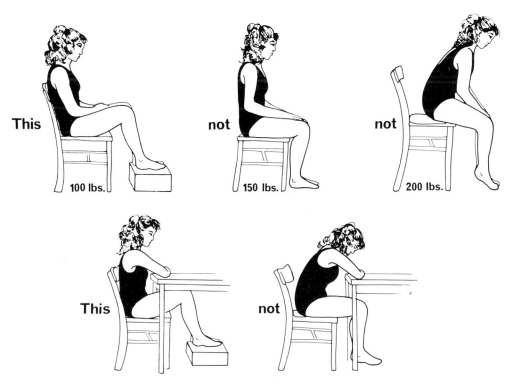

This 100 lbs.   **not** 150 lbs.   **not** 200 lbs.

This   **not**

Fig. 16-8C

One way to deal with this is to recognize the muscle tension when it starts to build and to learn to relax the muscles before the pain starts to get worse. It is also important to practice relaxing on a regular basis. The following steps may help:

1. Set aside 15 to 20 minutes of uninterrupted time, daily if possible. Use a quiet room away from telephone, television, or other distractions. Loosen clothing. Lie in the recommended resting position with hips and knees flexed, or sit with knees higher than hips (see Fig. 16-1 or 16-8C).

2. Close your eyes, or focus on a spot on the ceiling or wall. Concentrate and put all other things out of your mind.

3. Listen to your breathing. Concentrate on how smooth and regular it is. Place one hand just below the ribs. Your stomach should be rising and falling with your breathing. Continue to concentrate on your breathing. Take a slow, deep breath. As you breathe out feel the tension going out of your body and feel yourself relax. Think of letting yourself become heavy and relaxed. Feel your stomach area slowly rise and fill like a balloon. Feel the air enter your nose and lungs. Let the air out slowly. Feel your stomach area gently fall. Feel yourself relaxing as you breathe out.

4. As you continue deep relaxed breathing you may start to feel pleasantly warm and this is good. Improved blood circulation may raise your body temperature. Your legs and arms may feel heavy and relaxed. Try to remember this feeling. Teach your body to relax like this frequently during the day.

5. As you breathe in, tighten the right hand into a fist. Hold for 5 seconds thinking "my hand is tense." Then let go and let the hand go limp for three to four breaths. Do this three times and then repeat with the left hand.

6. Tighten the right hand into a fist, bend the elbow and move the fist to the shoulder. At the same time tighten the shoulder and neck muscles. Hold for 5 seconds and relax for three to four breaths. Do this three times and repeat with left side.

7. The muscles in the legs, back, and head can be tightened and relaxed in the same way as above.

8. Finish your relaxation session when you feel ready, but try to maintain some of that relaxed state as you open your eyes and get up.

Relaxation exercise should be done at least once a day. The result will be a healthier and happier patient.

Summary of Exercise Program

The exercise program should be split up between the first and second periods of instruction as best suits the patient. Four floor exercises should be taught during the first session, and the others should be taught during the second session. Swimming, aerobics and relaxation exercises should also be explained during the seond session.

The reader will note that most of the floor exercises are flexion exercises. It should be pointed out that some patients do not tolerate flexion exercises well and require more extention exercises. This is fully explained in Chapter 22.

BASIC BODY MECHANICS

Standing (Fig. 16-8A)

One foot forward, knees slightly bent; one foot up to change position.

To Sit (Fig. 16-8B)

Pelvic tilt; flex hips and knees; do not bend forward from the hips or waist. Lower yourself to the chair; use your hands if necessary. Sit on the front edge of the chair. Hold onto the back of the seat with your hands and pull yourself to the back of the seat. **To Get Up.** Reverse the procedure.

Sitting (Fig. 16-8C)

Sit slightly reclined, knees higher than hips, low back supported. Get close to work with chair, not with head.

Reaching (Fig. 16-8D)

Brushing Teeth (Fig. 16-8E)

Bend and rest knees or open cabinet door and put foot on low shelf or on a stool.

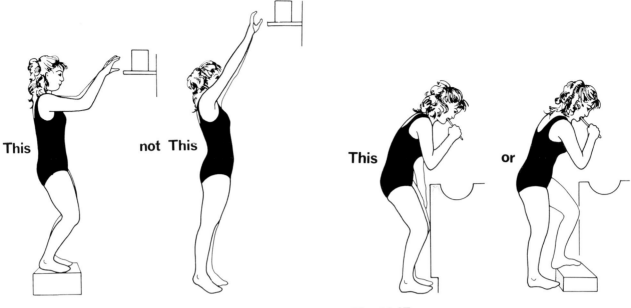

Fig. 16-8D

Fig. 16-8E

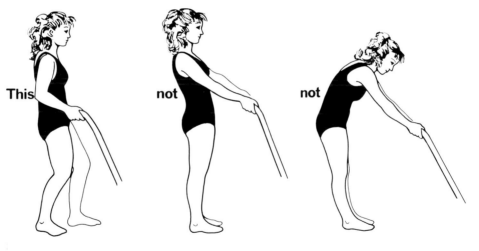

Fig. 16-8F

Weight Shift and Diagonal (Vacuuming) (Fig. 16-8F)

Left foot forward. Hold vacuum with right hand close to body. Take small step forward with left foot. Shift weight to right leg. Move forward with small steps and with rhythm.

Push More than Pull (Fig. 16-8G)

Lifting (Fig. 16-8H)

For light objects support body with one hand and lift opposite leg in air. Partial squat.

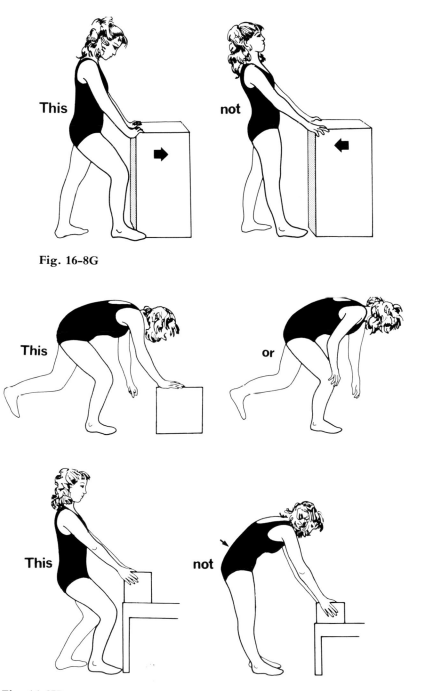

This　not

Fig. 16–8G

This　or

This　not

Fig. 16–8H

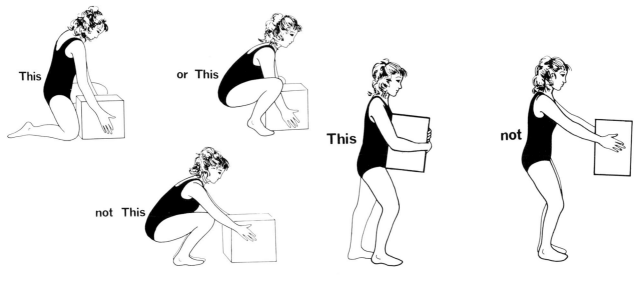

Fig. 16-8I

Fig. 16-8J

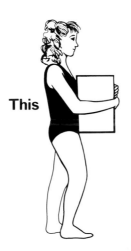

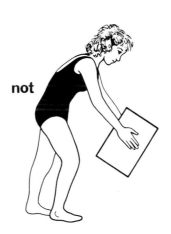

Fig. 16-8K

More Lifting (Fig. 16-8I)

For heavy objects full squat with one foot forward.

Keep Load Close (Fig. 16-8J)

Shift Weight to Back Leg Before Walking (Fig. 16-8K)

Recommended Sleeping Positions (Fig. 16-8L)

Getting in and out of Bed (Fig. 16-8M)

If your right side is more painful get in on the right side of the bed. (1) Sit on edge of bed with knees bent. (2) Let your head and trunk down onto the bed to lie on the right side and bring your legs onto the bed. (3) Roll carefully onto back with knees bent. (4) Reverse the procedure to get out of bed.

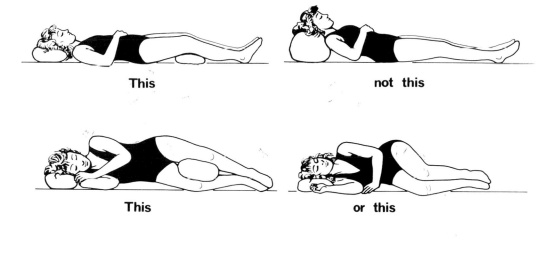

This   not this

This   or this

not this

Fig. 16–8L

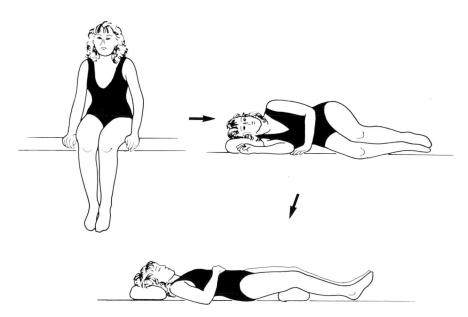

Fig. 16–8M

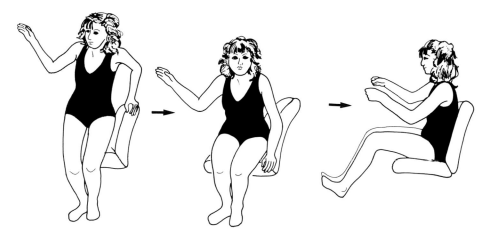

Fig. 16-8N

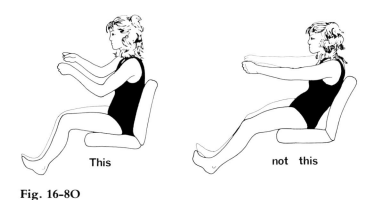

This   not this

Fig. 16-8O

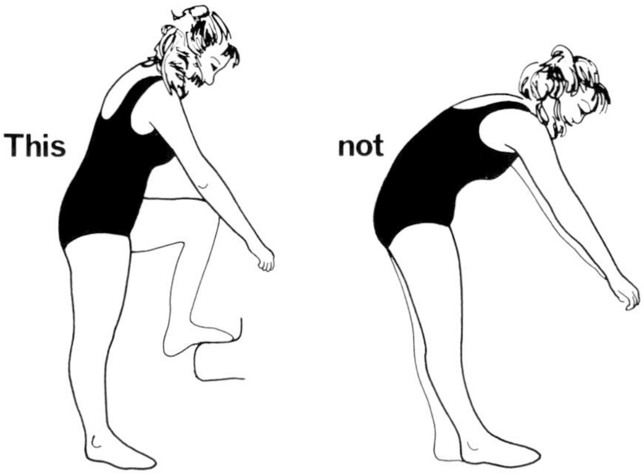

This   not

Fig. 16-8P

Getting in and out of Car (Fig. 16-8N)

Bend hips and knees with spine slightly flexed and lower yourself onto the seat facing the door. Use your hands on the door to help. Flex hips and knees further to bring your feet into the car. Using your hands, turn your whole body and legs as one unit to face forward in the car without twisting your low back. To get out of the car reverse the procedure.

Sitting in Car (Fig. 16-8O)

Do not attempt to drive your car when you have severe back pain.

Use Bumper on Car (Fig. 16-8P)

DOS AND DONT'S

When Your Back is Painful

SITTING

Avoid sitting. If you must sit: (1) Get up and move around every 20 minutes. (2) Use back and/or foot support. (3) Legs must not be straight out in front, as in sitting in bed, in the bathtub, or on the floor. (4) Use a small towel roll or magazine roll behind your low back. This will help straighten the curve in your low back. (5) Avoid leaning your trunk forward while sitting. (6) Sitting with poor posture is certain to aggravate your back pain. (7) When standing up, move to the edge of the chair; position one foot in front of the other; and use your legs to stand without leaning forward.

DRIVING

When your back is painful, try to avoid driving. As a passenger you can lie down on the back seat and bend your knees. When driving, bring the seat up close to the wheel so that your knees are slightly higher than your hips. Do not get so close to the wheel that you cannot turn it. Use a towel roll or magazine roll behind your low back. Stop frequently, for instance every 20 to 30 minutes, get out of the car and stretch. The hamstring stretch exercise is very helpful. Put foot on the rear bumper of the car (see Fig. 16-6G (2)).

BENDING FORWARD

When your back is painful try to avoid bending forward at the waist. Bending increases pressure on the disc. Think of this while performing all of your daily activities. Kneeling to make beds and to reach low levels is a good alternative when your back is painful.

LYING

A good firm support is desirable. The floor is too firm; a saggy mattress is too soft. When getting out of bed, turn to one side, draw your knees up and drop your feet over the edge. At the same time, push yourself up with your arms and avoid bending forward at the waist.

COUGHING AND SNEEZING

When your back is painful, stand up, if you can, and bend your knees. If a wall is handy, brace yourself against it. If you are sitting and cannot stand, lean back in your chair. Always avoid leaning forward at the waist. If possible, tighten your stomach muscles before you cough or sneeze.

When You Are Feeling Better

SITTING

Sit with a back support cushion. You may also maintain the same position with your own muscles. While you sit, do the pelvic tilt exercise for the low back to work out sore spots. Get up and move around every 20 to 30 minutes.

Recurrence

The next time you feel the warning signs of impending back pain:

1. Use the first aid technique—aspirin–ice–massage and stretching (AIM) to get rid of any muscle spasm.
2. Do the exercises that helped decrease the pain during the last episode.
3. If the first aid regimen every hour does not help significantly in the first 48 hours, or if you experience a different back or leg pain from that experienced before, see your doctor and follow his or her advice.

Summary of Basic Body Mechanics

Teaching patients with low back pain about basic body mechanics is most important. Knowing how to use the painful back correctly does more to get rid of the pain than anything else. As far as possible all the patients should do all the activities explained by the leader. Patients should be encouraged to ask questions all the way through the instruction.

Before the patients leave, the leader should once again emphasize the vital point that they are responsible for their own cure. This means hard work day after day, making the back school program part of their daily lives.

REVIEW OF KNOWLEDGE GAINED

The patient should return to back school 1 month after the second session of instruction (1) to test how much knowledge has been retained, (2) to make sure that the patient has been practicing the body mechan-

ics that were taught, and (3) to review any exercises and body mechanics that were found to be confusing or difficult.

A good approach is first to ask each patient what problems have been encountered and deal with these individually. It is difficult for some patients to realize that painful exercises must be reduced in number or avoided for a time. This point can be brought home by saying, "When driving your car and you come to a red light, you stop until the light changes to green. Pain is your red light. This red light tells you to stop what you are doing, to do less of the activity, or to modify it." The activity may be housework, work on the farm, or exercises.

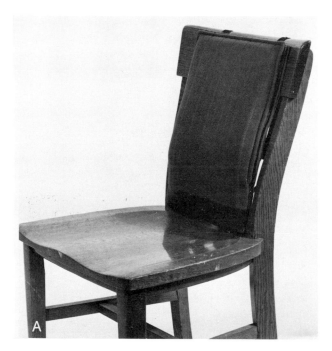

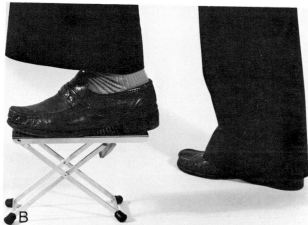

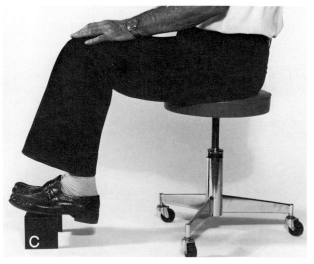

Fig. 16-9 Useful aids for back pain. **(A)** Spina-Bac, a firm, adjustable, portable cushion. **(B)** Back Easer footstool. **(C)** guitar-player's footstool, which serve to raise knees higher than hips.

SOME USEFUL AIDS

A Cushion for the Back

Many patients are helped by a firm cushion that can be carried around and placed behind the back in the chair at the office or home, in the car, on an aircraft, and in other similar situations. A recommended model is the Spina-Bac (Spina Bac, Fimax Inc., P.O. Box 595030, Miami, FL, 33159). The patient can adjust this to three different positions so that one cushion suits anyone. It can be fastened to the back of the chair with Velcro strips (Fig. 16-9A).

Foot Supports

A folding pocket footstool is useful for many people suffering from low back pain. When sitting in a chair, the patient should keep the knees slightly higher than the hips. The footstool is a simple way of achieving this. It is also helpful when standing to place one foot on a stool. This allows slight flexion of hip and knee and relaxes the low back. One type of stool is the Back Easer (Back Easer Footstool, T. Milburn Co., Ltd., D. Floor, 100 Front Street West, Toronto, M5J 1E3). A similar stool used by guitar players can be obtained at most stores that sell musical instruments (Fig. 16-9B, C).

ACKNOWLEDGMENTS

The author wishes to acknowledge her debt to Mrs Nancy Selby and her staff at the Spine Education Center, Dallas, Texas; Dr. Arthur White, St. Mary's Spine Center, San Francisco, California; Mrs. Lynne White, Health Education Systems Inc., Kentfield, California; and Dr. Hamilton Hall, The Canadian Back Institute, Toronto, Ontario, for their help and advice.

17
Manipulation

J. David Cassidy
William H. Kirkaldy-Willis

Manipulation is an art that requires much practice to acquire the necessary skill and competence. Few medical practitioners have the time or inclination to master it. This modality has much to offer the patient with low back pain, especially in the earlier stages during the phase of dysfunction. We have seen in previous chapters that the majority of patients are first seen while in this phase. Most practitioners of medicine, whether family physicians, or surgeons, will wish to refer their patients to a practitioner of manipulative therapy with whom they can cooperate, whose work they know, and whom they can trust. The physician who makes use of this resource will have many contented patients and save himself many headaches.

In this chapter we will ask and try to answer the following questions: What is manipulation? How dow it work? When is it indicated? What are the results of treatment? Because this book is written largely for medical practitioners, we will not attempt to describe the details of the technique. Those with a special interest should not only read textbooks on the subject but also be prepared to complete a full apprenticeship with one or more skilled practitioners before embarking on this method of treatment themselves.

WHAT IS MANIPULATION?

The definition given by Sandoz[1,2] is both clear and concise. A manipulation or lumbar invertebral joint adjustment is a passive manual maneuver during which the three-joint complex is suddenly carried beyond the normal physiological range of movement without exceeding the boundaries of anatomical integrity. The usual characteristic is a thrust—a brief, sudden, and carefully administered "impulsion" that is given at the end of the normal passive range of movement. It is usually accompanied by a cracking noise.

The stages of a manipulation are illustrated in Figure 17-1. The central arc on each side of the neutral position represents the range of active movement in one plane such as flexion-extension, lateral bending, or rotation. Passive movement increases the range of movement in both directions and at the end of this, when the slack is taken up, the practitioner feels a resistance, the elastic barrier of resistance. When mobilization is forced beyond this elastic barrier; a sudden yielding is felt; a cracking noise is perceived; and the range of movement is slightly increased beyond the physiological limit into the paraphysiological space. At this point a second final barrier of resis-

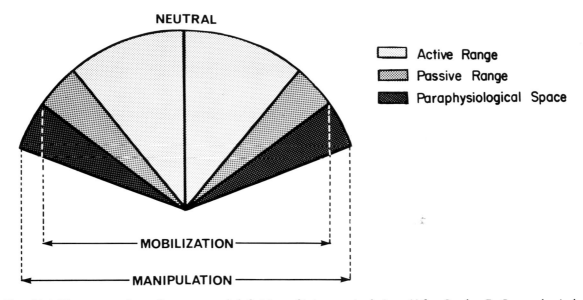

Fig. 17-1 The stages of an adjustment and definition of joint manipulation. (After Sandoz R: Some physical mechanisms and effects of spinal adjustments. Ann Swiss Chirop Assoc 6:91, 1976.)

tance is encountered, formed by the stretched ligaments and capsule; it is called the limit of anatomical integrity. Forcing movement beyond this point would damage the ligamanets and capsule.

The four zones distinguished in joint adjustment are (1) active movement, (2) passive movement, (3) paraphysiological zone, and (4) pathological zone of movement.

The two zones are the elastic barrier, overcome by a thrust without damage to joint structures, and the limit of anatomical integrity, which cannot be surpassed without injuring ligaments and capsule.

HOW DOES MANIPULATION WORK?

The Effect of Manipulation on a Normal Joint

Two British anatomists, Roston and Wheeler Haines,[3] published a paper in 1947 entitled "Cracking in the metacarpo-phalangeal joint." The three phalanges of the middle finger were wrapped in adhesive tape and the tape was attached to a spring dynamometer to indicate the degree of tension applied to the finger. A progressively increasing force was applied

to distract the metacarpophalangeal joint. Radiographs were taken at intervals to record changes in the joint space. In this experiment, the force was applied by a machine and not manually and by progressive traction rather than by a thrust, but the conditions may be considered comparable with those in a spinal adjustment.

The results of the experiment are shown in Figure 17-2. The tension is recorded on the abscissa and the separation of the cartilage surfaces on the ordinate. The initial separation of 1.8 mm is due to the thickness of the cartilages. The separation increases gradually up to a tension of 8 kg. At this point the surfaces jump to a separation of 4.7 mm and a cracking noise is heard. Increasing tension to 18 kg produces a further joint separation up to 5.4 mm. On reduction of the tension the joint surface separation is again approximately 2 mm, a distance slightly more than the initial separation of 1.8 mm. The ways in which the results of this experiment may be correlated with apophyseal joint manipulation are shown in Figure 17-3.

Three phenomena occur at the same time as the elastic barrier is passed: The articular surfaces separate suddenly; a cracking noise is heard; a radiolucent space appears within the joint. These occurrences can be explained as follows. Normally a small negative pressure is present in a joint space; it maintains the cartilage

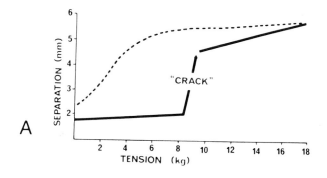

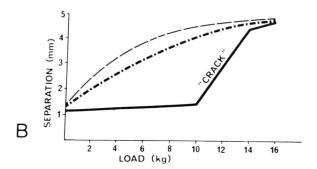

Fig. 17-2 (A) Effect of manipulation on a normal joint. A "crack" is heard at 9 kg of tension, with separation of the cartilage surfaces. Increasing tension produces some further separation of the surfaces. When the tension is released (the dotted line), the separation of the surfaces decreased but does not quite return to normal. (After Roston JB, Wheeler Haines RW: Cracking in the metacarpophalangeal joint. J Anat 81:165, 1947.) **(B)** Following the "crack" (lower solid line) the joint separation returns nearly to normal after 15 minutes (upper curve). On reloading immediately after "cracking," the joint separation follows the middle curve. No "crack" is heard. (Modified from Unsworth A, Dowson D, Wright V: Cracking joints, a bioengineering study of cavitation in the metacarpophalangeal joint. Ann Rheum Dis 30:348, 1971.)

surfaces in apposition and is one of the factors that maintain stability of the joint. With axial traction the synovial folds and capsule tends to invaginate toward the center of the joint.

When the joint surfaces are forced apart beyond the elastic barrier (to the limit of invagination of the soft tissues), the intra-articular pressure drops to a point where gas is suddenly liberated from the synovial fluid to form a bubble within the center of the joint space. As quickly as this bubble forms it collapses with an audible crack.[4] If tension is maintained across

the joint space, the gas will reform and can be seen on a radiograph (Fig. 17-4).[5] A refractory period of 20 min is required before the joint can be recracked. During this time the gases are slowly returned to solution in the synovial fluid. Analysis of the gas formed in the metacarpophalangeal joint by synovial fluid cavitation has shown that it consists of over 80% carbon dioxide.[4] Manipulation also stimulates the mechanoreceptors (see Chapter 5) with an effect both on the segmental muscles at the level of the intervertebral joint and on the pain mechanism (see Posterior Joint Syndrome, below).[2]

The Therapeutic Effect of Manipulation on the Abnormal Joint

Reference to the discussion of pathology and pathogenesis in Chapter 4 will make it clear that though we know much about the changes that take place, we still know very little about the way in which lumbar spinal disorders are initiated at the start of the degenerative process. Currently we know equally little about the effects of spinal adjustment. However, it is possible to postulate the ways in which this form of treatment may work in different spinal lesions.

POSTERIOR JOINT SYNDROME

In the posterior joint syndrome the joint may lock entrapping a synovial fold and a minor subluxation of facets may be present.[6] In acute back pain an arthrokinetic reflex results in a state of hypertonic contraction of paraspinal muscles splinting the posterior joints.[7] An adjustment (manipulation) that separates the articular surfaces may release entrapped synovial folds and stretch the segmental muscles initiating spindle mediated reflexes that relieve the state of hypertonicity and perhaps reduce a 1- or 2-mm subluxation.[8] In more chronic cases, manipulation might break intra-articular adhesions that have been observed in the posterior joints (see Chapter 4).[9] In both acute and chronic posterior joint syndrome, joint movement, previously restricted, is increased by the manipulation. Increased movement causes an increase in proprioceptive input to the spine, which has a reflex inhibition on the transmission of pain (see Chapter 5).[10]

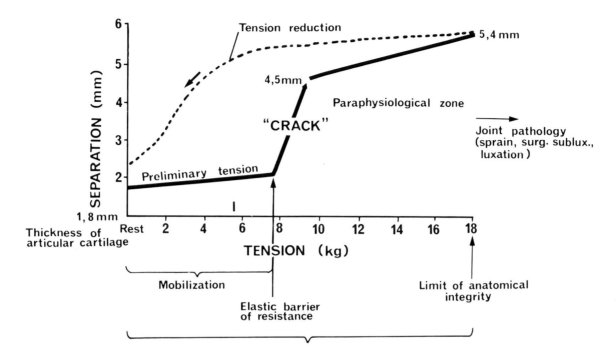

Fig. 17-3 Correlation of experiments described in Figs. 17-2 with intervertebral joint adjustment. (After Sandoz R: The significance of the manipulative crack and of other articular noises. Ann Swiss Chirop Assoc 4:47, 1969.)

SACROILIAC SYNDROME

In the sacroiliac syndrome local and reflex pain is present and movement is restricted. In our present state of knowledge it is difficult to envisage how synovium can be entrapped or how subluxation can occur in a joint that has very small range of movement. Adjustments directed specifically to this joint, however, often relieve the symptoms.

Possibly the effect is produced by stretching the posterior muscles, breaking intra-articular adhesions and relieving the joint fixation with the resultant stimulation of the surrounding mechanoreceptors.

QUADRATUS LUMBORUM SYNDROME

In the quadratus lumborum syndrome and other paraspinal myofascial syndromes, there is hypertonicity and a tender trigger point in the belly of the muscle. It is postulated that when the lesion is not treated quickly, fibrosis develops within the affected portion of the muscle. The thrust of the adjustment is directed to stretching the tight segment of muscle.

HERNIATION OF THE NUCLEUS PULPOSUS

Many theories have been propounded to explain the way in which manipulative adjustments may relieve the patient with this condition of back and leg pain. We are doubtful that manipulation can reduce a large disc herniation. Availability of the high resolution CT scanner and soft tissue imaging make it possible now to visualize accurately the site and size of a disc herniation and to assess the effects of different forms of treatment by repeat scanning after a period of time. Before long the physician should be in a position to say what form of treatment is most effective.

De Sèze[11,12] believes that lumbago develops because a fragment of the nucleus pulposus becomes incarcerated within an annular tear with resultant bulging of the annulus and pressure on the sinuvertebral nerve.

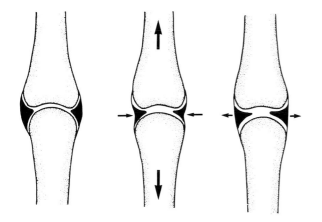

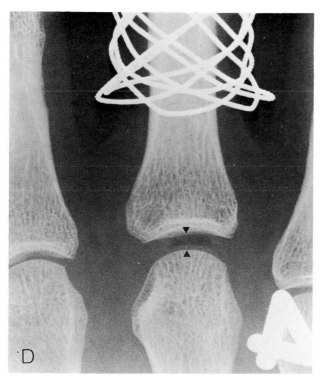

Fig. 17-4 (A–C) The effect of traction on the metacarpophalangeal joint. **(D)** Gas in joint space after manipulation of the metacarpophalangeal joint (arrows).

His adjustment exerts rotatory traction on the spine as follows: The lumbar spine is flexed with the patient lying on the side so that the disc space is opened posteriorly. The upper shoulder is rotated backward and the lower shoulder pulled forward. Lateral flexion

causes the disc space to open on the upper side. The shoulder girdle and the pelvis are further rotated in different directions to produce torsion. A thrust is delivered. The way in which de Sèze and others think that these manipulations work is shown in Figure 17-5.

Levernieux's experiments[13] on spines obtained at autopsy are of considerable interest. He injected an opaque dye into the disc, then placed the specimen in a traction device, and obtained radiographs before, during and after traction. When the disc was disrupted internally, the dye passed from front to back of the disc and sometimes protruded into the spinal canal. During traction the disc space became wider and the dye passed toward the center of the disc. When traction was discontinued, a part of the contrast medium was retained in the center of the disc (Fig. 17-6).

Chrisman et al[14] found that 51% of patients with sciatica improved clinically on side posture manipulation but that no change in the myelographic appearance occurred (Fig. 17-7).

Mathews and Yates,[15] using epidurography before and after manipulation in cases of acute lumbago, demonstrated that the bulge seen at the back of the disc was smaller in size following treatment.

Sandoz considers that traction for an internal derangement of the disc may aid in reducing sequestered

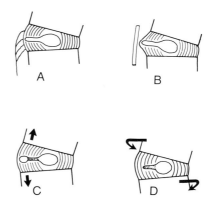

Fig. 17-5 Explanation of the way in which manipulation may reduce pressure of a disc herniation on a nerve. **(A)** Herniation with irritation of branches of sinuvertebral nerve. **(B)** Herniation with pressure on a spinal nerve. **(C)** Traction separates the vertebral bodies and allows the herniated material to return to the nucleus. **(D)** Rotation encourages further return of herniated material to the nucleus. (After de Sèze S: Les manipulations vertebral. Sem Hôp Paris 12313, 1955.)

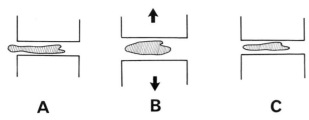

Fig. 17-6 Effect of traction after discography. **(A)** Disc herniation: dye protruding backwards (to the left). **(B)** On traction the protruding disc material returns to the centre of the disc. **(C)** On relaxing the traction the disc material tends to remain in the center of the disc. (After Levernieux J: Les tractions vertebrales. L'expansion, Paris, 1960.)

nuclear material but that it is difficult to see how traction can be of benefit in cases when the disc is extruded. He thinks that the aim of treatment should not be to reduce the herniation, but to ease the disco-radicular conflict. Figure 17-8 demonstrates the antalgic posture assumed for a herniation lateral to the nerve and for one medial to the nerve. He postulates that manipulation in the direction of this antalgic posture benefits the patient by shifting the inflamed nerve away from the herniation.[1,17]

We have to admit that most publications on the role of manipulation for a disc herniation deal mainly with theoretical concepts. On the other hand it is

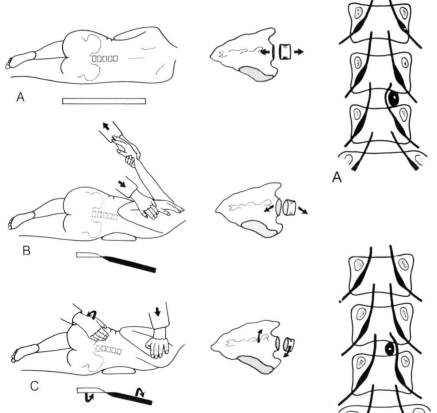

Fig. 17-7 The three stages of the mechanism of sideposture adjustment. **(A)** Flexing the plevis and thigh opens the disc space posteriorly. **(B)** The upper shoulder is rotated backward and the lower shoulder is rotated forward to create a turning moment. The pillow under the lower flank causes lateral flexion of the lumbar spine. The disc spaces are opened on the upper side. **(C)** Rotation of the pelvis and shoulder girdles in opposite directions produces a torque in the lumbar spine. The effect of this adjustment is a helicoidal traction exerted on the upper posterolateral portion of the motion segment.

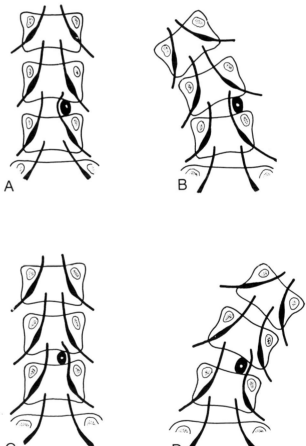

Fig. 17-8 Explanation of direction of scoliosis in patients with a disc herniation. **(A)** Herniation lateral to spinal nerve. **(B)** Bending (scoliosis) to the left moves the nerve on the right away from the herniation. **(C)** Herniation medial to spinal nerve. **(D)** Bending to the right moves the nerve away from the herniation and reduces the neurodisc conflict. (After Armstrong JR: Lumbar Disc Lesions. Livingstone, Edinburgh and London, 1965.)

not reasonable to condemn the procedure out of hand.

During the past 30 years the authors have not encountered any patient with a disc herniation who was made worse by manipulation. We have employed this modality of treatment in many cases of disc herniation where there are no signs of increasing neurological deficit or cauda equina syndrome. In most cases the manipulations relieve the back pain and muscle spasms but have little effect on the neurological status of the patient. In some cases nerve root tension is reduced, but it is difficult to relieve distal leg symptoms. Nwuga[16] has provided the only controlled clinical trial on the treatment of lumbar disc herniation by manipulation. He compared manipulation to conventional physiotherapy in patients with acute disc herniation. The manipulated group did significantly better on all measurement scales. Only 26% of the conventionally treated patients were able to return to work, whereas all manipulated patients returned to their work.

LATERAL CANAL STENOSIS WITH SPINAL NERVE ENTRAPMENT

The way in which this takes place by anterior subluxation and/or enlargement of a superior articular process has been described at length in Chapters 4, 10, and 11. In patients with dynamic recurrent lateral stenosis, adjustment of the spine into flexion and axial rotation in the pain-free direction open up the lateral canal and foramen and may be of benefit (Fig. 17-7). When the stenosis is fixed because gross degenerative changes have occurred, it is not easy to see how manipulation can be of assistance.[18]

CENTRAL STENOSIS

Manipulative treatment is less likely to be of benefit with increasing spinal stenosis. Nevertheless, it can be helpful in some patients and is worth a try in the early management of this syndrome. Flexion of the lumbar spine increases the diameter of the spinal canal. Impingement of posterior articular processes on the cauda equina may sometimes be reduced by flexion and rotation.

RETROSPONDYLOLISTHESIS

Retrospondylolisthesis is a common sequela of degenerative disease. This is reduced in flexion and accentuated in extension. Thus a manipulation—carried out with the patient lying on his side with the painful side uppermost—into flexion, opening up of the disc on the painful side, and rotation can be expected to help some patients.

DEGENERATIVE SPONDYLOLISTHESIS

The forward slip of the upper on the lower vertebra is accentuated in flexion. It is thus logical to think that manipulation into extension may be of assistance.

ISTHMIC SPONDYLOLISTHESIS

It is difficult to envisage the way in which this lesion can be alleviated by spinal manipulation. In many cases, however, spondylolisthesis is an incidental finding; and the cause for the patients pain is at another level. Frequently, spondylolisthesis is complicated by a posterior joint syndrome one level above the lesion or by a sacroiliac syndrome. Thus, improvement in the patient's symptoms results, not from any effect on posterior joints or disc at the level of the slip, but from the effect of manipulation on these other joints. In our experience, manipulation is a good first line of treatment in patients with spondylolisthesis.[19] We have seen patients who did not benefit from decompression and/or fusion but who were relieved of their back and leg pain by manipulation directed to the sacroiliac joint.

INSTABILITY

Patients with this phase of disease may expect temporary relief of back and leg pain. It is unreasonable to expect that relief will last for more than a short period of time. In some patients instability at the L4–5 level may be accompanied by dysfunction at the L3–4 or L5–S1 level and the latter may be helped considerably by manipulative adjustment.

THE EFFECT OF MANIPULATION ON THE MECHANORECEPTORS

Until now we have been concerned with the mechanical effect of manipulation on various clinical lesions and syndromes. While discussing the perception of pain in Chapter 5, we saw that stimulation of the mechanoreceptors, supplied by large fibers in the posterior joint capsule, the ligaments, and the annulus fibrosus had the effect of closing the gate for the perception of pain. It is reasonable to postulate that stimulating these sensory fibers by manipulation is a very important part of the way in which this modality is effective.

THE INDICATIONS FOR MANIPULATION

Some idea of these has been given as we discussed the ways in which we think manipulation affects the different lesions that were encountered. In defining the indications it is convenient to identify the categories in which manipulation is clearly and definitely the treatment of choice and those in which it is less clearly indicated.

Definite and Certain Indications

1. Dysfunction with a posterior joint and/or sacroiliac syndrome
2. Paraspinal muscle syndromes
3. Posterior joint or sacroiliac syndrome complicating isthmic spondylolisthesis

Less Certain Indications

1. Dysfunction complicating instability
2. Lateral canal stenosis (dynamic)
3. Dysfunction complicating degenerative stenosis
4. Disc herniation (small)

THE RESULTS OF TREATMENT

We recently completed a prospective observational study of spinal manipulative therapy in 283 patients with chronic low back and leg pain.[20] This patient population was taken from the university low back pain clinic, and all patients were disabled at the start of treatment. The patient's response to treatment was assessed by an independent observer and based on the patient's impression of pain relief and loss of disability. The results were graded as follows:

Grade I. Symptom free and with no restrictions for work or other activities

Grade II. Mild constant pain or intermittent pain with no restrictions for work or other activities
Grade III. Improved but restricted in their activities by pain
Grade IV. Constant severe pain. Symptoms not significantly affected by manipulation

The results, calculated separately for each of the conditions treated, are given in Tables 17-1 to 17-7; they are summarized in Table 17-8.

It is important to point out, first, that these patients are a select group taken from a specialized low back pain clinic, reserved for patients who have not responded to simple conservative measures; second, that they had all suffered from low back pain for

Table 17-1 Sacroiliac Syndrome

Number of patients	69
Average duration of symptoms	7.9 years
Length of follow-up (av)	10.3 months
Results	
Grade I	72%
Grade II	20%
Grade III	3%
Grade IV	4%

Table 17-2 Posterior Joint Syndrome

Number of patients	54
Average duration of symptoms	5.6 years
Length of follow-up (av)	9.2 months
Results	
Grade I	64%
Grade II	15%
Grade III	9%
Grade IV	12%

Table 17-3 Combined Posterior Joint and Sacroiliac Syndrome

Number of patients	48
Average duration of symptoms	9.8 years
Length of follow-up (av)	13.9 months
Results	
Grade I	67%
GradeII	21%
Grade III	6%
Grade IV	6%

Table 17-4 Posterior Joint and/or Sacroiliac Joint Syndrome with Lumbar Instability

Number of patients	31
Average duration of symptoms	7.7 years
Length of follow up (av)	8.0 months
Results	
Grade I	26%
Grade II	19%
Grade III	29%
Grade IV	26%

Table 17-5 Fixed Lateral Entrapment

Number of patients	60
Average duration of symptoms	7.2 years
Length of follow up (av)	14.0 months
Results	
Grade I	25%
Grade II	25%
Grade III	17%
Grade IV	33%

Table 17-6 Dynamic Lateral Entrapment

Number of patients	10
Average duration of symptoms	11.5 years
Length of follow up (av)	12.6 months
Results	
Grade I	40%
Grade II	10%
Grade III	20%
Grade IV	30%

Table 17-7 Central Stenosis

Number of patients	11
Average duration of symptoms	16.9 years
Length of follow up (av)	7.0 months
Results	
Grade I	18%
Grade II	18%
Grade III	18%
Grade IV	46%

Table 17-8 Statistical Summary

Patient Status	Improved	Not Improved
No previous operation	157	58
Previous operations	44	24
Proximal leg symptoms	70	15
Distal leg symptoms	77	51
No leg symptoms	54	16
Mild degenerative changes	107	35
Severe degenerative changes	89	45

ulation, yet many experienced an increase in pain during the first week of treatment. It is important to reassure patients that the initial discomfort is only temporary. It has been our experience that anything less than a 2-week regimen of daily treatment is inadequate for chronic back pain patients. Furthermore, if no improvement occurs by the end of 2 weeks, manipulation is not likely to be of benefit.

Comment

The best results were obtained in patients with dysfunction due to a posterior joint or sacroiliac syndrome or a combination of these. Some patients with instability were improved. The authors believe that improvement was due to treatment of dysfunction that was present with the instability. Fifty percent of patients with lateral entrapment were markedly improved and as a result did not require operation. Thirty-six percent of patients with central stenosis were significantly improved. These were patients who were not fit for operation. It is evident that many patients, especially those in the phase of dysfunction, were greatly improved by this form of treatment.

CONCLUSION

Assessment of the results of treatment shows that manipulation has very considerable value in carefully selected patients. It is essential to make an accurate diagnosis before embarking on treatment. This includes defining both the phase and the clinical lesion. The most definite indication is to treat dysfunction. The majority of patients seen are in this phase.

many years and, third, that they were in Grade IV (disabled by pain) at the start of treatment.

All patients were given a 2- to 3-week regimen of daily spinal manipulations by an experienced chiropractor (JDC). No patient was made worse by manip-

No patient in this series was made worse by manipulation though in some patients it was discontinued because it was not helping the patient.

From the discussion of the natural history of the degenerative process (Ch. 1), it will be appreciated that this process is often a continuing one and therefore we cannot expect a permanent cure from manipulation or from any other modality, including operation.

ACKNOWLEDGMENT

The authors would like to acknowledge the assistance of Drs. M. McGregor, G.E. Potter, A. Grice, R. Gitelman, and R.A. Milne for their assistance in assessing manipulative therapy.

REFERENCES

1. Sandoz R: Some physical mechanisms and effects of spinal adjustments. Ann Swiss Chirop Assoc 6:91, 1976
2. Sandoz, R: Some reflex phenomena associated with spinal derangements and adjustments. Ann Swiss Chirop Assoc 7:45, 1981
3. Roston JB, Wheeler Haines R: Cracking in the metacarpophalangeal joint. J Anat 81:165, 1947
4. Unsworth A, Dowson D, Wright V: Cracking joints. A bioengineering study of cavitation in the metacarpophalangeal joint. Ann Rheum Dis 30:348, 1971
5. Cassidy JD, Mierau DR, Noftal F, et al: A quantitative study of joint mobilization and manipulation. Presented to the Back Pain Research Society, Boscombe, Bournemouth, Nov. 1, 1985
6. Giles LGF: Lumbo-sacral and cervical zygapophyseal joint inclusions. Manual Med 2:89, 1986
7. Wyke BD: Articular neurology and manipulative therapy. In Glasgow EF, Twomey LT, Scull ER, Kleynhans AM (eds): Aspects of Manipulative Therapy. Churchill Livingstone, New York, 1985.
8. Buerger AA: Experimental neuromuscular models of spinal manual techniques. Manual Med 1:10, 1983
9. Kirkaldy-Willis WH, Heithoff KB, Tchang S, et al: Lumbar spondylosis and stenosis: correlation of pathological anatomy with high resolution computed tomographic scanning. In Post MJD (ed): Computed Tomography of the Spine. Williams & Wilkins, Baltimore, 1984
10. Terret ACJ, Vernon H: Manipulation and pain tolerance: a controlled study of the effect of spinal manipulation on paraspinal cutaneous pain tolerance levels. Am J Phys Med 63:217, 1984
11. de Sèze S: Les accidents de la deterioation structurale du disque. Sem Hop Paris 1:2267, 1955
12. de Sèze S: Les attitudes antalgique dans la sciatique discoradiculaire commune. Sem Hop Paris 1:2291, 1955
13. Levernieux J: Les tractions vertebrales. L'expansion, Paris, 1960
14. Chisman OD, Mittnacht A, Snook GA: A study of the results following rotatory manipulation in the lumbar intervertebral disc syndrome. J Bone Joint Surg 46A:517, 1964
15. Mathews JA, Yates AH: Reduction of lumbar disc prolapse by manipulation. Br Med J 3:695, 1969
16. Nwuga VCB: Relative therapeutic efficacy of vertebral manipulation and conventional treatment in back pain management. Am J Phys Med 61:273, 1982
17. Armstrong JR: Lumbar Disc Lesions. Churchill Livingstone, Edinburgh, 1965
18. Mior SA, Cassidy JD: Lateral nerve root entrapment: pathological, clinical and manipulative considerations. J Can Chiro Assoc 26:13, 1982
19. Cassidy JD, Potter GE, Kirkaldy-Willis WH: Manipulative management of back pain patients with spondylolisthesis. J Can Chiro Assoc 22:15, 1978
20. Cassidy JD, Kirkaldy-Willis WH, McGregor M: Spinal manipulation for the treatment of chronic low back and leg pain: an observational trial. In Buerger AA, Greenman PE (eds): Empirical Approaches to the Validation of Manipulative Therapy. Charles C Thomas, Springfield, IL, 1985

18
Supports and Braces

William H. Kirkaldy-Willis

The aim of treatment is restoration of function and activity with regained movement and freedom from pain. Therefore, rigid braces and casts are rarely used. This chapter describes the following types of support:

1. The original Elasticon garment (Camp 400).
2. The new Elasticon garment for women (Camp 455).
3. The new Elasticon garment for men. (Camp 465).
4. The Lumbosacral corset for elderly patients with generalized spondylosis.
5. The chair back brace employed in elderly patients with advanced spondylosis and sometimes following spinal fusion.
6. The Scotch cast jacket spica, applied for 3 months to immobilize the lumbar and lumbosacral spine after a spinal fusion.

THE ORIGINAL ELASTICON GARMENT*

For the past 15 years the author has used an elastic type of supporting garment, the Elasticon, to treat patients with acute, subacute, and chronic low back

---

*Manufactured by Camp Company, Trenton, Ontario, Canada and by Camp International Inc., Jackson, Michigan, U.S.A.

strains and disc herniations and has found it to be of considerable help to them. This garment has also been used by patients recovering from surgery for disc herniation and central and lateral spinal stenosis. It is complementary to a program of instruction in low back care and exercises.

While rigid supports and braces have their place in treating fractures, infections, neoplasms, osteoporosis, marked generalized degenerative spondylosis, and scoliosis, the situation is entirely different in low back pain that is caused by repeated minor trauma and to many localized degenerative lesions.

In treating painful conditions of other joints, such as shoulder, hip, or knee, it is well recognized that freedom from pain closely depends on a return to near normal movement. A stiff joint that is not ankylosed is frequently a painful joint. In treating strains and injuries to the lumbar spine the desirability of obtaining near normal movement has not generally been appreciated.

Physicians and others skilled in techniques of mobilizing the lumbar spine are well aware of the benefit of returning normal movement to a stiff and painful three-joint complex at one level. And so is the patient. In discussing the role of the Elasticon, emphasis is placed on both the need for some support and the desirability of allowing almost full spinal movement during treatment, as tolerated by the patient. The degree of comfort that is obtained is considerable, equivalent to that supplied by a tensor bandage for minor injury to the collateral ligaments of the knee.

297

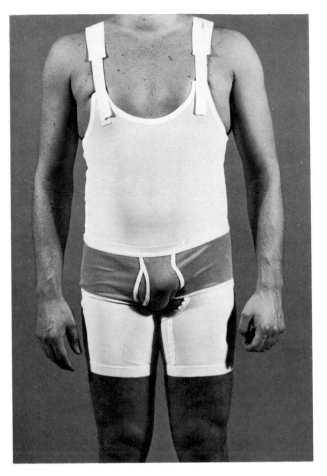

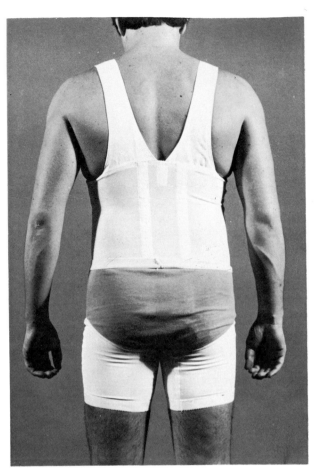

Fig. 18-1 The Elasticon from the front. Note the two shoulder straps fastened with Velcro strips. These can be adjusted to make the garment fit more loosely or more tightly.

Fig. 18-2 The Elasticon from behind. Note the two spiro-flex metal strips, one on each side of the midline.

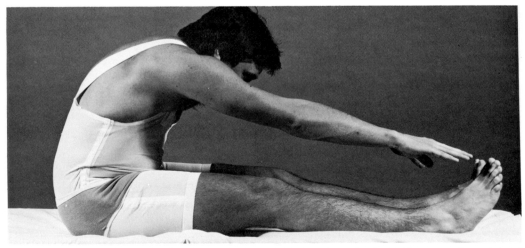

Fig. 18-3 Full movements of the spine are possible while wearing Elasticon; thus muscle activity is not impeded.

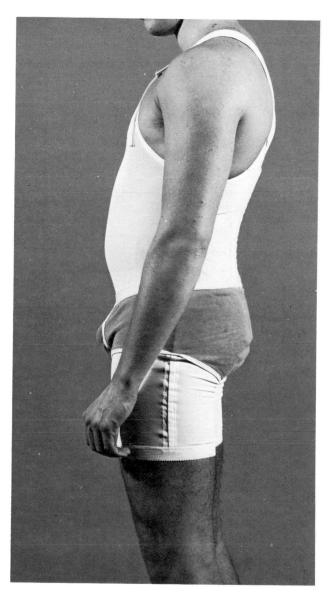

Fig. 18-4 Side view of the patient. Note the lumbar lordosis.

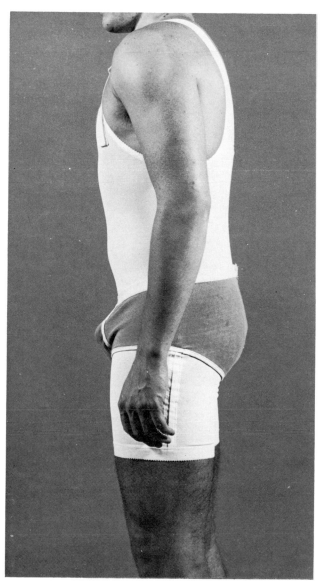

Fig. 18-5 Side view of patient. The lordosis is corrected by pelvic tilting. The Elasticon helps to pull in the abdominal muscles.

Description of Original Elasticon Garment

Designed to resemble a garment rather than a corset, the Elasticon is made of two-way stretch lycra spandex material. It is supplied in four sizes. The essential components are:

1. An encircling cylinder of two way stretch material extending from the nipple line to the level of the greater trochanter

2. Two spiroflex spring supports sited on either side of the midline at the back

3. Two thigh pieces reaching halfway from hip to knee to prevent the bottom of the cyclinder from rolling up

4. Two shoulder straps, fastened by velcro strips on each side in front, to prevent the top of the cylinder from rolling down and to allow adjustment of the garment

5. The length of the main elastic supporting cylinder is longer in front than at the back. This tends to draw the lumbar spine into flexion (Figs. 18-1 to 18-5).

THE NEW ELASTICON GARMENT

The Women's Garment

The principles are the same as those employed in the original Elasticon. The garment (Fig. 18-6, right) is made of the same type of two-way stretch elastic material. It has two spiroflex spring supports on each side at the back. (Fig. 18-7, right). These can be removed if so desired as less support is required. There is a simple mechanism for opening and closing the garment in the crotch for toilet purposes.

The Men's Garment

The new Elasticon for men is essentially the same as the old Elasticon (Camp 400) with two important modifications. (1) Two pieces of the elastic material pass over the shoulders doing away with the more cumbersome Velcro straps. (2) The garment reaches no farther than the junction of groin and thigh, thus abolishing the need for the thigh pieces, which some patients have found uncomfortable. It has similar spiroflex supports to the Camp 455 on each side at the back. These can be removed as less support is needed. (Fig. 18-6 left and Fig. 18-7 left). The garment has a simple snap mechanism in the crotch for toilet purposes.

The Ways in Which the Elasticon Functions

1. It gives support to the painful area, spread over several segments above and below the site of pain.
2. It helps the patient to look upon the lumbar spine as a unit.
3. The elastic material exerts pressure on the abdomen. This tends to reduce the lumbar lordosis and to increase the intra-abdominal pressure.
4. It permits almost full movement of the lumbar spine in all directions and thus allows full muscle activity.

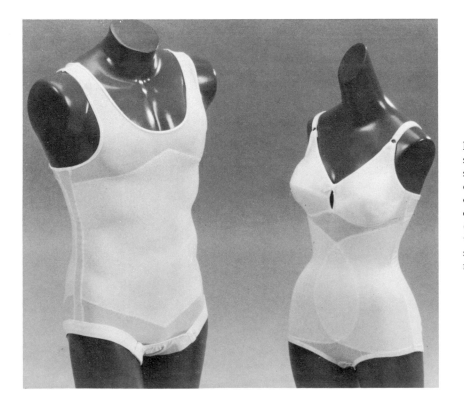

Fig. 18-6 (Left) New Elasticon support for men. Note (1) The two shoulder straps (2) The garment does not extend beyond the junction of groin and thigh. (3) Snap fasteners in the crotch for toilet purposes. (Right) New Elasticon support for women. The main features are the same as in that for men with the necessary differences.

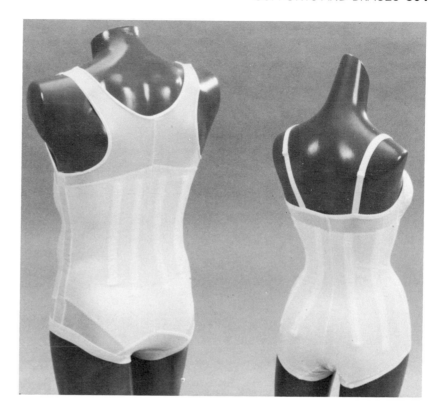

Fig. 18-7 (Left) New Elasticon support for men, back view. Note the four spiroflex supports, two on each side of the midline. (Right) New Elasticon support for women, back view. Note again the four spiroflex supports, two on each side of the midline.

5. The result is that the patient experiences increased comfort and is reassured without developing dependence on the garment.

6. It enables the patient to increase activity more quickly and to indulge in activities that would otherwise not be possible without pain.

Discussion

The majority of patients for whom the Elasticon is prescribed find it considerably helpful.

Those recovering from an acute low back strain, from a herniation of the nucleus pulposus, or from a discectomy find that they can pursue their activities of daily living more easily, with more confidence and less pain. Among these activities are getting in and out of a car and taking long car or plane journeys. Initially, it is more effective for such patients to carry out pelvic tilting and exercises to strengthen the abdominal muscles while wearing the garment. Most patients gradually discard the support after 3 to 5 months, wearing it only for long journeys by car, for golf or tennis, or during a particularly arduous day of work. A few patients continue to wear the garment indefinitely. This does no harm because almost full muscle activity is still possible.

Other patients suffering from generalized degenerative disease of the lumbar spine and those who have had a decompression for spinal stenosis often continue to wear the Elasticon indefinitely.

The present design of the Elasticon makes it very suitable for men. Women sometimes prefer a light elastic body stocking. This is almost as effective, though it has no spiroflex spring supports at the back.

THE LUMBOSACRAL CORSET

This garment is made of elastic material with cotton front and back panels. It extends from about 7 inches above the waist line to 2 inches above the greater trochanter. It encircles the lower chest and abdomen. It is fastened by snap fasteners in front (Fig. 18-8.)

This type of corset reduces the movement of the lumbar and lumbosacral spine but does not eliminate movement completely.

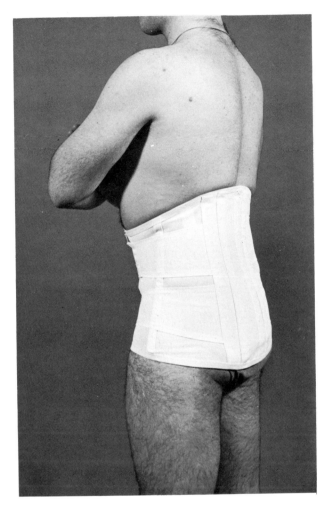

Fig. 18-8 The lumbosacral corset viewed from behind and from the side.

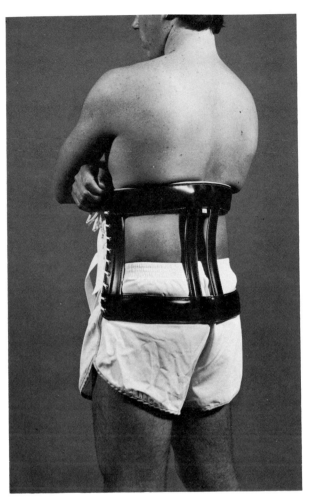

Fig. 18-9 The chair back brace viewed from behind and from the side.

In the writer's experience it is useful in two situations: (1) For elderly patients with generalized spondylosis that results in low back pain. The reduction of movement gives relief from the pain, and lack of muscle activity is no great disadvantage in such patients. (2) For patients after spinal fusion who have been immobilized in a body jacket for 3 months and require further protection.

THE CHAIR BACK BRACE

This support is more rigid than the lumbosacral corset. It is made of slightly malleable metal, covered by leather or similar synthetic material, fastened by buckles in front and tightened by laces or stays (Fig. 18-9). It is employed in the same situations as the lumbosacral corset (see the preceding section) but when more rigid and complete immobilization is deemed advisable. The upper part of the lumbar spine is more completely immobilized than the lower. The immobilization produced by this support is not in the writer's opinion sufficient to treat a patient during the first 3 months following a spinal fusion.

THE LIGHT CAST JACKET SPICA

This is made in the cast room from "light cast" bandages. It encircles the chest and abdomen from the nipple line to the groin. One hip and one thigh

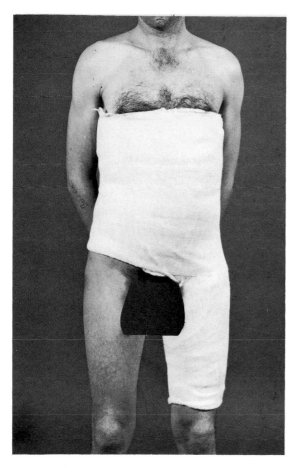

Fig. 18-10 The light cast jacket spica seen from the front.

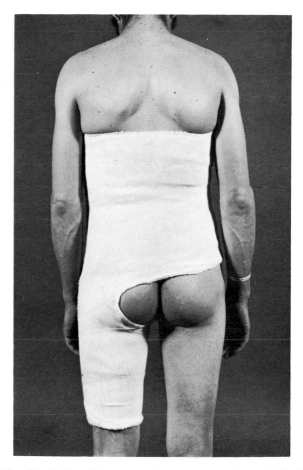

Fig. 18-11 The light cast jacket spica seen from behind.

are incorporated as far as the knee. A jacket spica made from this material is lighter, stronger, and more durable than one made with plaster of paris bandages (Figs. 18-10 and 18-11).

This type of cast is employed after all lumbar or lumbosacral spinal fusion operations and is worn for 3 months to produce the highest possible rate of fusion by almost complete immobilization.

19
Gravity Lumbar Reduction

Charles V. Burton

In August 1986 the Associated Press published an estimate that the annual cost of back pain in the United States was approaching $81 billion dollars.[1] In the state of Minnesota where low back problems represent 30% of worker's compensation claims and account for about 60% of total expenditures, the magnitude of this entity as the most inefficient single application of health care dollars in our present system becomes evident.

A substantial portion of low back care costs reflects surgical therapy. It should not come as a surprise to find accumulating data that many patients coming to surgery could have been effectively treated by less stringent means when one considers that the average spine surgeon is usually neither trained in nor knowledgeable about conservative spinal therapy. Actually in some of the present socialized health care systems, surgery is routinely performed on almost all cases of low back pain. This serves more as a reflection of local economic conditions rather than appropriate therapy for the patient.

These observations make clear that a greater understanding and effort is called for in addressing the ubiquitous problem of low back pain. As a neurosurgeon specializing in comprehensive lumbar spinal care, I believe that the greatest single need is for early education and preventive programs. The next need is for more productive approaches to the initial management of acute low back pain, particularly in societies enmeshed in third party payer, worker's compensation, and legal concerns.

A number of centers are now expert in the salvage of chronic low back pain and failed back surgery syndrome patients. The real challenge for the future is to prevent these situations from occurring in the first place by focusing on better initial management of acute cases. In this regard it is appropriate to review a most rational and appropriate commentary which has been provided by the State of Minnesota in its 1985 "Employer's Guide" to the Worker's Compensation System:

> The initial few weeks after an injury are a critical period. The importance of close case management, early aggressive mobilization, and early return to work cannot be overemphasized. Bed rest and other passive treatments should be kept to the absolute minimum. Early protected mobilization of the injured body part, combined with a gradual, progressive increase in activities in a controlled, supervised manner gives the best result.

The particular liability of excessive bed rest in managing low back pain was recently addressed by Deyo et al.[2] who observed in acute low back pain patients (with mechanical syndromes and no neurological deficit) that those with 2 days of bed rest versus 7 days missed 45% less work time over the subsequent 3-month follow-up.

Recently a Canadian television special on low back care referred to the Institute for Low Back Care and the Low Back Clinic of the Sister Kenny Institute as a "low back supermarket." As the supermarket "manager" this author has particularly appreciated the unique dilemma of having to select patient care from a myriad of skilled health care professionals providing many sophisticated therapies. Such extensive resources can actually represent a confusing liability. The real challenge for society is to design realistic conservative management programs for acute low back pain patients that are effective, low in cost, and appropriate for use on a widespread basis by unsophisticated health care professionals.

AXIAL TRACTION

The recognition that some spinal disorders were amenable to therapy and that axial traction could be beneficial is a concept that can be traced to the ancient Egyptian Edwin Smith Papyrus dated to the 17th century B.C.[3] In this modern world even though axial spinal traction is routinely employed in physical therapy, chiropractic, osteopathy, and medicine effective lumbar traction continues to be an elusive quarry. Lancourt[4] pointed out in a recent review that lumbar traction is no better than a homeopathic remedy when used with the usual 15 to 30 pounds of weight and that 65 to 70 pounds of traction, not dissipated by friction, is required to influence meaningfully the lumbar spine.

In addition to the actual amount of force applied, the *method* by which it is employed is also of importance as too acute an influence can be the cause of tissue injury. The difference between therapy and injury may, at times, be only a fine line. Unlike the cervical spine where paravertebral muscle bulk is minimal, the heavy lumbar paravertebral musculature normally exerts significant resistance to distraction.

In recent years a number of inversion devices of the hanging head variety for exercise and physical fitness have emerged, associated with some (at times most remarkable) claims regarding lumbar therapy. Although the latter claim has not yet been demonstrated and remains unlikely from the biomechanical standpoint, the basic value of anti-gravity exercise

in the prevention of low back disorders can not be overlooked.

The lumbar disc is a unique structure in many ways. It is vascular only during infancy and is dependent afterwards on the diffusion of nutrients from adjacent vertebrae across the endplate. This phenomenon occurs most prominently during sleep. We are all shorter at night and taller when we awake in the morning. The relaxation of musculature and decrease in loading creates a "bellows-like" phenomenon, which appears to enhance the diffusion of nutrients across the disc endplate (Fig. 19-1). The reverse phenomenon has been demonstrated by dynamic high pressure intradiscal injection studies performed by my associate Dr. Charles Ray. He has shown that under increased pressure conditions intradiscal dye can directly pass through the intact endplate and enter into the adjacent spinal venous system. The simple influence of acute changes in body position on loading has been demonstrated by Nachemson.[5] He has shown that discal loading decreases by a factor of 5 from the standing to supine positions.

I suggest that during episodes of discal decompression when nutrition is enhanced and discal volume increases this is also the phase when healing occurs. Although this remains to be demonstrated experimentally, it seems logical to assume that the deposition of reparative collagen in the natural healing of

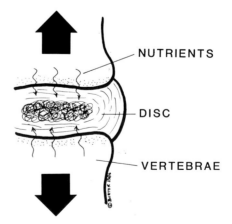

Fig. 19-1 The distraction produced by axial traction probably creates a favorable diffusion gradient tending to enhance disc nutrition across the endplate and thus promote the natural healing process.

annular tears and fissures would be enhanced under these conditions.

THE SISTER KENNY INSTITUTE GRAVITY LUMBAR REDUCTION THERAPY PROGRAM

Since the introduction by Walter Dandy[6] in 1929 of the concept of lumbar disc herniation, its differentiation from lumbar tumor and its surgical removal, later popularized by Mixter and Barr[7], have been often considered routine surgical fare. It is only in recent years that less stringent means of successful therapy have entered into the general medical and surgical consciousness. When one considers that no less an authority than Finneson[8] has determined, in one series of 94 patients who experienced failed back surgery, that in 81% the "original surgery was not indicated," the need to focus on cost-effective conservative low back care becomes all the more compelling.

The Sister Kenny Institute Gravity Lumbar Reduction Therapy Program (GLRTP) was first introduced into clinical use in 1976 after a 2-year development period.[9] At that time its primary use was for the conservative therapy of acute contained disc herniations. The rib cage served as the point of fixation made possible by a specially designed vest-harness. The lower 40% of body weight served as the distractive force. This was gradually loaded by increasing the angle of tilt over a period of days to allow patients to acclimate and for the force to be applied in a gradual and progressive manner. A number of different means to apply axial traction to the lumbar spine are presently available. It is important to recognize that force applied too suddenly is capable of producing tissue injury rather than benefit.

For the first 10 years of clinical use, GLRTP was applied and studied on an inpatient basis. After successfully initiating therapy and instruction in the hospital patients would then be discharged, return to normal life and work activities, and continue to maintain traction for 1 hour twice a day at home with a lightweight traction frame.

The original theory regarding the mechanism of action of head-up gravity traction was that the distractive force would create negative pressure within the abnormal disc and allow sufficient reduction of the herniation to allow both spinal nerve decompression and natural healing of the abnormal disc. More specifically it was felt that through the daily intermittent use of this treatment modality reparative beta collagen deposition would be enhanced. After 10 years of clinical use and study of GLRTP at our institute, about 500 hospitals in the United States, and hospitals in other countries it appears that the original predictions have been substantiated and a great deal of additional important knowledge has been gained.

The original focus of GLRTP has been on the treatment of acute contained disc herniations (Fig. 19-2) clearly recognizing that patients with neurological emergencies (e.g., profound neurological deficit such as complete foot drop or bowel or bladder impairment) are considered to be immediate surgical rather than conservative therapy candidates. It is interesting to note that gravity traction has also turned out to be an excellent means of identifying patients with noncontained discs (Fig. 19-3), as these patients typically experience dramatically increased leg pain within the first 48 hours of traction. We consider noncontained disc herniations to be surgical problems.

At the 1985 Challenge of the Lumbar Spine Meeting in Minneapolis my associate Richard Salib presented a GLRTP survey review based on 212 inpatient cases of documented disc herniation treated at the institute for low back care over a 3-year period and followed from 1 to 3 years (Table 19-1). These data have provided some interesting insights regarding acute and chronic populations. At a tertiary referral center such as ours we see many problem cases but very few in the acute stage. The best results were in the acute private patients who experienced a 78% good-to-excellent result while the worst results (21% good-to-excellent) represented the chronic worker's compensation/litigation group from gravity traction. Although the acute private patient group in this study was small, reports from other institutions and countries confirm a 70% to 80% good-to-excellent results for larger groups of patients in this category.

Because the majority of patients referred to the institute for low back care are difficult or problem cases we see many chronic cases. Because of this our use of GLRTP on chronic cases of musculoligamentous pain indicated poor results, and we discouraged others from implementing it in this situation. Only in recent years have other groups demonstrated that when used acutely for musculoligamentous pain,

CONTAINED DISCS

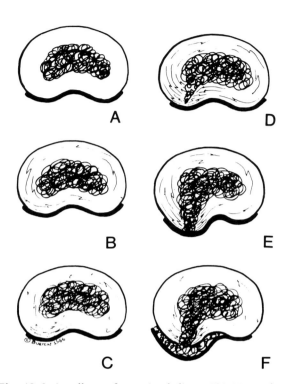

Fig. 19-2 A gallery of contained discs. **(A)** Normal configuration. **(B)** Scattered annular tears from torsional stress. The heavy black posterior line represents the posterior longitudinal ligament-disc capsule complex (PLDC) and is shown prominently only because of its anatomical significance (rather than its true thickness, which is quite small). **(C)** Multiple annular tears have begun to coalesce in the posterolateral aspect and a radial fissure is starting. **(D)** The radial tear has occurred and nuclear material is extruding into it. Nuclear material has now protruded into the radial tear **(E)** but has not passed the annulus. This disc is clearly herniated and, depending on the nature of the spinal canal and surrounding anatomical structures, the proximal spinal nerve can be either displaced or compressed. **(F)** The nuclear material has now been extruded past the annulus but is still contained by the PLDC. This situation is sometimes referred to as a roof disc.

GLRTP is highly effective in reducing spasm and inflammation and also promoting collagen repair in the plane of the muscle or ligament action rather than being deposited as randomized scar tissue.

These data on the successful acute application of GLRTP when associated with the identified need to reduce bed rest and initiate early mobilization of the patient make clear that gravity traction will have a much more important future role in early aggressive conservative therapy. The window of opportunity in dealing with acute low back and leg pain is clearly within the first few weeks following onset of pain. Elizabeth Hepper, Director of the Low Back Club, which uses GLRTP on an outpatient basis, has coined the term "nova" to describe this important phase. For acute musculoligamentous injuries nova is 1 week following onset of pain and for acute disc herniations

NON-CONTAINED DISCS

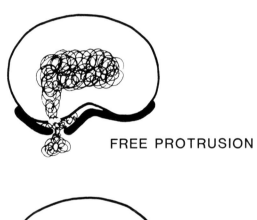

FREE PROTRUSION

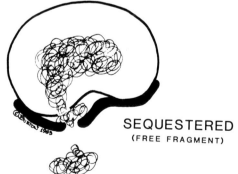

SEQUESTERED
(FREE FRAGMENT)

Fig. 19-3 When discal material extrudes through the PLDC, the disc is considered to be noncontained. This has become an important therapeutic determination as its identification suggests that surgical therapy is most appropriate for the patient given adequate clinical and neurological justification. As long as the nuclear herniation is connected to the disc itself, a free protrusion is present. When there is no connection a sequestered or free fragment disc herniation is identified.

Table 19-1 Gravity Lumbar Reduction Inpatient Traction: Results for Documented Lumbar Disc Herniation

| | Results (%) | | |
Lumbar Disc Herniation	Good/ Exc	Fair	Poor
Acute disc herniation (19 patients)			
Private insurance	78		
		0	22
Worker's comp/litigation	70	0	30
Total	74	0	26
Chronic disc herniation (145 patients)			
Private insurance	47.8	6.7	45.5
Worker's comp/litigation	21	12	67
Total	34.4	9.4	56.3

Retrospective review. Data based on recovery of 94% of patients contacted. Acute disc herniation defined as symptomatic for 6 weeks or less. Follow-up period 1–4 years.

it is 2 weeks. There is presently little doubt but that nova represents a key identification regarding future back therapy. The low back club program focuses on nova patients and offers a comprehensive acute therapy program designed to return clients rapidly to normal activities. For those patients who are so acute that they can not stand or ambulate, hospitalization for 48 hours is often required for cool down, which involves parenteral anti-inflammatory and analgesic medications.

Such modern, cost-effective, conservative management programs designed to address musculoligamentous and discogenic pain satisfy an important sociological need. Recent national statistics indicate that the present average direct medical cost of treating a patient with musculoligamentous pain is $5,000; the cost for treating a patient with a herniated disc is $23,000. Actual costs are considerably higher since they must also reflect lost wages, lost productivity, insurance payments, and job retraining.

During the past 10 years gravity traction has been successfully used in a small number of special applications including progressive scoliosis, spondylolisthesis, and early lateral spinal stenosis. A particularly interesting case involved a young and physically fit man who developed multilevel, unilateral lateral spinal stenosis at the concavity of lumbar scoliosis. He was not improved by gravity traction alone, and it was felt that fusion would only place strain on adjacent segments and create a domino failure pattern. Following localized multilevel decompression of the impaired exiting spinal nerves, he returned to daily use of gravity traction. This use of traction in association with surgery has been highly successful.

At this time our radiological consultants under the direction of Kenneth Heithoff have performed about 40,000 high resolution CT and MRI lumbar scans. It is now an unusual experience for an institute surgeon to find, at surgery, a condition other than the one predicted by the clinical examination and imaging studies.[10–12] This highly accurate and sophisticated imaging information has essentially relegated myelography to a minor role in our practice. Almost all new patients are seen on an outpatient basis with CT being performed prior to examination. In this way the clinical information can be immediately combined with the imaging data producing a time-efficient, comparatively low cost, and highly accurate diagnosis. It is important to emphasize that a surgical decision must be made on clinical grounds alone. An abnormality seen on imaging and not confirmed by the clinical examination is not an indication for surgery.[13] The advent of imaging has allowed us to not only "fine tune" the nature of a herniated disc but also to follow, in serial fashion, its response to therapy as well as the progression of those phenomena that represent the normal healing process.[14] In this way each patient can serve as his or her own control.

It is fair to observe that the great enthusiasm in the United States for chemonucleolysis as a panacea for disc herniation has cooled rather remarkably. The major reason for this has been the very visible group of devastating neurological complications, which appear to have reflected technical inexperience as well as lack of appreciation of the limitations of the technique itself. Chemonucleolysis does not appear to be indicated in patients with noncontained discs, lateral entrapment syndromes characterized by lateral spinal stenosis, or segmental instability. Our experience suggests that many patients following chemonucleolysis trade their leg pain for accentuated back pain reflecting the sudden reduction of disc volume and the stress placed on buckling annulus and facet joints.

Yet, careful patient selection and use of chemonucleolysis continues to produce reasonable results.

Following chemonucleolysis a disc is more "plastic" and deformable. I have used gravity traction following chemonucleolysis to restore segmental alignment and moderate the severe degree of discal collapse, but the series at this point is too small to draw any statistically valid conclusions. Although the increasingly high efficacy of surgery tends progressively to discourage chemonucleolysis it remains reasonable as an alternative to GLRTP for some patients who can not use it because of obesity, cardiopulmonary disease, or chest harness intolerance due to a number of different reasons.

Technique

The GLRTP program is now administered in both the inpatient as well as the outpatient modes. There is always a desire on the part of clinicians to use a new therapeutic modality on those who have failed to improve with other therapies. This inclination has led to GLRTP being initially used on previously operated, chronic, and obese patients where a poor result is almost guaranteed. The more physically fit and acute the patient the more successful the endeavor.

INPATIENT

The inpatient program is now used for more complicated or demanding cases where more intense physician observation and support is required. Following hospital admission patients are fitted with a chest harness, and placed in a self-controlled electrical tilt bed (Fig. 19-4). Starting at 30° elevation and progressing initially at 5°/day then 10°/day, each patient completes a total of 4 hours of traction/day in multiple episodes (typically 30 minutes). The usual goal is to reach 70° traction in the hospital and continue the second (maintenance) phase at 60°. Progressing to 90° is always an option for the highly motivated and fit patient. Use of a safety strap system is required in all patients at all times. While in the hospital patients are exercised and exposed to therapeutic swimming. They are now allowed nonaggravating activities between episodes of traction rather than complete bed rest.

An important component of the inpatient program is education through publications, audiovisuals, and

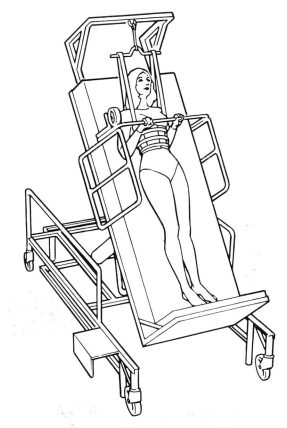

Fig. 19-4 Gravity traction is initiated by fitting the patient with a specially designed chest harness and using a patient-controlled electrically operated tilt bed. The traction angle is gradually increased according to patient tolerance. In outpatient programs the tilt bed is used only for a short term, and patients are then transferred into maintenance units. The safety strap system is not shown in this illustration. (Courtesy of the Institute for Low Back Care, Minneapolis.)

low back school as well as instruction by our physical, occupational, and recreational therapists. Continuing fitness, better posture and nutrition, exercise, and use of appropriate body dynamics and mechanics remain the individual's best bet at enhancing their prognosis.

Gravity traction produces tenderness of the rib cage in almost all patients within the first few days. This is alleviated by local massage after removing the vest. Approximately 5° of patients find the traction too uncomfortable to continue. Initial accentuation of back pain is normal, but accentuation of leg pain suggests the presence of a free fragment disc herniation (noncontained). During inpatient therapy the physician has the unique opportunity of monitoring patient's reaction to the stress of initiating gravity traction, which requires significant effort. More meaningful information regarding the patient's psychological makeup and response to stress is conveyed by this than any psychological test ever developed.

The maintenance phase begins when the patient leaves the hospital. Prior to this they are provided with a maintenance frame (Figs. 19-5 and 19-6) and instructed in its use. Typical maintenance is at either 60° or 90°. (A recent patient required 90° because she lived aboard a world traveling motor yacht.) This phase usually continues for about 3 months but in special cases can be for longer periods with recommended traction time being 1 hour twice a day. It

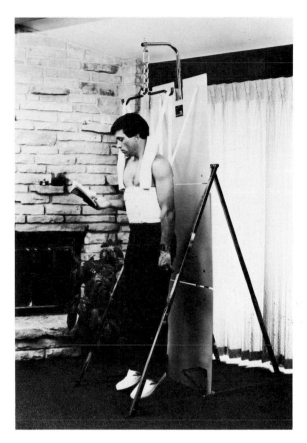

Fig. 19-6 The 90° free-standing gravity traction unit. If an attic or basement is convenient patients can affix traction and safety strap bolts and eyelets and hang directly from these. (Courtesy of Camp International, Jackson, MI.)

is most important that once patients have left the hospital they return to normal activities and gainful employment. Progress is assessed at outpatient clinic follow-up visits.

Outpatient

In the first edition of this book GLRTP therapy for acute lumbosacral strain was identified as an investigational area. Since then accumulating experience in clinics in which acute patients are routinely seen has continued to suggest that this is a prime application in addition to acute contained disc herniation. A prototype outpatient GLRTP based program "the Low Back Club" has been established as a "user friendly" establishment at the Sister Kenny Institute. Intended for nova class patients who are ambulatory,

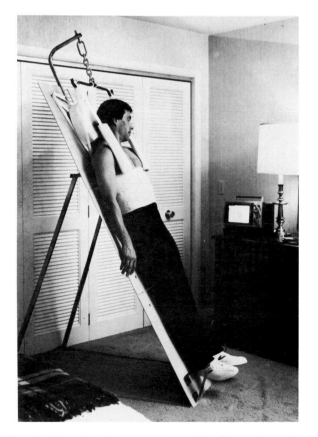

Fig. 19-5 A 60° maintenance unit. This allows the patient to continue traction at home while returning to normal activities. (Courtesy of Camp International, Jackson, MI.)

this comprehensive therapy and educational program provides 5 days of gravity traction at the club and maintenance as required. The key element is returning this nova patient to normal activities and employment before compensation, legal, incapacitation, and learned pain behavior problems can start. This active approach to the low back problem represents a meaningful, realistic, and practical answer to the enormous present liability of low back cost and needless human suffering.

Efficacy

In addition to clinical observation it has been possible with the GLRTP program to allow, through the use of imaging, patients to serve as their own controls (Figs. 19-7 and 19-8) and to confirm what has been theoretically predicted (Fig. 19-9). Long-term, good-to-excellent results can be expected in 70° to 80° of appropriately selected acute contained disc herniation patients. For this patient group, the GLRTP program is the safest, least expensive therapeutic modality available.

Continuing experience and study in using gravity traction as a primary means of managing acute musculoligamentous injuries has been most encouraging.

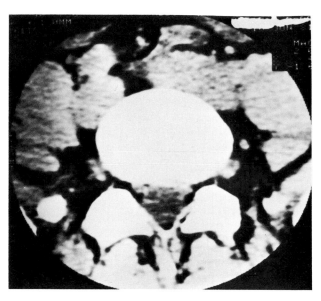

Fig. 19-8 Following 8 months of gravity traction therapy the repeat CT scan confirms the resolution of abnormal neurological findings and the relief of pain. In this manner patients can serve as their own controls. This particular patient had been referred to the institute for surgical discectomy.

This application will be a primary focus of attention and data collection in the next few years.

Contraindications and Precautions

GLRTP is contraindicated for patients whose obesity precludes use of a chest harness; patients with pulmonary disease in whom the harness would compromise function; patients with some types of cardiovascular disease; and some patients who have had previous abdominal surgery or hiatus hernia, where abdominal compression produces significant pain. Gravity traction has been extensively studied in patients with the failed back surgery syndrome. In only a few cases has improvement been noted. Based on these data it can not be recommended as a basic application unless there is an acute disc herniation at an unoperated spinal level.

Generally, the optimal candidates are within the first five decades of life. A safety strap system must be used at all times. Should leg pain be significantly accentuated by traction discontinuance and further patient evaluation is called for.

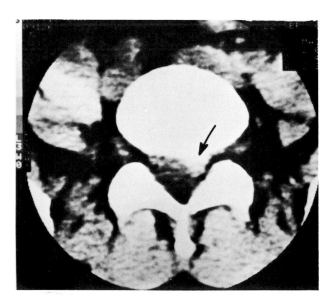

Fig. 19-7 A large disc-contained herniation projecting into the spinal canal and compressing the traversing S1 nerve root is identified by the arrow.

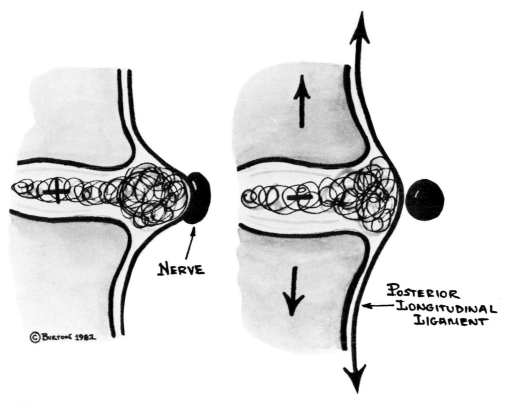

NERVE

POSTERIOR
LONGITUDINAL
LIGAMENT

©BURTON 1982

Fig. 19-9 CT shows that the application of axial traction on the vertebrae, annulus fibrosus, and longitudinal ligaments causes the protruding disc to diminish in volume but rarely to return to its normal state. The clinical problem relates to distension of annular and ligamentous dorsal ramus nerve fibers and spinal nerve compression. It is believed, on the basis of biomechanical calculation, that significant intradiscal negative pressures may be produced. The intermittent reduction appears to allow reparative processes to reestablish support.

Complications

Potential complications relate to the misuse of components or loss of support during traction. The safety strap system and the published instructions for use should be strictly followed. In the 10 years of clinical use, no noteworthy patient morbidity has occurred in patients treated at our institute.

Summary

The Sister Kenny Institute GLRTP continues to represent a safe, cost-effective, and increasingly more valuable means of treating acute patients with low back and leg pain. With the development of outpatient programs there is accumulating evidence that this approach is rational for the routine therapy of large patient populations in both developed and underdeveloped countries and promises to become an important means of decreasing the inappropriately great cost burden that low back care presently represents.

ACKNOWLEDGMENTS

The continuing documentation and improvement of the Sister Kenny Institute Gravity Lumbar Reduction Therapy Program has involved the combined efforts of the staffs of the Institute for Low Back Care, Sister Kenny Institute, Abbott-Northwestern Hospital, the Low Back Club of Minneapolis, and Camp International. Particular appreciation is expressed to Gail Nida, R.N., Elizabeth Hepper, and

Joyce Mueller, R.N. for their efforts on the patient's behalf; Kenneth Heithoff M.D. and his associates for the wonders of CT and MRI spinal imaging, and to William H. Kirkaldy-Willis, M.D., who has served us all as friend, medical pioneer, and mentor. His devotion to excellence in understanding and treating the lumbar spine has been an important inspiration.

REFERENCES

1. Annual costs of back pain approaching $81 billion. Minneapolis Tribune. August 21, 1986
2. Deyo RA, Diehl AK, Rosenthal M: How many days of bed rest for acute low back pain? JAMA 315:1064, 1986
3. Wilkins RH: Neurosurgical Classics. Johnson Reprint Corp., New York, 1965
4. Lancourt JE: Traction techniques for low back pain. J Musculoskel Med April, 1986. pp. 44
5. Nachemson A: The load on lumbar discs in different positions of the body. Clin Orthop 45:107, 1966
6. Dandy WE: Loose cartilage from intervertebral disc simulating tumor of the spinal cord. Arch Surg 19:660, 1929
7. Mixter WJ, Barr JA: Rupture of the intervertebra disc with involvement of the spinal canal. N Eng J Med 210, 1934
8. Finneson BE: Low Back Pain. 2nd Ed. JB Lippincott, Philadelphia, 1980
9. Burton C, Nida G: The Sister Kenny Institute Gravity Lumbar Reduction Therapy Program. Publication No. 731. Sister Kenny Institute, Minneapolis, 1982
10. Heithoff KB: High resolution computed tomography in the differential diagnosis of soft-tissue pathology of the lumbar spine. In Genant HK, Chafetz N, Helms CA (eds): Computed Tomography of the Lumbar Spine. University of California Press, San Francisco, 1982
11. Heithoff KB: Pathogenesis and high resolution computed tomographic scanning of direct bony impingement syndromes of the lumbar spine. Edited by Genant HK, Chafetz N, Helms CA (eds): Computed Tomography of the Lumbar Spine. University of California Press, San Francisco, 1982
12. Heithoff KB, Burton CV: CT evaluation of the failed back surgery syndrome. Orthop Clin North Am 16:417, 1985
13. Burton CV: Successful surgical management of lateral spinal stenosis. In Stauffer ES (ed): Instructional Course Lectures, The American Academy of Orthopaedic Surgeons. CV Mosby, St. Louis, 1985
14. Kirkaldy-Willis WH, Wedge JH, Yong-Hing K, et al: Pathology and pathogenesis of lumbar spondylosis and stenosis. Spine 3:319, 1978

20
Surgical Techniques

Ken Yong-Hing

Although operations on the lumbar spine for backache are not difficult to master, there is no place for the occasional spinal surgeon. This is not because exceptional technical expertise is required but rather because of the more difficult and important aspect of selecting the correct patients and operations in a complex syndrome that often affects demanding patients. In addition, not all surgeons have the temperament required for maneuvering in the small deep space between two laminae.

The desired goal of the operation—decompression, fusion, or both—has been dealt with in Chapter 15. The means of achieving the goal and the surgical approach and technique will be described here. Certain assumptions will be made: (1) An accurate diagnosis has been made. (2) Proper conservative treatment has failed. (3) The patient has been correctly selected as suitable for operation.

The principles of operating on the lumbar spine are the same two as for any operation: to deal with the lesion that causes the symptoms and to prevent intraoperative and postoperative complications.

PREVENTION OF COMPLICATIONS

Complications are prevented by careful technique, a clear knowledge of the anatomy of the spinal canal, and especially a constant awareness of all the possible complications.

Nerve Root Damage

A good surgical exposure helps to prevent accidental damage to nerve roots and makes strenuous retraction of the roots unnecessary. We do not recommend routine extensive exposures by making long incisions; stripping four or five vertebrae of paraspinal muscles; or excising several laminae, ligaments, and posterior joints because such exposures increase the risk of late instability and adhesions. We aim for the minimum exposure necessary to thoroughly explore the spinal canal and safely execute the planned procedure.

We previously recommended exploring the lateral recess on the asymptomatic side at the time of a discectomy. If lateral stenosis was present, we recommended prophylactic decompression to prevent spinal nerve entrapment from the inevitable settling of the disc space after the disc was excised. This routine bilateral exploration is now unnecessary if the CT scan demonstrates a normal lateral recess on the asymptomatic side.

If only one side is to be explored, the spinous process can be cut at its base and retracted to increase the view of the depths of the canal (see following) without sacrificing the process and interspinous ligaments (Fig. 20-1).[1]

Magnifying glasses and an operating headlamp with adjustable focus are recommended during that part of the operation in which the nerve root is being exposed, manipulated, and decompressed.

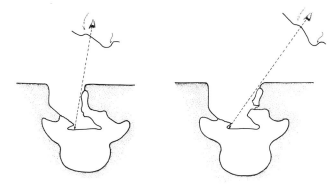

Fig. 20-1 Osteotomy and displacement of the spinous process improves the view during unilateral exposure.

Bleeding

Excessive bleeding can convert a straightforward operation into an awful "snatch and grab" exercise because only intermittent glimpses of the nerve roots are obtained. Bleeding must be diminished by properly positioning the patient (see following) and injecting a hemostatic solution. Elevation of the paraspinal muscles should be meticulously subperiosteal and care must be taken to cauterize the muscular branches of the lumbar arteries as they are encountered.[2] Bipolar diathermy should be tested on subcutaneous fat and adjusted before it is used on epidural vessels, and then only after the dura and nerve root are retracted away from its tip. Temporary packing with patties and Gelfoam in the epidural space further controls bleeding and increases the exposure in the spinal canal. Routine hypotensive anesthesia is unnecessary, but blood should be available for replacement if difficulty is predicted. We recommend cross matching 1 or more liters for reexplorations and spinal fusions.

Wrong Side and Level

To avoid operating on the wrong side or the wrong level the surgeon should develop and routinely practice a series of checks. I check the recorded notes, myelogram, and CT scan; and I doublecheck the side with my first assistant before starting. To avoid operating on the wrong level I routinely expose the sacrum and identify it by both visual examination and palpation. I apply a Kocher forceps to the L5 spinous process to elicit movement in relation to S1. Occasionally, I also obtain a lateral x-ray with the Kocher

forceps on a spinous process to confirm the level. I always do this if a transitional vertebra is present and when operating on the upper lumbar spine.

Damage to Dura and Large Vessels

At the start of the operation the x-ray films should be examined for defects in the posterior elements (spina bifida occulta); if defects are present, special care should be taken to avoid accidental penetration into the spinal canal during elevation of the paraspinal muscles. The dorsal surface of the normal sacrum can be surprisingly thin and easily penetrated. During both the first entry into the canal and excision of the ligamentum flavum the dura should be protected from the scalpel blade with patties or a blunt dissector.

Damaging the aorta, vena cava, and iliac vessels is a risk during discectomy from a posterior approach, and the dura and nerve roots are at risk during discectomy from an anterior approach. These serious complications are avoided by constant awareness of the depth of any instrument that is placed in the disc space. The average midline anteroposterior (AP) diameter of the lumbar disc space is 2.5 to 3.0 cm, but laterally this measurement is smaller. Use of curettes and rongeurs with marks on the metal at graduated intervals are recommended. Placing a red mark at 2.5 cm is a good safety precaution. During the maneuvers in the disc space, the "feel" of the instrument on the bone of the endplate will avoid penetration beyond the confines of the annulus (Figs. 20-2 and 20-3).

Postoperative Adhesions

Gentle handling and retraction of the tissues in the spinal canal decrease the risk of postoperative adhesions and arachnoiditis. Control of bleeding by bipolar diathermy during the operation and removing hematoma by a closed suction drain in the first 2 days following surgery decrease the severity of this complication. Free fat grafts measuring 0.5 to 1.0 cm in thickness are taken from subcutaneous fat either at the edge of the incision or, rarely, from a separate buttock incision and are placed over the exposed dura.[3] Two to four absorbable sutures are placed through the edge of the graft and nearby soft tissues to hold the graft against the dura and prevent its displacement. Langenskiold and Valle[4] demonstrated

Fig. 20-2 Disc removal. Avoid damaging the nerve by inserting the pituitary forceps with its jaws closed. Avoid damaging the great vessels by referring to depth mark scored on forceps.

the fat grafts, by CT, in patients 18 years after discectomy. All Gelfoam used for temporary packing is removed before the wound is closed (Fig. 20-4).

Wound Infections

Routine prophylactic antibiotics are unnecessary. We give high-dose intraoperative broad-spectrum intravenous antibiotics during the more difficult and longer procedures, if a break in aseptic technique occurs, or during reexplorations that were previously infected. No antibiotic is given after completion of the operation. At intervals during the operation and before wound closure the entire wound is irrigated with a dilute antibiotic-saline solution.

SURGICAL APPROACHES

The lumbar spine can be approached from in front or from behind (Fig. 20-5).[5]

Anterior Transperitoneal Approach

This approach can be used for L5–S1 fusion. It should be remembered that the level of bifurcation of the aorta is not always the same. Fusion at L4–L5 through this approach is more difficult and the anterior extraperitoneal approach is preferred. The transperitoneal approach can also be used for osteomyelitis and for tumors involving the L5 or S1 vertebral bodies.[6]

As with the retroperitoneal approach the transperitoneal approach cannot be used if decompression of the neural elements is necessary. It involves all the hazards of a laparotomy. The real risk of sterility (not impotence) due to retrograde ejaculation is unknown. Also unknown is the relative risk of this complication in the transperitoneal as compared with the retroperitoneal route. The risk seems to have been exaggerated in earlier publications.[7,8]

General anesthesia with muscle relaxation is used.

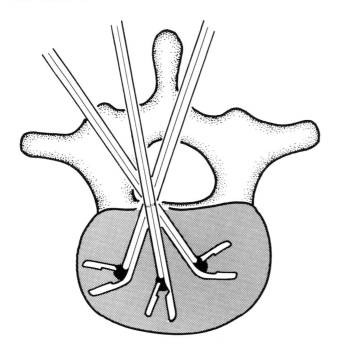

Fig. 20-3 Use straight and angled pituitary forceps with marks on metal to indicate a measured depth.

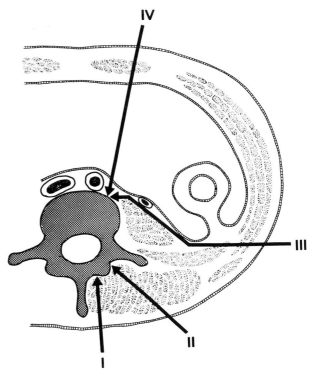

Fig. 20-5 Surgical approaches. (I) Posterior midline. (II) Posterolateral. (III) Anterioir extraperitoneal. (IV) Anterior transperitoneal. (After Rathke FW, Schlegel KF: Surgery of the Spine. WB Saunders. Philadelphia, 1979.)

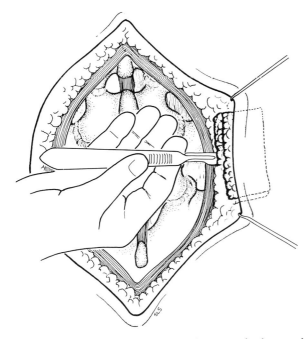

Fig. 20-4 Free fat graft taken from the wound edge used to cover the dura and prevent adhesions.

The patient is positioned supine, 10 to 15° head down (to displace the intestines cephalad and to decrease venous bleeding) with a 5 to 10° break in the table at the level of the iliac crests in order to displace the spine nearer to the anterior abdominal wall (Fig. 20-6).

A midline longitudinal, paramedian, or Pfannenstiel incision is made. If a midline incision is used, the anterior peritoneum is split with the linea alba. The intestines are packed off cranially and laterally with saline-soaked packs behind abdominal retractors. The bifurcation of the aorta and, below it, the sacral promontory are identified (Fig. 20-7).

Anterior Extraperitoneal Approach

This approach provides wide exposure and all operations of the vertebral bodies and discs from L2 to S1 can be accomplished through it. It is better than the transperitoneal approach for interbody fusion if

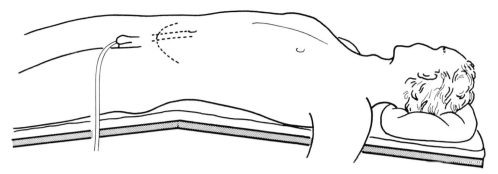

Fig. 20-6 Anterior transperitoneal approach. Note 10° head down position and 10° break in table. The choice of incisions is shown.

both the L4–L5 space and the L5–S1 space are to be fused. It has the advantage that an iliac bone graft can be taken through the same skin incision. Care must be extended to protect the aorta on the left side, the inferior vena cava on the right side, and—proceeding more distally on both sides—the common

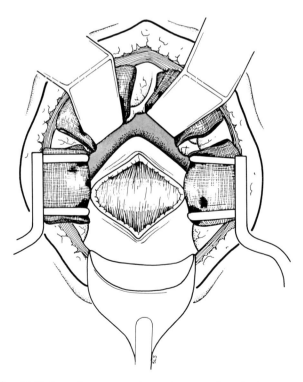

Fig. 20-7 Anterior transperitoneal approach. The bifurcation of the aorta and, below it, the sacral promontory are identified. The peritoneum is split vertically to avoid injuring the presacral plexus.

iliac vessels. In the presence of an inflammatory process the ureter may adhere to the scar tissue and require careful dissection.[6–8]

General anesthesia supplemented by muscle relaxants is used. For the upper lumbar spine the patient is placed in the left lateral position with the right hip and knee flexed and the left extremity straight. The table is broken at 10° at the level of the iliac crests and in addition is tilted 10° head down to displace the intestines cranially and decrease bleeding (Fig. 20-8). To approach the lower lumbar spine the supine position is used and again the table is broken 10° at the iliac crests and tilted 10° head down (Fig. 20-9).

All or part of an oblique incision extending from the anterior to the posterior midline is employed. The line of incision is midway between the umbilicus and symphysis pubis and midway between the costal margin and iliac crest. Alternatively, the lower lumbar spine may be approached by a paramedian incision.

The external oblique aponeurosis and muscle are divided in the direction of their fibers. The internal oblique is divided transversely in the line of the incision. The transverse abdominis is carefully nicked to avoid cutting the peritoneum, which is then pushed away from the abdominal wall and vertebral bodies with blunt dissection using a swab-on-forceps. Any perforation of the peritoneum should be repaired immediately to prevent extension of the tear or omission of this repair later on. The ureter is reflected medially with the peritoneum. Three columns formed by the aorta, vertebral bodies, and the psoas muscle come into view (Figs. 20-10 to 20-13).

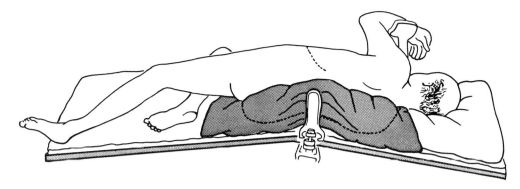

Fig. 20-8 Anterior extraperitoneal approach. Positioning and skin incision for operations on the upper lumbar levels.

Posterolateral Approach

The posterolateral approach provides good exposure of the transverse process and pars interarticularis.[9] We recommend it for posterolateral fusion in spondylolisthesis. Decompression of the nerve roots is easily accomplished through this approach. Access to the posterolateral quadrant of the vertebral body and disc space after osteotomy of the transverse process is possible but very restricted. Operating anterior to the plane of the transverse process endangers the aorta, vena cava, or common iliac vessels depending on the side and level.

The patient is anesthetized, intubated, and positioned prone as for a posterior midline approach (see following). The subcutaneous fat and paraspinal muscles are infiltrated with a hemostatic solution in the line of the planned incision. A longitudinal incision is made 5 to 7 cm lateral to the midline, and the dorsolumbar fascia is incised in line with the incision.

Retraction is made easier by extending the fascial incision in J-fashion (Figs. 20-14, 20-15). The lateral third of the paraspinal muscle mass is then split longitudinally, generally in line with the muscle fibers, by a combination of blunt dissection and diathermy knife (Fig. 20-16). Careful attention should be given to controlling bleeding muscle branches as they are encountered, if a continuous ooze is to be avoided.

An alternative is to make the skin incision a little more lateral and make the deep dissection between the paraspinal muscle mass and quadratus lumborum. This is not recommended, since it offers no advantage and poor exposure.

A large periosteal elevator is used to strip the muscles from the transverse process laterally and the posterior joint and lamina medially. For limited procedures on the posterolateral quadrant of the vertebral body and disc, the anterior surface of the transverse process is carefully stripped of periosteum with an elevator, taking care to keep the instrument in contact

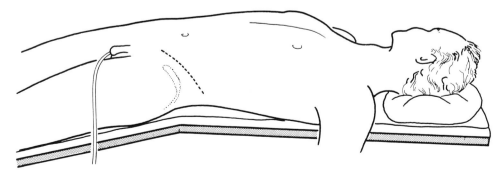

Fig. 20-9 Anterior extraperitoneal approach. Positioning and skin incision for operations on the lower lumbar levels.

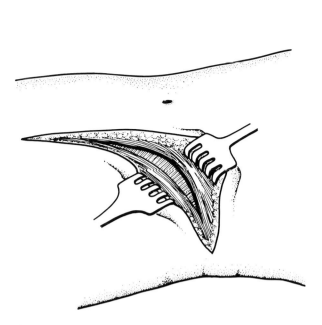

Fig. 20-10 External oblique aponeurosis and muscle fibers are incised in line of incision. (After Rathke FW, Schlegel KF: Surgery of the Spine. WB Saunders, Philadelphia, 1979.)

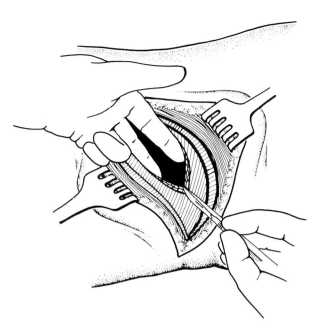

Fig. 20-12 Transversus abdominis is divided taking care not to cut the peritoneum.

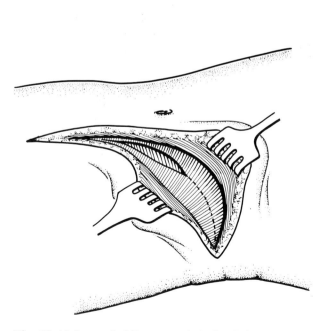

Fig. 20-11 Internal oblique muscle is divided transversely. (After Rathke FW, Schlegel KF: Surgery of the Spine. WB Saunders, Philadelphia, 1979.)

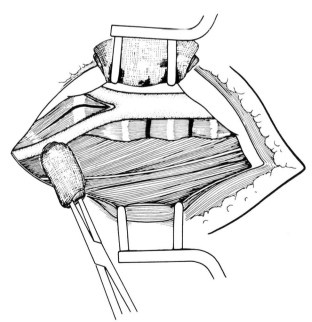

Fig. 20-13 Three columns formed by the aorta, vertebral bodies, and the psoas muscle. The ureter is pushed medially with the peritoneum. The genitofemoral nerve is seen on the psoas muscle.

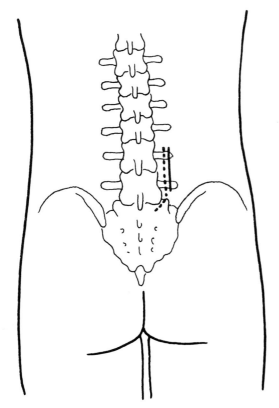

Fig. 20-14 Posterolateral approach. Skin (solid line) and fascial (broken line) incisions.

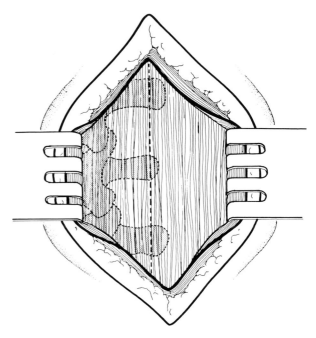

Fig. 20-15 Posterolateral approach. The dorsilumbar fascia is incised (dotted line).

with bone throughout the maneuver (Fig. 20-17). The transverse process is excised to its base with rongeurs or a guarded osteotome. The posterolateral aspect of the vertebral body comes into view when a long retractor is inserted and braced against the lateral surface of the vertebral body (Figs. 20-18 and 20-19).

Posterior Midline Approach

The posterior elements, transverse processes, spinal canal, disc space, and vertebral bodies can be exposed for discectomy, laminectomy, partial facetectomy, posterolateral fusion, or posterior interbody fusion by using the posterior midline approach.

Operations through this approach are carried out under general anesthesia and endotracheal intubation. Several positions—sitting, lateral, knee-to-chest (rabbit position)—have been used but we prefer the semi-flexed prone position on a modified Hastings frame.

We continue to experiment with other positions, frames, and bolsters, but we have found none as satisfactory as the Hastings frame.[10]

The original Hastings frame was made of wood. We use a simplified metal version with the patient in the same position as Hastings described, i.e., with the knees and hips flexed 110 to 120°. The patient's weight is borne on the chest—which rests on a firm padded washable cube—the buttocks, and the knees. The spine should be 10° head down. The advantages of this position and frame are that the dependent position of the abdomen, together with the 10° head-down position, serves to decrease the pressure in the vena cava and to minimize epidural bleeding. The spine is slightly flexed to increase the interlaminar space. The knees and hips are not in such an excessively flexed position as to predispose to deep vein thrombosis (Fig. 20-20).

Special precautions are important to prevent serious complications.
1. Avoid pressure on the eyes to prevent blindness.
2. Avoid excessive neck extension or rotation to prevent nerve root or spinal cord injury.
3. Avoid pressure over the ulnar nerve at the elbow and peroneal nerve at the knee to prevent paralysis.

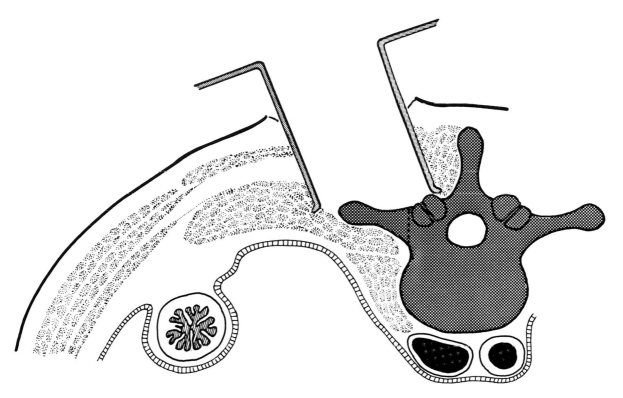

Fig. 20-16 Retraction and exposure. The transverse process may be osteotomized (dotted line) to approach the posterolateral quadrant of the disk or vertebral bodies for limited procedures.

4. Avoid excessive abduction of the shoulders to prevent brachial plexus traction injury.

The patient may move on bolsters and frames during the operation. We have had one case of femoral nerve palsy caused by pressure of blanket bolsters in the groin. Fortunately, this disappeared spontaneously after 4 days. Bolsters probably increase the risk of deep vein thrombosis by pressing on the femoral vein.

Crock's sausage is an excellent and versatile bolster that is useful for patients with special problems such as stiff joints in the lower extremities or gross obesity. It is economically made and consists of a plastic-covered roll of firm material that can be bent into a U-shape. The bend in the U supports the sternum and clavicles. The roll is thick enough to allow the obese abdomen to be dependent. A break in the table at the level of the iliac crests reduces the lumbar lordosis (Fig. 20-21).

A midline longitudinal incision that is centered over the level to be explored is made. Only as many laminae as necessary to safely complete the planned procedure are exposed. For example, the L4 to S1 laminae are exposed for L5–S1 discectomy. The subcutaneous fat and paraspinal muscles are infiltrated with a hemostatic solution using 22-gauge 6-inch needles. First, the skin is infiltrated through two punctures. It is then incised to expose the deep fascia and is retracted with self-retaining Gelpi retractors. The paraspinal muscles are then infiltrated by inserting the needles 5 cm lateral to the spinous processes in fanlike directions. The needle is inserted level with the spinous process deep enough to strike the posterior joint or transverse process and then retracted 1 cm before the injection is started. The injection is continued as the needle is withdrawn. This is repeated at every level that is to be exposed and on both sides for bilateral approaches. This technique avoids puncturing the skin in more than two places. The deep fascia is longitudinally incised close to the spinous processes to be exposed. A large periosteal elevator is inserted against the surface of the spinous process and the

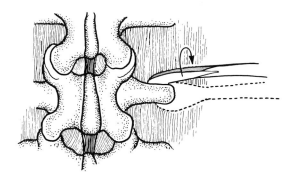

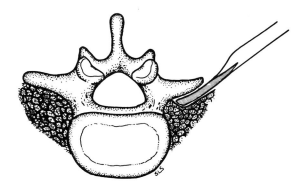

Fig. 20-17 The anterior surface of the transverse process is carefully stripped of periosteum.

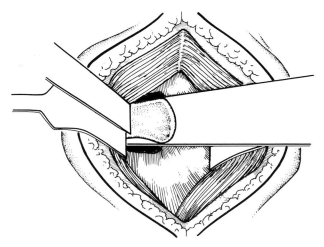

Fig. 20-18 The anterior structures are protected and the transverse process is osteotomised at its base. (After Rathke FW, Schlegel KF: Surgery of the Spine. WB Saunders, Philadelphia, 1979.)

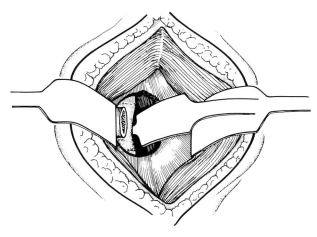

Fig. 20-19 The lateral surfaces of the vertebral body and disc are exposed. A blunt ended Hohmann retractor is braced against the vertebral body and protects the great vessels.

muscles are stripped subperiosteally. With the elevator held in one hand to stretch the musculotendenous fibers of origin, they are divided close to the bone with a scalpel in the other hand. The spinous processes should be exposed distally-to-proximally because the orientation of the muscle fibers that originate from the spinous processes facilitates this maneuver. A gauze pack is inserted and the elevator is used to push the pack and muscles laterally to expose the posterior joints. This step is repeated at each level and on both sides in bilateral exposures. A good habit to cultivate is to insert no more than one pack for each spinous process—making sure to remove the same number in the next step. The packs are removed

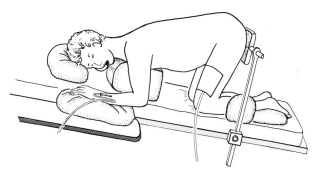

Fig. 20-20 The modified Hastings frame. Take care to prevent injury to the eyes, cervical spine, brachial plexus, ulnar nerve, and peroneal nerve (see text).

on the side to be explored and half the lamina on the opposite side (see Fig. 20-1).

The L5–S1 junction is then identified by visual examination, palpation, probing with a blunt dissector, forcibly moving the L5 spinous process, and, in many cases, a lateral x-ray with a metal marker on the L5 spinous process.

DISCECTOMY

Central and lateral stenosis may be present in association with a disc herniation.[11] If present, the stenoses are dealt with as discussed below after the herniation is excised. If a CT scan has shown normal central and lateral canals, the exploration is confined to the side of the herniation with or without osteotomy of the spinous process. If central or lateral stenosis is present, a bilateral approach is made and the stenosis dealt with as described below. In the event that no CT scan is available, the myelogram will also determine if central stenosis is present. However, the possibility of missing lateral stenosis on the asymptomatic side is real and we recommend bilateral exploration, intraoperative measurement of the lateral recesses with graduated probes, and lateral decompression if the canals are narrow. The CT scan is obviously invaluable in avoiding unnecessary bilateral explorations.

Technique

A posterior midline approach is made and the level to be explored is identified. The upper edge of the ligamentum flavum is partly detached from its attachment to the anterior surface of the upper lamina with a curette using a controlled scraping and pushing motion. The exposed lower edge of this lamina is then excised using Kerrison rongeurs. The safest place to start the incision into the ligamentum flavum is in the midline where it is tented away from the underlying dura. A small patty or narrow dissector is then inserted through the opening to displace anteriorly and protect the dura and epidural fat. The ligamentum flavum is then excised in one piece to expose the interlaminar space on one side. The opening is widened by excising one third of the superior and inferior laminae. Pressing gently on the dura with a blunt dissector may detect the fullness caused by a disc

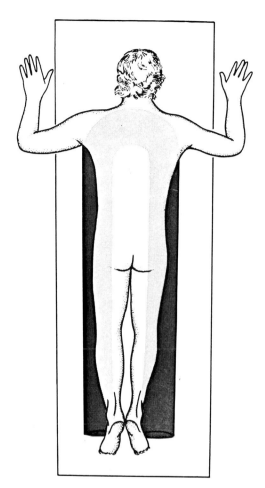

Fig. 20-21 Crock's sausage. A useful bolster for patients with stiff lower extremity joints or obesity.

and Gelpi self-retaining retractors inserted. Bleeders in muscle are cauterized. Fat, torn periosteum, and frayed tags of muscle are removed to denude completely the laminae and ligamenta flava in the entire field. A bone rongeur is best suited for this step. This procedure is repeated on both sides for bilateral exposures.

For a unilateral exploration in obese or muscular patients the surgeon's view can be improved by temporary displacement of the spinous process.[1] The spinous process is osteotomized, with a curved osteotome and mallet, where the process flares outward at the apex of the spinal canal. One or more spinous processes may be osteotomized. Gelpi retractors placed on the interspinous ligaments displace the spinous process or processes to expose both the lamina herniation felt through two thicknesses of dura. The surgeon dons headlight and magnifying glasses and with a bayonet nontoothed forceps and a blunt Penfield dissector explores the lateral recess. The nerve root lying medial to the pedicle is identified and retracted. Any difficulty retracting the root suggests that it is compressed by a disc herniation or entrapped in a narrowed lateral recess. Care should be taken not to confuse a nerve root stretched over an anteriorly placed herniation for the bulge of the herniation itself. The best precaution is always to confidently identify the nerve root before incising the presumed annulus fibrosus (Fig. 20-22). Epidural vessels are cauterized with bipolar diathermy at a low setting, taking care not to diathermize the nearby dura or nerve root inadvertently. Patties can be packed anterior and lateral to the dura both proximally and distally in the canal to control bleeding further and to retract the dura. Once the nerve root is confidently identified, it is retracted and a cruciate incision is made in the bulging annulus. The loose fragments of disc material are extracted with pituitary rongeurs. To avoid accidental avulsion of the root in the jaws of the rongeur, the latter is inserted through the annulus incision with the jaws closed and opened only when it is in the disc space. To avoid accidental damage to the retroperitoneal great vessels, the surgeon should take the special precautions described above. Ring curettes are inserted to scrape the endplates gently and the procedure with pituitary rongeurs is repeated (Figs. 20-2 and 20-3).

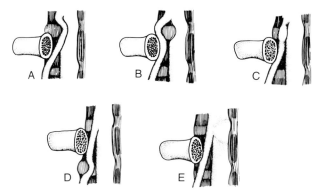

Fig. 20-22 The disc herniation may lie in one of several positions. Always identify the nerve root before incising the presumed herniation.

The nerve root should be freely mobile and easily retracted. Difficulty retracting the root may indicate that residual compression by migrated disc material or lateral stenosis is present, and a search should be made by probing the canal and foramen proximally and distally. The method of enlarging the lateral recess and foramen is described below.

At intervals throughout the procedure the entire wound is irrigated with a topical antibiotic diluted in saline. All patties, Gelfoam, and packs are removed and a free fat graft is placed over the exposed dura and sutured loosely to nearby soft tissue such as a posterior joint capsule. A closed suction tube drain is placed deep to the muscles and brought through a stab incision in the skin. A water-tight closure of the edges of the dorsilumbar fascia is made with interrupted sutures of absorbable material. Another tube drain is placed in the subcutaneous fat, which is apposed with a layer of absorbable sutures. The skin is closed with subcuticular absorbable material.

Postoperative Care

A neurological examination is carried out in the recovery room and any new deficit noted. The findings serve as a baseline. The patient is nursed supine for 24 hours. Intramuscular narcotic analgesics and antiemetics are given as required. Difficulty with micturition is frequent in males and if simple measures fail, a small catheter is inserted to be removed in 2 to 3 days. On the second postoperative day the patient is stood up at the bed side twice for 5 minutes each time. Thereafter, the patient stands and walks for increasing periods that are interspersed with rest periods in bed. The wound dressing is not removed unless excessive pain, tenderness, or fever raises the suspicion that a wound infection is present. The drains are removed without disturbing the dressing on the second postoperative day. The patient can usually go home by the tenth day after surgery, often earlier. No braces are prescribed.

The patient starts low back exercises (pelvic tilting and half sit-ups) at this stage and is seen at 4- to 6-week intervals initially. Light work is started at 6 to 8 weeks and heavy work at 12 to 16 weeks. Patients are encouraged to continue daily exercises indefinitely.

CENTRAL CANAL DECOMPRESSION

The narrowed central canal is unroofed by a wide laminectomy that extends laterally on both sides as far as the facet joints. The number of laminae to be excised is determined by the clinical picture, the number of narrow levels seen on the CT scan or myelogram, and the reestablishment of normal dural pulsation during the operation.

In severe central spinal stenosis, the nerve roots of the cauda equina are tightly crowded within the dura in a small bony canal. In addition the interlaminar spaces are narrow and the bone is hard. The risk of damaging the cauda equina by clumsy probing, excessively large instruments, or tight packing is great.

Technique

A posterior midline approach is made and the paravertebral muscles are elevated on both sides of all the vertebrae with narrow canals. Starting with the most distally involved vertebra, the spinous process is excised with angled double-action bone shears. The epidural space is entered by incisinig the ligamentum flavum as described for discectomy. If the canal is exceedingly small, the lamina is excised piecemeal. First the posterior cortex of the lamina is removed, leaving the thin anterior cortex intact. A toothed rongeur or high speed burr makes this step easy. The anterior cortex is then removed piecemeal with small Kerrison rongeurs. This precaution is important in central stenosis because of the crowded space, the small amount of epidural fat present and the dramatic immediate bulging of the dura as more of the lamina is excised. This procedure is repeated for all the vertebrae with narrowed canals (Figs. 20-23 and 20-24).

The wound is then irrigated with antibiotic diluted in saline and a free fat graft is loosely sutured to cover the exposed dura. The wound is drained and closed as described for discectomy (Fig. 20-25).

Postoperative Care

Care is the same as after discectomy, but these patients experience less discomfort in the immediate postoperative period and so require less analgesia.

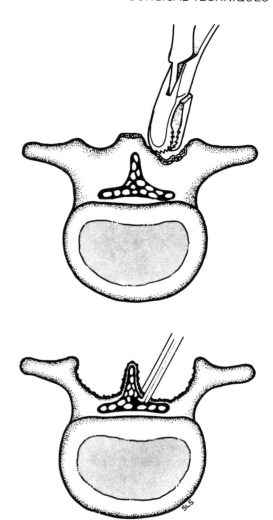

Fig. 20-23 Central spinal stenosis. Thin the thick hard lamina with a toothed rongeur before using a Kerrison rongeur. This prevents damage to the nerve roots, which are crowded into a small canal.

LATERAL CANAL DECOMPRESSION

When lateral stenosis is present on one side, the opposite side is often narrowed enough to cause symptoms or, if asymptomatic, to require prophylactic decompression. At any one level four nerve roots (two pairs) should be explored.[11] For example, at the L5-S1 level exploration should include the pair

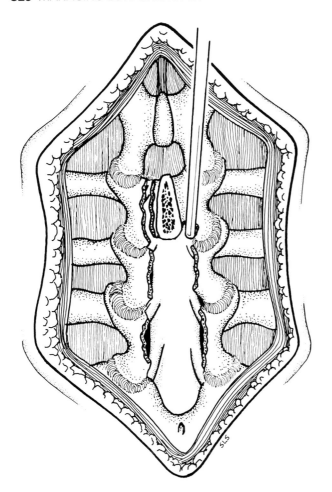

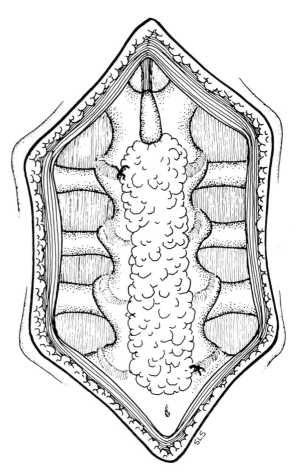

Fig. 20-24 Three level laminectomy for central spinal stenosis.

Fig. 20-25 A free fat graft is loosely sutured to prevent its displacement.

of L5 "exiting" and the pair of S1 "transversing" roots. Blunt-ended probes measuring 3,4,5, and 6 mm are used to measure the diameter of the lateral recesses and the foramina. The L5 roots are decompressed by excising the tips of the superior articular processes of S1 vertebrae and the S1 roots are decompressed by bilateral partial medial facetectomy (Fig. 20-26).

Technique

A posterior midline approach is made. The paraspinal muscles are elevated bilaterally and the involved intervertebral space identified. The ligamentum flavum is excised and the interlaminar space widened by excision of the upper and lower lamina edges and spinous processes.

The medial third of the inferior articular process is cut with a narrow osteotome and mallet or with a high speed burr. This step exposes the joint cartilage on the superior articular process. The medial third of the superior articular process is osteotomized with the same osteotome while the nerve is retracted and a flat dissector is placed in the recess to protect the nerve from injury. While the nerve is still being retracted, the most lateral part of the recess is widened by shaving the anterior surface of the superior articular process with a curette or high speed burr. The size of the recess is remeasured and if still narrow, it is widened further. The same procedure is repeated on the opposite side (Figs. 20-27 and 20-29).

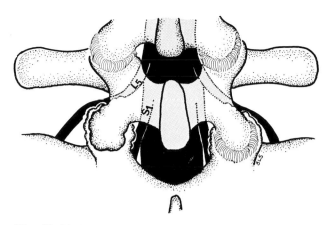

Fig. 20-26 At any one level four nerve roots (two pairs) can be explored.

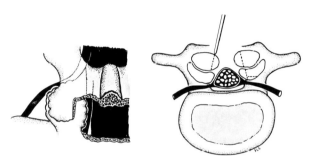

Fig. 20-27 The medial third of the L5 inferior articular process is osteotomized.

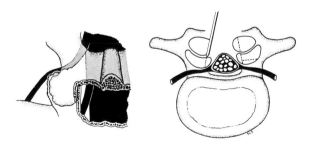

Fig. 20-28 The medial third of the S1 superior articular process is osteotomized. The nerve root should be retracted and protected.

On occasion the major narrowing is at the foramen. Further decompression should be effected by excising the lower medial edge of the pedicle with the use of the curette, Kerrison rongeurs, or high speed burr.

The exiting nerve is explored by excising more

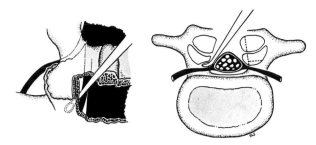

Fig. 20-29 The anterior surface of the S1 superior articular process (roof of the lateral recess) is shaved with a curette.

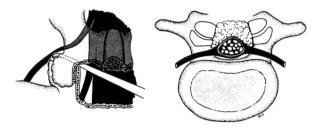

Fig. 20-30 The tip of the S1 superior articular process is removed to decompress the exiting L5 nerve. A free fat graft is loosely sutured to cover the dura.

of the inferior edge of the upper lamina. The nerve root should be seen exiting at the tip of superior articular process. In the event that the tip of the superior articular process is entrapping the exiting root the tip is excised with a curette or burr to permit free passage of the nerve (Fig. 20-30).

The wound is irrigated at intervals during and at the completion of the operation with antibiotic diluted in saline. A free fat graft is positioned to cover exposed dura and loosely sutured to nearby soft tissue such as a posterior joint capsule. The wound is drained and closed as for discectomy.

Postoperative Care

Care is the same as that described for discectomy.

REEXPLORATIONS

Reexplorations after previous surgery through the same approach can be pleasantly simple or exceedingly difficult. The scar may be tough enough to require a new scalpel blade after every few scalpel strokes. Heterotrophic bone in the scar is occasionally present. The dura may adhere densely to the laminectomy membrane and may tear easily. A few precautions should be observed and a few tips may simplify the operation.

Technique

Blood should be cross-matched in case excessive bleeding occurs. The preoperative plain x-ray films should be studied to determine the extent of previous laminectomies and the myelogram should be searched for postsurgical pseudomeningoceles so that problems can be anticipated.

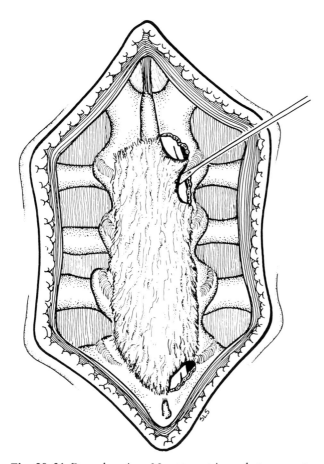

Fig. 20–31 Reexploration. No attempt is made to separate the laminectomy membrane from the dura. The nerve roots are dissected out by starting at the proximal, distal, and lateral edges of the membrane.

The original skin incision is used. The deep fascia is incised. The deep dissection is started in relatively normal tissues proximal, distal, and lateral to the previous laminectomy. Attention is directed at the most distal *intact* vertebra, which is stripped of muscles with an elevator. The same is done for the *intact* lamina just proximal to the previous laminectomy. The approximate depth of the dura below the laminectomy membrane can then be estimated, and the scar is incised down to this level without cutting the dura, for the length of the laminectomy. The blunt elevator is used to extend the dissection laterally to just beyond the lateral bony limit of the previous laminectomy, whether this is the lamina, posterior facets, or pedicle. Attention is directed at the lateral edge of the laminectomy membrane where the dissection becomes subperiosteal. The dissector is used to push the laminectomy membrane and encased dura off the sides of the bony canal. Roots often encased in scar tissue are exposed by blunt dissection using a Penfield dissector. The root and dura can then be retracted to expose the disc. No attempt should be made to separate the central part of the laminectomy membrane from the dura, since this is unnecessary and increases the risk of tearing the dura (Fig. 20-31).

Discectomy, lateral decompression, central decompression, pseudarthrosis repair is now carried out.

Postoperative Care

No special care is necessary.

SPONDYLOLISTHESIS

The surgical treatment of spondylolisthesis depends on several factors (Table 20-1).
1. Age
2. Degree of slip
3. Presence or absence of leg symptoms
4. Integrity of the disc above the proposed fusion
   We concur with Wiltse's and Jackson's experience in regard to the need for decompression in some adults but rarely in children and adolescents.[12] We do fusion alone, or decompression and fusion, but rarely a decompression alone.

In the more severe degrees of slip it is technically difficult to place grafts for posterolateral fusion be-

Table 20-1 Surgical Treatment of Isthmic Spondylolisthesis

Age	Leg Symptoms	Grade	Operation
Child	Yes	I, II	Fusion L5-S1
		III, IV	Fusion L4-S1
	No	I, II	Fusion L5-S1
		III, IV	Fusion L4-S1
Adult	Yes	I, II	Decompression and fusion L5-S1
		III, IV	Decompression and fusion L4-S1
	No	I, II	Fusion L5-S1
		III, IV	Fusion L4-S1

tween the L5 and S1 posterior elements and transverse processes. The pseudarthrosis rate for one-level fusion is unacceptably high, so we extend the fusion to L4.

The method of decompression is different for a posterior midline and posterolateral approach. In a midline approach we excise the entire "rattler"—a spinous process, laminae, and pars defect. It is extremely important to excise the mass of fibrous tissue, cartilage, and bone on the cephalad side of the pars defect. We do this with a high speed burr or with osteotome and mallet. At completion of the decompression the pair of exiting nerve roots should be easily visible from behind without the need for retraction. In a bilateral paraspinal approach the pair of exiting roots are decompressed by excising the fibrous tissue and approximately 0.5 cm of bone on either side of the defect without excising the entire lamina and spinous process, or rattler (Fig. 20-32).

In the adult for whom a one-level fusion is being

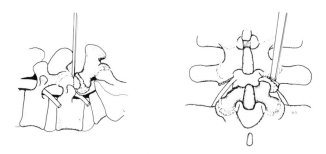

Fig. 20-32 Decompression for spondylolisthesis. Removing the rattler is optional, but the fibrous tissue and bone proximal to the pars defect must be excised in order to decompress the nerve.

considered, a discogram of the next proximal disc should be obtained and if it is abnormal, the fusion should be extended to include this level. Instability, lateral stenosis, and disc herniation at this level should be searched for on stress radiograms and the CT scan.

We have not attempted to reduce the subluxation. The results of posterior interbody fusion for spondylolisthesis in our hands have been disappointing because of a high rate of pseudarthrosis.[13]

SPINAL FUSION

The principles for successful arthrodesis apply to the spine as much as elsewhere.
1. Large areas of decorticated bone must be present at the site.
2. Cancellous bone graft must be abundant.
3. Bone contact and compression are desirable.
4. Immobilization must be prolonged until fusion has taken place.

Posterolateral Fusion

TECHNIQUES

If a posterior midline approach is used, a transverse cut is made in the dorsilumbar fascia without cutting the underlying paraspinal muscles. This facilitates the strong retraction that is necessary to expose the transverse processes as far as their tips. At the end of the operation, this transverse facial incision is repaired and seems to cause no detectable defect (Fig. 20-33). Bone graft is taken from the posterior iliac crest through a separate oblique or transverse incision. In muscular or obese individuals this approach offers a restricted view and is not recommended. Instead a bilateral paraspinal approach is used, and one of the two incisions is used to harvest the bone graft from the posterior iliac crest. Thereafter the operation is the same. This approach is highly recommended.

The posterior articular and transverse processes are completely denuded of periosteum with an elevator. Care should be exercised during this procedure to avoid damaging the posterior joint at the level above the planned fusion. The dissection should extend to the tips of the transverse processes and should be kept in a plane posterior to the transverse processes, except for one maneuver that will now be described.

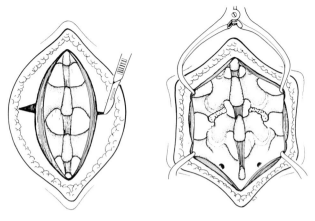

Fig. 20-33 Posterolateral fusion. A transverse cut in the dorsilumbar fascia permits strong retraction of the muscles to expose the transverse processes. The cuts are repaired before wound closure.

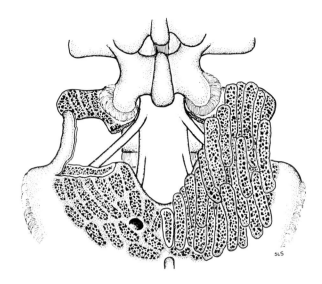

Fig. 20-34 Posterolateral fusion. (Left) Avoid damaging the posterior joint and sacroiliac joint during decortication. (Right) Avoid placing bone graft on exposed nerves.

Once the posterior surface of the transverse process is stripped, the anterior surface is stripped using a flat elevator with a peeling action starting at the superior edge of the transverse process. The instrument is kept constantly flat against the surface of the process. This extra stripping provides more bare bone and stimulates more new bone formation. However, the temptation to place bone graft anterior to the transverse processes should be resisted (Fig. 20-17). A sharp, curved gauge is used to raise "shingles" of cortico-cancellous bone on the posterior surface of the transverse process. The same process of denuding and shingling is done to the upper and posterior surface of the sacrum far laterally without interfering with the capsule of the sacroiliac joint. A generous block of bone is elevated from the flat upper surface of the lateral sacral mass. The graft is made long enough to span 2.5 cm to the L5 transverse process when it is hinged on itself. Free cancellous bone graft is then placed over and between the denuded surfaces. If a midline approach was used, a free fat graft is carefully trimmed, positioned, and sutured over the exposed dura to prevent encroachment onto the bone graft (Fig. 20-34).

POSTOPERATIVE CARE

The postoperative care is the same as after discectomy up to the tenth day. Then the sutures are removed and a body spika that extends from nipples down to the thigh on one side but permits free hip flexion on the other is applied with the patient standing. All patients should be able to walk in the spika with a cane or crutches. The spika is worn for 12 weeks and then a chair back brace is worn during the day until fusion occurs—usually an additional 8 weeks.

Posterior Lumbar Interbody Fusion

Cloward[13] published clear step-by-step illustrations of this procedure, but we suggest that anyone planning to do this operation should first be taught by observing a practiced operator. He has designed a set of instruments, many of which are indispensable for the operation. The operation takes a long time, especially when autogenous bone graft is taken at the same session. Lin[14] has described minor modifications to Cloward's operation.

The advantage of this operation over anterior interbody fusion is that either discectomy or decompression can be done through the same approach as the fusion. At least theoretically it is advantageous for the bone graft to be under compression. The possibility of posterior migration of the graft with serious consequence cannot be ignored, although this seems rare.

More epidural dissection, retraction, and cauterization is required than for other operations. The average spinal surgeon seeing the procedure for the first time may be taken aback by the amount of cauterization that is necessary to make the procedure possible. Postoperative perineural fibrosis is probably severe after the Cloward technique, but any role it may have in causing symptoms is uncertain. It may not be of consequence if a successful fusion eliminates movement at the operated level. Our experience does not allow us to recommend this procedure. Other authors report good results.

TECHNIQUE

This description is a little different from that of Cloward. The patient is positioned prone and an oversized bone graft is taken from the posterior iliac crest through a transverse incision. Use an oscillating power saw rather than osteotome to avoid cracks that weaken the graft. A posterior midline approach using a midline skin incision is made. If the fusion follows excision of a disc herniation, the canal is approached through the interlaminar space. For spondylolisthesis, the approach is made after the "rattler" has been excised. In either case we completely excise the ligamentum flavum.

When the operation is for disc disease, the interlaminar space is widened by removal of the superior and inferior margins of the adjacent laminae, partial medial facetectomy, and retraction with a laminar spreader. Epidural vessels are liberally cauterized and the charred remains are excised with scissors. A self-retaining nerve root retractor is placed on the root and dura, which are retracted to the midline.. The cauterized vessels are pushed aside to expose the annulus anteriorly. Bleeding vessels are pushed off with patties and packed temporarily with Gelfoam behind more patties. It is important not to proceed further until good hemostasis and good exposure of the annulus are obtained (Fig. 20-35). A rectangle of annulus is excised. The bony ledge or shelf of the posterior superior margin of the lower vertebral body that "overhangs" the interspace is removed with a narrow osteotome. The endplates and disc material are removed with alternate use of straight and curved osteotomes, curettes, and pituitary rongeurs. Bleeding from the endplates can be extensive and can require temporary packing with Gelfoam or Surgicel (Figs. 20-36 to 20-41). Blocks of cortico-cancellous bone

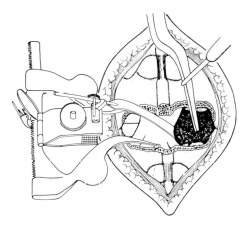

Fig. 20-35 Posterior lumbar interbody fusion. Epidural vessels are cauterized with cutting diathermy set at a low current. (After Cloward RB: The Cloward technique. In Finneson BE (ed): Low Back Pain. 2nd Ed. JB Lippincott, Philadelphia, 1980.)

taken from the iliac crest are cut to the measured size of the "disc space" and jammed into the space. The first grafts are moved medially to enlarge the laterally adjacent space so that the second or third graft can be inserted. This maneuver is carried out with a pair of blunt ended "chisels" using three maneuvers. The same is repeated on the opposite side. A free fat graft is sutured to nearby soft tissue to cover the dura (Figs. 20-42 to 20-47).

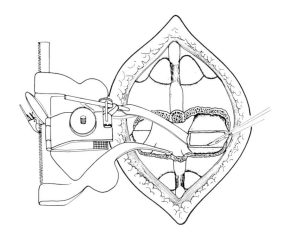

Fig. 20-36 Posterior lumbar interbody fusion. A window of posterior longitudinal ligament and annulus is excised. (After Cloward RB: The Cloward technique. In Fenneson BE (ed): Low Back Pain. 2nd Ed. JB Lippincott, Philadelphia, 1980.)

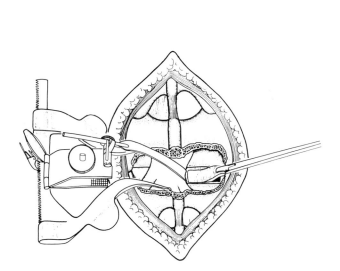

Fig. 20-37 Posterior lumbar interbody fusion. (After Cloward RB: The Cloward technique. In Finneson BE (ed): Low Back Pain. 2nd Ed. JB Lippincott, Philadelphia, 1980.)

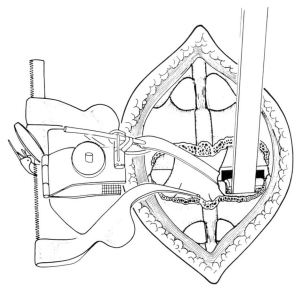

Fig. 20-39 The superior edge of the lower vertebra is removed. (After Cloward RB: The Cloward technique. In Finneson BE (ed): Low Back Pain. 2nd Ed. JB Lippincott, Philadelphia, 1980.)

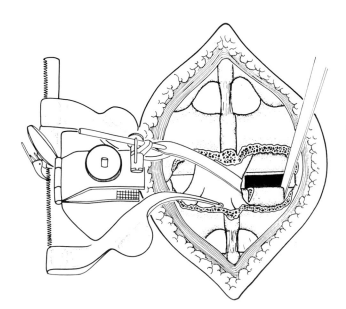

Fig. 20-38 Vertical cuts in the superior edge of the lower vertebra. (After Cloward RB: The Cloward technique. In Finneson BE (ed): Low Back Pain. 2nd Ed. JB Lippincott, Philadelphia, 1980.)

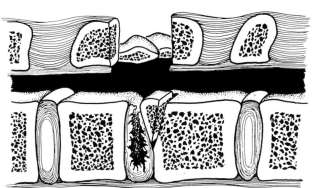

Fig. 20-40 The wedge of removed bone is shown. (After Cloward RB: The Cloward technique. In Finneson BE (ed): Low Back Pain. 2nd Ed. JB Lippincott, Philadelphia, 1980.)

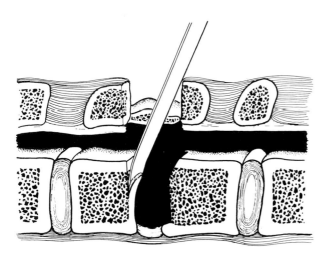

Fig. 20-41 A curved osteotome is used to remove the end-plates. (After Cloward RB. The Cloward technique. In Fenneson BE (ed): Low Back Pain. 2nd Ed. JB Lippincott, Philadelphia, 1980.)

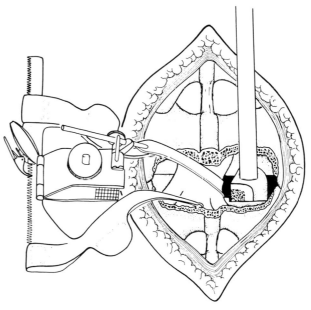

Fig. 20-43 A slightly oversized graft is punched into the Space. (After Cloward RB: The Cloward technique. In Finneson BE (ed): Low Back Pain. 2nd Ed. JB Lippincott, Philadelphia, 1980.)

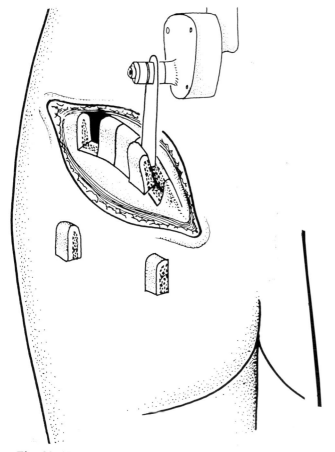

Fig. 20-42 Oversized partial and full thickness cortico-cancellous bone graft is removed with an oscillating saw through a separate skin incision.

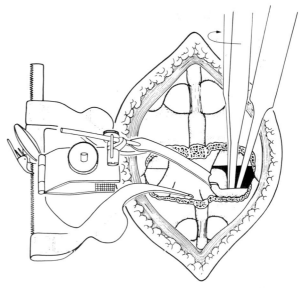

Fig. 20-44 The graft is moved medially with Cloward's blunt chisels.

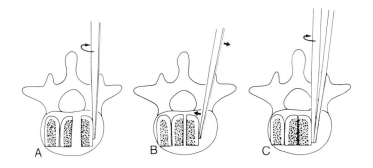

Fig. 20-45 Techniques for moving the graft medially. **(A)** Twisting. **(B)** Levering. **(C)** Twisting with a second chisel.

POSTOPERATIVE CARE

Cloward does not recommend braces or casts when the procedure is for disc disease and recommends a chair type steel brace for 30 days for spondylolisthesis.

Anterior Interbody Fusion

TECHNIQUE

The help of two good assistants is important. An anterior retroperitoneal or transperitoneal approach is made. The aorta and its bifurcation are identified. When L5–S1 fusion is planned, two long narrow blunt-ended retractors are placed, one to retract the common iliac vessel and viscera to the right and the other to retract the iliac vessels to the left. The disc excision and grafting are carried out between these two retractors, which protect the vessels from damage. A flap of anterior longitudinal ligament and anterior annulus fibrosis hinged on the right is raised

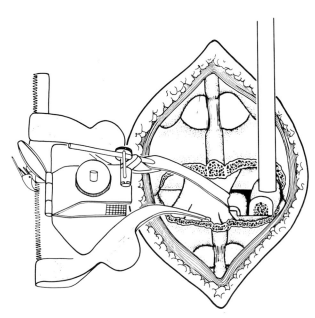

Fig. 20-46 A second or third graft is punched into the space. (After Cloward RB: The Cloward technique. In Finneson BE (ed): Low Back Pain. 2nd Ed. JB Lippincott, Philadelphia, 1980.)

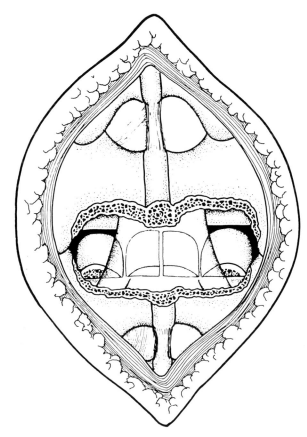

Fig. 20-47 The completed operation. (After Cloward RB: The Cloward technique. In Finneson BE (ed): Low Back Pain. 2nd Ed. JB Lippincott, Philadelphia, 1980.)

with a scalpel. When the disc space is extremely narrow, this step is impossible and instead a horizontal incision in the annulus is made (Fig. 20-48). The disc material is removed piecemeal under direct vision with curettes and pituitary rongeurs as far posterior as the posterior longitudinal ligament. Work on the bone is postponed until the disc is completely cleared posteriorly and laterally. The endplates are then excised to bleeding cancellous bone using straight and curved osteotomes. Bleeding may be brisk and the space may have to be packed temporarily with Gelfoam or Surgicel (Fig. 20-49). Full thickness iliac crest grafts are then punched into the space. During their insertion, they are guided and stabilized by punches that are placed into the disc space to fill openings not yet filled with graft. Once the last graft is in place, all the grafts are counter-sunk 2 to 3 mm deep to the anterior edge of the vertebral body, and the break in the table is straightened to hold the grafts in between the vertebral bodies. The flap of anterior ligament and annulus is replaced and sutured with heavy Dexon (Figs. 20-50 and 20-51).

To fuse L4–L5 or L3–L4 the lumbar spinal vessels above the below the disc are identified and ligated. The same retractors are used, one to retract to the right and protect the aorta and the other to retract the viscera in a cephalad direction. The disc excision and bone grafting are the same as described for the L5–S1 level.

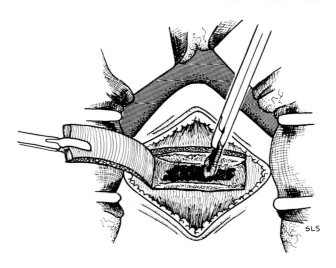

Fig. 20-49 The disc is removed piecemeal under direct vision with pituitary forceps. The endplates are removed with curved osteotomes.

At the end of the procedure the retroperitoneal space is drained with a closed suction tube drain and the abdominal muscle layers are closed with interrupted Dexon sutures.

POSTOPERATIVE CARE

A nasogastric tube is routinely inserted and oral intake is delayed until bowel sounds return or flatus has been passed. The care is the same as for discectomy

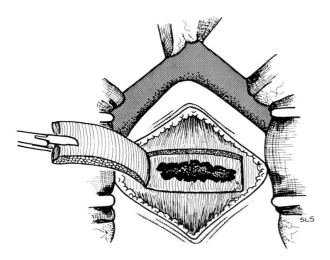

Fig. 20-48 Anterior interbody fusion. A window of annulus is incised and hinged to the patient's right.

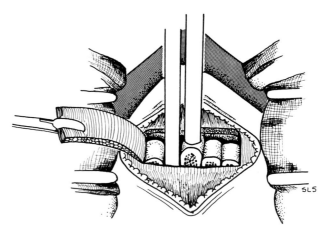

Fig. 20-50 Slightly oversized cortico-cancellous bone grafts are punched into the space. Punches in the unfilled spaces prevent the grafts from tilting during their insertion.

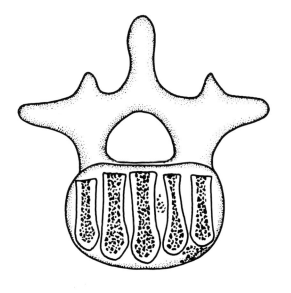

DISCOGRAPHY

The indications for diagnostic lumbar disc injections are controversial. The most common indication is for a discogram-CT, or discogram enhanced CT, in cases that are clinically suspicious of a disc herniation but have an equivocal or negative CT. The next most common indication we find is to assess the condition of the disc above a proposed spinal fusion (Fig. 20-52).

The resistance to the injection, the volume of fluid accepted, the x-ray appearance, and CT are reliable criteria for differentiating between a normal and abnormal disc. We have not found any reliable indicators for distinguishing if a particular abnormal disc causes the complaints. In our experience, the patient's reports of pain on injection of saline, contrast fluid,

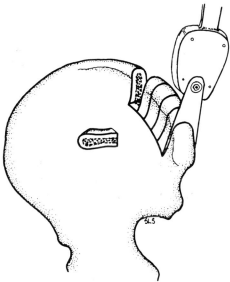

Fig. 20-51 Bone grafts are cut with a power saw to prevent cracks and are counter sunk behind the edge of the intervertebral space.

except that a plaster spika that immobilizes the hip on one side is fitted to be worn continuously for 12 weeks. If the fit of the graft in the interspace is judged insecure, the patient is kept horizontal in an ordinary bed for 6 weeks. Log-rolling 45° each way is permitted. The patient is then permitted to walk in a plaster spika for 6 weeks.

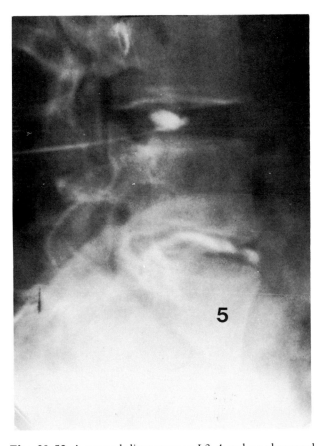

Fig. 20-52 A normal discogram at L3–4 and an abnormal discogram at L4–5. A fusion was planned for L5–S1 spondylolisthesis, but was extended one level higher.

or local anesthetic have not been as reliable as other authors claim.[15–17]

An abnormal disc accepts the injection with small resistance, a quality that is quickly learned after only a few injections. The abnormal disc accepts more than 0.5 ml of fluid. Radiographs show that the contrast is confined to the center of the normal disc, though the shape may vary. The dye tracks extensively into the periphery of the abnormal disc, and outside the confines of the disc if the annulus is ruptured (Fig. 20-52).

Technique

After the patient is mildly sedated, the procedure is carried out in the radiology department under local anesthesia with aseptic technique and two-plane x-ray fluoroscopy guidance. It is helpful to have an articulated spine in the room at the time. The posterolateral extradural approach is easy and is used routinely unless difficulty is encountered, when the transdural approach is used. For either approach, the patient is positioned on the side with a folded sheet placed under the flank to straighten the spine. The position is adjusted so that a true lateral and anteroposterior view of the spine is obtained before starting.

In the posterolateral approach, a 6-inch 18-gauge needle is inserted 8 cm lateral to the midline and is angled 45 to 60° toward the midline at the level of the disc. For the more difficult L5–S1 level it is often necessary to pierce the skin further from the midline (9 to 10 cm to avoid striking the posterior joint, which is larger and in a more lateral position. However, the iliac crest usually prevents more lateral needle placement.

The "bent needle" technique is useful if difficulty is encountered at the L5–S1 level. A 4-inch 18-gauge needle is inserted 10 cm lateral to the midline and 60° to the sagittal plane. The needle is advanced and adjusted so that its tip is adjacent to the posterior aspect of the disc space. A 6-inch 22-gauge needle is then introduced through the lumen of the 18-gauge needle. The terminal ¾ inch of the 22-gauge needle is first bent so that the bevel lies on the convex side of the curve; thus when it emerges from the 18-gauge needle, it curves towards the disc space.

The needle direction is adjusted as necessary to place the tip equidistant from pedicles on the AP view and in the center of the disc equidistant from the endplates on the lateral view. When the needle direction is to be changed, the needle tip must be withdrawn close to the skin before it is redirected and reinserted (Fig. 20-53). Renografin 60 is injected, and the fluoroscope is used to check that sufficient dye for a good image has been injected. The needle is removed and permanent lateral and AP films are made. The latter is taken with the patient supine with hips and knees flexed and the x-ray beam directed 20° cephalad. CT can be carried out up to 6 hours later.

In the posterior transdural approach, a 4-inch 18-gauge needle is inserted between the two spinous processes in the midline and advanced as far as the ligamentum flavum. The direction is adjusted as necessary. A 6-inch 22-gauge needle is passed through the shorter needle and its tip is advanced through the two layers of dura and into the disc. The remainder of the procedure is as described for the posterolateral approach.

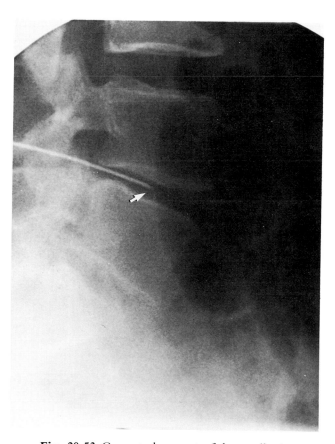

Fig. 20-53 Correct placement of the needle tip.

CHEMONUCLEOLYSIS

Complications following chymopapain injection are rare, unpredictable, and potentially lethal. A repeat chymopapain injection is contraindicated in patients who have been injected previously.

Technique

Early on we gave the injection in the operating room under general anesthesia with endotracheal intubation. McCulloch[19] reported his large experience of chemonucleolysis under local anesthesia. Anaphylactic shock can be diagnosed more rapidly in a conscious patient, and it can be treated more easily in the absence of the pharmacological effect of general anesthetic agents. We changed to using local anesthesia in our center.

Aseptic technique and two-plane image intensifier guidance are used. The posterolateral extradural approach (as described above for discography) is always used to avoid penetrating the dura and prevent leakage of chymopapain into the subarachnoid space. Preparations are made before injection to treat a possible anaphylactic reaction. A secure intravenous line is established and pulse rate and blood pressure are monitored. Hydrocortisone, epinephrine, aminophylline, and diphenhydramine are immediately available. An anaesthetist with intubation and ventilation equipment must be present during the injection.

The use of contrast material is kept to a minimum. Only a drop or two is injected to confirm needle placement before the chymopapain injection. The chymopapain must be refrigerated up to the time of mixing with distilled water that has been at room temperature. The mixed solution must be used immediately and cannot be stored. The dosage is 4000 U or 2 ml per disc, injected over 3 to 4 minutes.

Postoperative Care

The patient is encouraged to be as active as pain permits. A stiff canvas corset, oral analgesics, and antiinflammatory drugs are prescribed. Many patients require a few days of in-hospital care and a few may require intramuscular narcotic analgesics.

SELECTIVE NERVE ROOT INJECTION

It is technically possible to inject all lumbar nerves and the first sacral nerve. This procedure is occasionally helpful to identify which particular spinal nerve is the cause of leg pain in patients who have no objective neurological deficit. It is especially useful in patients with vague symptoms and CT scan findings of borderline lateral stenosis at two or more levels. The L4, L5, and S1 nerves are the ones most commonly injected.

Information is obtained by irritating the nerve with the needle tip and contrast medium and then blocking the nerve with local anesthetic. The success in finding the target nerve is confirmed by a clear radiculogram and by a sensory or motor deficit that corresponds to the particular nerve. This requires repeated reexamination before and after each nerve block. The most reliable evidence is quadriceps weakness for L3, knee jerk loss for L4, weak toe extension for L5, and ankle jerk loss for S1. We have not been able to obtain reliable information concerning the nature of the particular pathological process from the dye outline or pattern.[20]

Before and after each root is injected, the patient is questioned and examined. In addition to sensory and motor tests, the range of spinal movement and straight leg raising is tested each time. This requires reprepping and redraping the skin before each nerve is injected in turn. A great deal of patience and cooperation is required from the patient.

Technique

The procedure is carried out in the radiology department with two-plane image intensifier guidance under local anesthesia. Excessive preoperative sedation may reduce the patient's cooperation and invalidate the information. The patient is positioned prone with two folded sheets under the hips.

The needle placement is the same for all the lumbar nerves. The L5 nerve may require a technique similar to the "bent needle" technique described above. A 22-gauge needle is introduced 3 to 4 cm lateral to the midline, level with the spinous process. The needle is directed at 90° to the skin surface toward the base of the transverse process. When the needle is

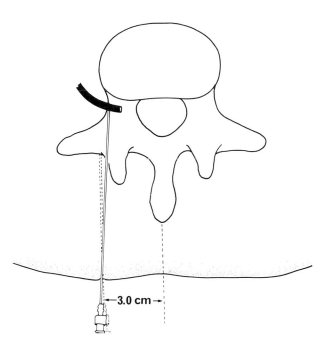

Fig. 20-54 Technique of selective lumbar spinal nerve block. (See text.)

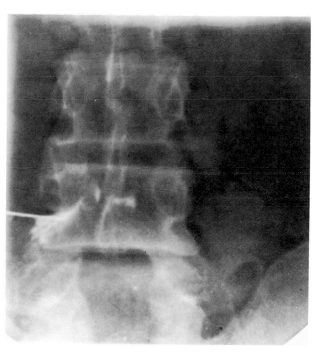

Fig. 20-56 L4 spinal nerve block. Needle placement and a radiculogram are shown.

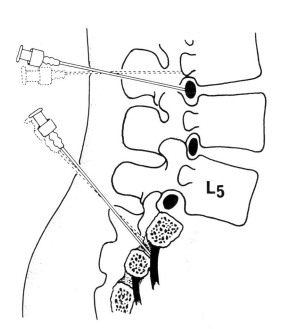

Fig. 20-55 Technique of selective third lumbar spinal nerve and first sacral nerve block. The sacrum has been cut away in a sagittal plane through its anterior and posterior foramina.

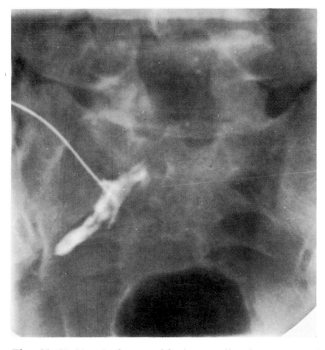

Fig. 20-57 S1 spinal nerve block. Needle placement and a radiculogram are shown. Patient had a previous L5 laminectomy.

felt to strike the transverse process, the position is confirmed on AP and lateral views. The needle is retracted 1 cm and redirected caudad and medially. The needle tip is felt and seen to advance anterior to the transverse process and into the intervertebral foramen (Figs. 20-54 and 20-55). The patient may experience radiating leg pain, and he is questioned about its character and distribution. Lateral and AP views should confirm that the needle tip is located immediately inferior to the pedicle. A 1 or 2 ml of 60% Conray is injected and the patient may experience pain again. AP films are taken and 2 to 3 ml of 1% lidocaine are injected. The leg pain disappears and the patient is stood up and examined (Fig. 20-56).

The S1 nerve requires a different approach through the S1 posterior foramen of the sacrum. The image intensifier and needle are directed 45° caudad to allow for the backward tilt of the sacrum. This view superimposes the posterior on the anterior sacral foramina to produce a clearer image. The needle is introduced 2 to 2.5 cm lateral to the midline, level with the L5 spinous process. It is directed 45° caudad to contact the edge of the posterior sacral foramen. The needle is adjusted to enter the foramen, then advanced 2 cm so that its tip lies in the anterior foramen. X-ray confirmation is made and the contrast and local anesthetic are injected as described above (Figs. 20-55 to 20-57).

No special postoperative care is necessary.

POSTERIOR JOINT INJECTION

Injecting the posterior joints is an easy procedure. The injection is placed around the joint capsule and sometimes probably into the joint cavity. At least two pairs and usually three pairs of joints are routinely injected, each with 12.5 mg prednisolone acetate (Meticortelone) and 5 ml of 0.25% bupivacaine (Marcaine).

The injection is carried out as an outpatient proce-

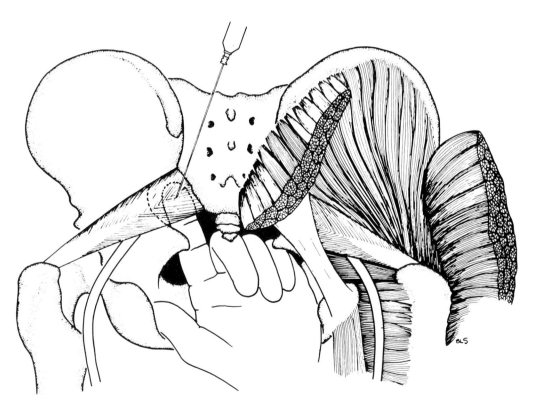

Fig. 20-58 Technique of piriformis injection. (After Wyant GM: Chronic pain syndromes and their treatment. III. The piriformis syndrome. Can Anaesth Soc J 20:305, 1979.)

dure in the radiology department under local anesthesia with fluoroscopy guidance. The patient is placed in the lateral position with folded sheets under the flank to straighten the spine. The skin entry points are infiltrated with a local anesthetic. A 4-inch 18-gauge needle is inserted level with the interspinous space 5 to 6 cm lateral to the midline. The needle is directed 60° to the skin towards the posterior joints until the needle tip encounters the bone of a facet. The needle tip position is confirmed with fluoroscopy. All the needles are positioned before the injection is made. If a needle has to be repositioned, its tip is retracted near to the skin before it is redirected and reinserted.

PIRIFORMIS INJECTION

The injection is placed in the belly of the piriformis muscle, just lateral to the edge of the sacrum and medial to the course of the sciatic nerve. Prednisolone acetate (Meticortelone) 25 to 50 mg and 0.25% plain bupivacaine 3 to 5 ml are injected under aseptic technique as an outpatient procedure.[21]

The patient is positioned on his side, with hips and knees flexed and the affected side uppermost. The skin is prepped and all drugs are drawn up in syringes before the next step. The physician then inserts the index finger of his (or her) nondominant hand into the rectum and palpates the lateral edge of the sacrum high in the sciatic notch. This will be the site of maximum tenderness. With the dominant hand, a 6-inch 20-gauge needle is directed perpendicular to the skin at a point on the buttock skin overlying the finger pulp in the rectum. The needle is advanced to stop 2 to 3 cm short of the finger pulp and the injection placed there. If the needle hub is repeatedly wiggled as it is advanced, the movement of the needle tip will be felt by the finger placed in the rectum, and in this way the physician can safely estimate the distance of the needle from the finger and avoid penetrating the rectal mucosa (Fig. 20-58).

REFERENCES

1. Yong-Hing K, Kirkaldy-Willis WH: Osteotomy of lumbar spinous process to increase surgical exposure. Clin Orthop 134: 218, 1978

2. Macnab I, Dall D: The blood supply of the lumbar spine and its application to the technique of intertransverse lumbar fusion. J Bone Joint Surg 53B: 628, 1971

3. Yong-Hing K, Reilly J, de Korompay V, Kirkaldy-Willis WH: Prevention of nerve root adhesions after laminectomy. Spine 5: 59, 1980

4. Langenskiold A, Vallem: Epidurally placed free fat grafts visualized by CT scanning. Spine 10: 97, 1985

5. Rathke FW, Schlegel KF: Surgery of the Spine. WB Saunders, Philadelphia, 1979

6. Kirkaldy-Willis WH, Thomas G: Anterior approaches in the diagnosis and treatment of infections of the vertebral bodies. J Bone Joint Surg 47A: 87, 1965.

7. Crock HV: Anterior lumbar interbody fusion: indications for its use and notes on surgical technique. Clin Orthop 165: 157, 1982

8. Goldner LJ, Wood KE, Urbaniak JR: Anterior lumbar discectomy and interbody fusion: indications and technique. In Schmidek HH, Sweet WH (eds): Current Techniques in Operative Neurosurgery. Grune and Stratton, Orlando, 1977

9. Wiltse LL: The paraspinal sacrospinalis-splitting approach to the lumbar spine. Clin Orthop 91: 48, 1973

10. Hastings DE: A simple frame for operations on the lumbar spine. Can J Surf 12: 251, 1968

11. Kirkaldy-Willis WH, Wedge JH, Yong-Hing K, Tchang S, deKorompay V, Shannon R: Lumbar spinal nerve lateral entrapment. Clin Orthop 169: 171, 1982

12. Wiltse LL, Jackson DW: Treatment of spondylolisthesis and spondylolysis in children. Clin Orthop 117: 92, 1972

13. Cloward RB: The Cloward technique. In Finneson BE (ed): Low Back Pain, 2nd Ed. JB Lippincott, Philadelphia, 1980

14. Lin PM: A technical modification of Clowards posterior interbody fusion. Neurosurgery 1: 118, 1977

15. Cloward RB: Discography: technique, indications and evaluation of the normal and abnormal intervertebral disc. Am J Roent 68: 552, 1952

16. Simmons EH, Segil CM: An evaluation of discography is the localization of symptomatic levels in discogenic disease of the spine. Clin. Orthop 108: 57, 1975

17. Wiley JJ, Macnab I, Wortzman G: Lumbar discography and its clinical applications. Can J Surg 11: 280, 1968

18. McCulloch JA, Waddel G: Lateral lumbar discography. Am J Rad 51: 498, 1978

19. McCulloch JA: Chemonucleolysis: experience with 2000 cases. Clin Orthop 146: 128, 1980

20. Tajima T, Furukawa K, Kuramochi E: Selective lumbosacral radiculography and block. Spine 5: 68, 1980

21. Wyant GM: Chronic pain syndromes and their treatment, III. The piriformis syndrome. Canad Anaesth Soc J 26: 305, 1979

21
Physical Therapy

Arlis McQuarrie

The most important role of physical therapy in the multidisciplinary approach to the management of low back pain is the assessment of functional capacity, specific joint mobility, patterns of muscle action, and treatment including patient education, specific exercises, specific joint mobilization, and manipulation.

Integral to this approach is the involvement of the patient as an active participant in the treatment program. This is particularly important in treating difficult longstanding low back pain problems. The therapist must build patient confidence in the ability to regain an ever increasing measure of functional activity.

In all instances the patient is taught to assume some responsibility for his or her program. This can be achieved by planning appropriate modification of activity, using correct biomechanics, improving physical fitness and exercise tolerance, and setting up sensible limits to daily activity. Therapist supervision of the program emphasizes the importance of the active role of the patient, and ensures progression of activity. A specific exercise program should be planned to encourage preparation for returning to work.

It cannot be stressed too much that throughout treatment the emphasis is on function and not on relief of pain. Very often as the functional capacity and level of fitness of the patient improve, pain diminishes.

ASSESSMENT OF FUNCTION

The functional assessment is done with considerable attention to detail. This includes postural control, the performance of specific daily activities, exercise tolerance, daily activity level tolerance, the length and frequency of rest periods, and the patient's perception of those activities that are possible and those that are harmful. It is useful to have the patient keep a diary of the amount and type of daily activity accomplished.

Integral to this is an assessment of pain behavior, the degree of confidence in choosing and performing various activities, and the patient's understanding of the back problem and the reasonable limitations that it imposes. The therapist is in a position to gain an understanding of social, economic, and emotional problems.

As a preparation for achieving functional improvement, the therapist will assess muscle flexibility and strength, patterns of muscle action and specific joint mobility (Fig. 21-1).

PHYSICAL THERAPY TREATMENT

A number of modalities commonly used by the therapist in treating low back pain are in fact primarily adjunctive and are employed mainly as a preparation

345

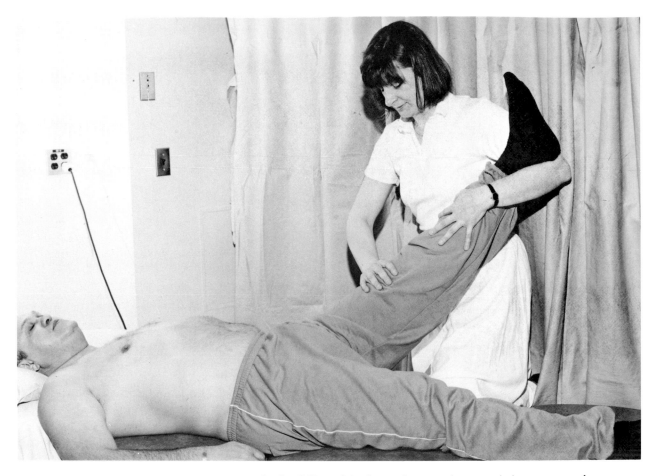

Fig. 21-1 Hamstring flexibility. Testing the flexibility of the hamstring muscle group is important and must be done with careful positioning.

for active measures. These modalities, such as heat and cold, traction, transcutaneous electrical nerve stimulation, ultrasound, diathermy and mobilization, are passive forms of treatment.

Active measures include exercise, biofeedback, postural control, and activities of daily living. Emphasis is placed on active restoration of function rather than on passive pain control.

RELAXATION AND PAIN CONTROL

Heat and Cold

These are available in a number of different forms. They include hot packs, cold packs, cryotherapy machines, short wave diathermy, ultrasound, infra-

red, and hot and cold whirlpool baths. These measures, together with massage are frequently used to reduce muscle spasm, increase soft tissue extensibility, induce a feeling of well being and relaxation, and reduce pain. They may also be used in the control of edema and inflammation from mechanical causes. Their effects have been described elsewhere.[1] They are used both before and after exercise and mobilization to improve performance of activity and reduce any irritating effects of treatment. The use of these passive measures alone does not usually effect a permanent beneficial change in the patient's condition.

Ice is usually the modality of choice in managing acute injuries or recent exacerbations of a chronic condition. In other cases the decision as to whether heat or ice should be used is a personal one. Most therapists believe that ice produces better relaxation of muscle spasm and better reduction of pain. The application of heat or cold should include a judicious choice of resting position for the patient.

Transcutaneous Electrical Nerve Stimulation

This treatment is noninvasive. It provides a current for sensory stimulation to block pain. There are primarily two ways in which it can be applied, each specific to a suggested mechanism of action or physiological response that results in pain reduction.[2]

The first method is often called a conventional high frequency TENS application. This method employs a continuous output with a frequency usually between 80 to 150 cycles/sec. This high frequency TENS application stimulates the large sensory afferent fibers whose input, at the dorsal horn level, results in selective blockage of nociceptive input from unmyelinated and small myelinated sensory afferent fibers.

The electrode placement for conventional high frequency TENS application is commonly in the vicinity of the painful area, in a 'crossfire' technique, or on related paravertebral segments and their dermatomal distribution (Fig. 21-2).

Low frequency TENS applied in a 'burst' mode is the second common method of application. This uses a frequency of two to four cycles/second with a train of impulses (usually seven) to each 'burst.' Some evidence suggests that this method of stimulation results in a release of endorphins in the central nervous system.[3] The suggested electrode placement for this mode is usually over acupuncture or trigger points.

A word of caution is needed. TENS has been so well marketed and publicized that it can be prescribed too often and used at the expense of more definitive treatment. It should not be used in the absence of a satisfactory working diagnosis. It can mask pain that is an indicator of a more sinister condition such as a malignant lesion.

Patient education in the use of TENS is necessary to insure maximum benefit and appropriate activity levels. It requires patience to try out various types of application and a good working knowledge of the variety of modes of application available to gain maximum benefit. It is used as an adjunctive measure to active forms of therapy.

Ultrasound

Depending on the application chosen, ultrasound primarily will result in a thermal heating effect, a mechanical effect, or a combination of these.[4] Ultrasound is sometimes helpful in relieving spasm and in decreasing the mechanical inflammatory response

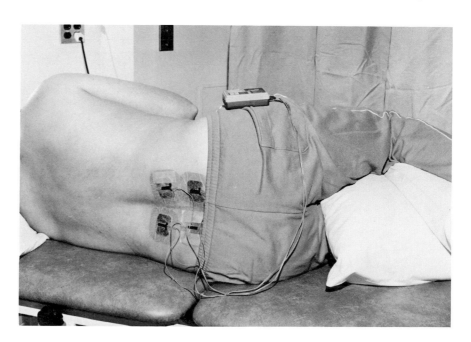

Fig. 21-2 TENS may be used as a preparation for exercise and activity, as a method of controlling pain while practicing correct body mechanics or performing activity, and as an adjunct to relaxation and good resting postures.

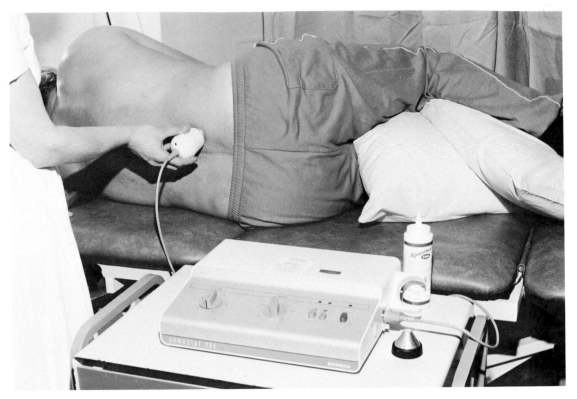

Fig. 21-3 Ultrasound. In the treatment of low back pain ultrasound may provide a deep heating effect, relaxation of muscle spasm, pain control, and improved extensibility of soft tissue.

over well-defined lesions such as a posterior joint or sacroiliac joint syndrome or associated multifidus muscle syndrome. It is not useful when used in a broad-sweeping nonspecific way and where the pathology is poorly defined. Ultrasound has limited usefulness in the treatment of spinal disorders (Fig. 21-3).

Mobilization

Specific passive mobilization techniques are frequently used in physical therapy to assess joint movement, to restore joint movement, to provide for pain control, to improve joint lubrication, and to relax muscle spasm.[5] The patient is positioned carefully to allow for movement at a specific spinal segment. The therapist may choose to reproduce passively a single movement or combinations of flexion, extension, rotation, and lateral flexion at that spinal segment. The amount of movement is carefully graded to reproduce the range of movement desired at a specific spinal segment. The mobilization chosen may be gentle oscillations or stretch and thrust techniques, depending on the specific joint dysfunction.

EXERCISE

Exercise is one of the most important contributions that a physical therapy program can make in the management of low back pain. It is particularly important in helping patients with severe longstanding low back pain. In many cases, the program should include both flexion and extension exercises, exercises for stretching tight contracted muscles, exercises for strengthening weak muscles, postural control exercises, and exercises for musculoskeletal dysfunction at a distance from the spine. In the latter case dysfunction of hamstrings, calf muscles or muscles in the neck or shoulder girdle may contribute to the low back pain.

Aerobic fitness is of great importance both from the physical and the emotional point of view. Increased cardiovascular fitness provides more stamina for daily activity and delays the onset of fatigue.

Different elements need to be emphasized in the exercise program depending on the type, severity, and stage of back pain. Any program needs to be reviewed regularly for reinforcement, correct application, and progression. Exercise programs for low back pain frequently fail, not because the wrong exercise was prescribed, but because the therapist's instructions were misunderstood or not carried out correctly. Other causes of failure include a lack of compliance on the part of the patient or a lack of progression to the point at which exercise contributes to improvement in the activities of daily living in a functional way.

Flexion and Extension Exercises

Although generally regarded as an important element of any physical therapy program, exercise is often neglected because of the controversy surrounding exercise for low back pain. One of the most prominent current controversies is that of flexion versus extension exercise. There are proponents of both of these methods. Both flexion and extension exercises play a vital role in the recovery of movement, strength, and function. At different stages in treatment it is often wise to include elements of each.

Extension is most useful when maintaining or increasing the lumbar lordosis, decreases pain and centralizes radiating symptoms and signs. This is often useful when the source of the pain comes from tears mainly in the posterior or posterolateral annulus (Fig. 21-4). In this instance, repetition of slow, controlled hyperextension, with the patient lying prone or standing, to the point of a feeling of stretching or mild discomfort is advocated by McKenzie.[6] A patient, characterized by a relatively flat lumbar spine when standing, loss of the ability to extend, who improves with repeated hyperextension, is probably a candidate for a predominately extension exercise program. Often the patient's history of factors that aggravate and alleviate the symptoms form an important indicator as to whether flexion or extension is indicated. At the beginning of treatment, the patient should be examined for the presence or absence of a postural list. When present this must be corrected before hyperextension exercises can be beneficial (Fig. 21-5). For discussion of the 'extension principle' in greater detail the reader is referred to the work of McKenzie[6,7]

Flexion is thought to be more beneficial in treating paravertebral muscle and posterior facet syndromes. This usually includes pelvic tilting, the strengthening

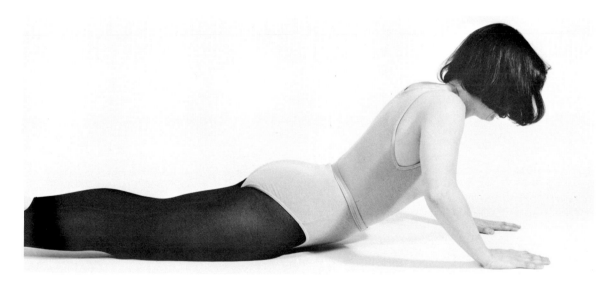

Fig. 21-4 Passive hyperextension. The patient performs a press up with the arms while maintaining relaxed low back and gluteal muscles. This controlled passive hyperextension stretch is thought to assist reduction of a posterior bulging disc.

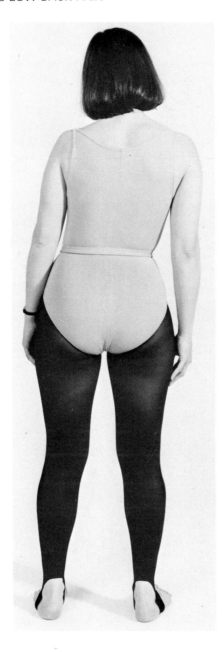

Fig. 21-5 The postural list is usually described as a list, tilt, or lateral shift. The patient should be examined for a postural list, which will appear as laterally displaced shoulders relative to the pelvis when observed from behind. Approximately 9 out of 10 subjects exhibiting a shift move away from the painful side.

of abdominal muscles, including the oblique muscles, together with stretching of the low back extensors and the hip flexors. Traditional pelvic tilting exercises require simultaneous contraction of abdominal and gluteal muscles to rotate the pelvis posteriorly and thus reduce a lumbar lordosis. Flexion exercises are most appropriate for patients with an exaggerated lumbar lordosis and tight contracted hip flexors and lumbar extensors (Figs. 21-6 and 21-7).

Altered Patterns of Muscle Contraction

Altered patterns of muscle recruitment in chronic low back pain have been clearly delineated by Janda.[8] One of the most common of these is the overuse and early recruitment of the low back extensors and scapular stabilizers to produce hip extension. The result of this is disuse atrophy and weakness of the gluteal muscles. This can be tested with prone hip

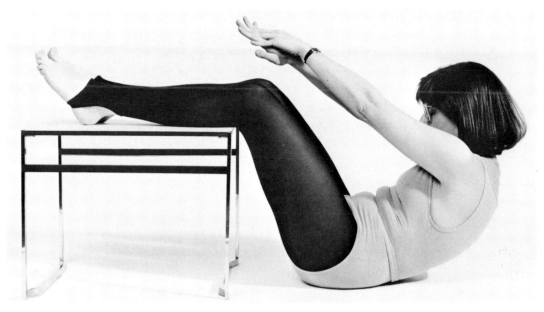

Fig. 21-6 Sit-ups. A useful exercise to strengthen abdominal muscles, while inhibiting activity of the hip flexors, is to do a curl up with the legs supported in hip and knee flexion. The patient is instructed to press the heels down and actively contract the hamstring muscles before starting the curl up.

extension to observe sequential recruitment of muscle groups. Another common pattern associated with low back pain is overuse of the hip flexors and weakness of the abdominals. Therefore any exercise program for low back pain should start with an assessment of patterns of muscle recruitment. It is frequently important to retrain the gluteal muscles and inhibit overuse of the lumbar extensors, a maladaptive pattern of muscle action. (Fig. 21-8).

Shortened muscle groups are commonly present in patients with low back pain. It is often necessary to stretch hamstrings, calf muscles, the iliotibial tract, piriformis, quadratus lumborum, hip adductors, hip flexors and low back extensors. Janda[9] has also drawn

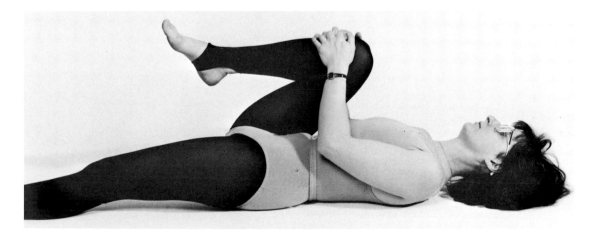

Fig. 21-7 Hip flexor stretch. A relatively safe and easy hip flexor stretch, with pelvic control, is done with the patient lying supine. One leg is fully flexed while pressing the straight leg into extension. This is a good initial exercise to stretch hip flexors.

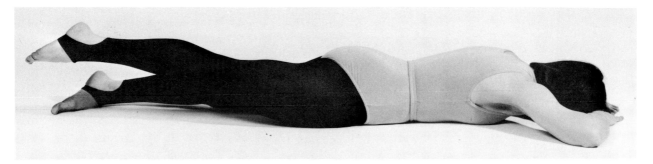

Fig. 21-8 Gluteal strength. An exercise to strengthen the gluteal muscles is done with the patient prone. The patient is instructed to lift the leg straight up a few inches while contracting the gluteal muscles. Care must be taken not to hyperextend the lumbar spine. This exercise can also be used as a test for the pattern of muscle recruitment during hip extension.

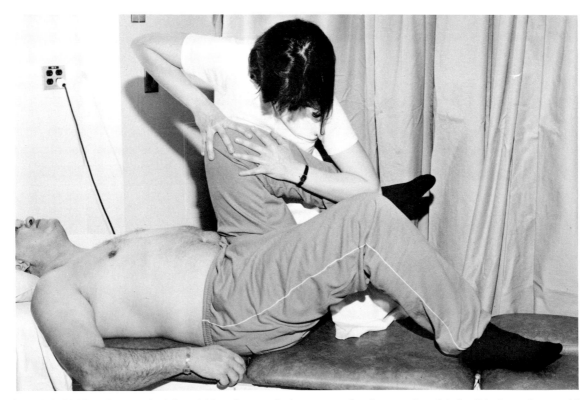

Fig. 21-9 Piriformis stretch. The piriformis muscle is commonly shortened and inflexible in patients with problems of the low back and pelvis. Specific stretching combined with inhibitory contraction and relaxation techniques may be an important part of the treatment program.

attention to the fact that tight, contracted muscle groups reciprocally inhibit their antagonists. It is therefore very difficult to strengthen a particular muscle group if the opposing groups of muscles are shortened. Common examples of this phenomenon related to low back pain include tight hip flexors with weak gluteal muscles and tight lumbar spine extensors with weak abdominals. Therefore, it is most efficient to stretch tight shortened muscle groups before any attempt is made to strengthen their antagonists (Fig. 21-9).

Postural Control

Postural control is habitual and unconscious. Low back pain may be the result of habitual poor posture. Alternatively the development of poor posture may be a compensatory action following an attack of low back pain. Postural correction of the lumbar spine does not only involve posterior pelvic tilting, although this is a common misinterpretation. Positioning of the pelvis is an integral component of postural correction and the basis on which the correct position of the rest of the spine is frequently built.

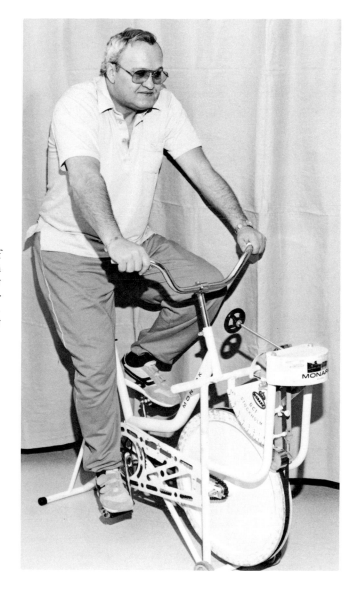

Fig. 21-10 The bicycle. There are many forms of safe, effective exercise to improve aerobic fitness in patients with low back pain. Aerobic fitness is now thought to be an important component of rehabilitation from low back pain and should be encouraged. Correct positioning during aerobic exercise activity is mandatory.

Depending on the postural fault present, the functional position of the pelvis may involve either backward or forward pelvic tilting. The habitual postural stance must be carefully assessed for each patient to determine the appropriate pelvic correction required. Maintenance of a normal lumbar lordosis is the desired result.

Postural malalignment frequently also includes a protracted shoulder girdle, shortened pectoral muscles, weak scapular retractors, protrusion of the chin, overuse of the trapezii, and weakness of the deep neck flexors.

Aerobic Fitness

It is now becoming apparent that aerobic fitness is an important factor in recovery of function following onset of low back pain. A patient education program should include advice and encouragement toward achieving aerobic fitness. This can be done in many ways. Some of these are brisk walking, swimming, cycling, and cross country skiing. A new trend is the development of nonimpact aerobic classes. These reduce jarring and jolting activities and are very suitable for many people with low back problems. It is important that these classes be taught by certified instuctors who understand the appropriate spinal mechanics. Patients should be screened for medical problems that would contraindicate referral to an aerobic class. Patients must be fully instructed in the correct application, intensity, and posture when employing any of these suggested activities (Fig. 21-10).

LOW BACK SCHOOL

Patient education is best satisfied by attendance at a low back school.[10] Patients must be encouraged to participate actively in a low back school by performing correct mechanics with activities of daily living, practicing dynamic and static postural control, learning relaxation techniques, and participating in discussion with therapists and other patients. This type of discussion centers round the management of pain and choice of appropriate activity.

The low back school augments and reinforces individual treatment. It should not be used as a substitute for specific treatment. Optimally patients should attend back school after a specific assessment is done to determine individual needs. Exercises and body mechanics taught at back school can then be modified when necessary to reinforce treatment priorities such as flexion versus extension. It helps the patient to gain confidence in dealing with his or her back pain by providing as much knowledge as possible about the way in which the back functions. For this reason it is imperative that trained health professionals contribute to the program.

If possible some of the personnel chosen to assist with the class should have personal knowledge of dealing with low back pain, so that they can relate to the patients' problems.

Those participating in back school should be observed closely for correct body mechanics. Any necessary corrections should be taught immediately. A knowledgeable physical or occupational therapist should be present to assure this.

REFERENCES

1. Lehmann JF: Therapeutic Heat and Cold. 3rd Ed. Williams & Wilkins, Baltimore, 1982.
2. Mannheimer JS, Lampe GN: Clinical transcutaneous electrical nerve stimulation. FA Davis, Philadelphia, 1985.
3. Mannheimer C, Carlson AC: The analgesic effect of transcutaneous electrical nerve stimulation in patients with rheumatoid arthritis. A comparative study of different pulse patterns. Pain, 6: 329, 1979.
4. Scott PM: Clayton's electrotherapy and actinotherapy. 7th Ed. Williams & Wilkins, Baltimore, 1975.
5. Paris SV: Mobilisation of the spine. Phys Ther, 59: 988, 1979.
6. McKenzie RA: Treat your own back. 3rd Ed. Spinal Publications Ltd, Waikenae, New Zealand, 1985.
7. McKenzie RA: The lumbar spine, mechanical diagnosis and therapy. Spinal Publications Ltd, Waikenae, New Zealand, 1981.
8. Janda V: Muscle function testing. Butterworth, Toronto, 1983.
9. Janda V: Postural and phasic muscles in the pathogenesis of low back pain. Proceedings of the XIth Congress of the International Society for Rehabilitation of the Disabled, Dublin, 1969.
10. Porter RW, Paris SV: The role of back education in the prevention and treatment of back pain. Proceedings of the Vth International Conference of the International Federation of Orthopaedic Manipulative Therapists, Vancouver, 1984.

22

Psychological Treatment of Back Pain and Associated Problems

A. J. Roy Cameron
Larry F. Shepel
Eldon Tunks

Many psychological treatments for pain and disability have been developed recently.[1–4] Rather than attempting an exhaustive review, we shall present only basic information about psychological treatment approaches. Our goals are to describe very briefly the sorts of treatments psychologists or psychiatrists offer, and, as far as possible, to provide suggestions for management that can be implemented by physicians or surgeons.

Pain is a complex experience that incorporates sensory, behavioral, cognitive, and emotional elements. Therapeutic change in any of these domains may have a salutary effect. For heuristic purposes, we shall organize our chapter by considering in turn treatments designed to modify (1) sensory, (2) behavioral, (3) cognitive, and (4) emotional aspects of pain and disability. In practice, of course, this compartmentalization is quite artificial, since any given treatment is likely to have a complex effect. For instance, patients who learn to reduce sensory discomfort may

well report concomitant improvement in behavior, attitudes, and emotional state.

The most realistic goal of treatment often is to enable patients to cope more effectively with continuing discomfort and disability. It is frequently not possible to achieve the ideal outcome of complete, permanent relief. It is important to recognize this at the outset in order to avoid inflated expectations that may lead to disappointment and an unwarranted sense of failure. Learning to live more comfortably and normally is a good outcome, even if residual problems are present.

Many of the treatment techniques described below are educational in nature. The aim is to help patients find ways to help themselves. In general, this involves helping them learn how to avoid self-defeating patterns of thought and behavior, to respond more adaptively, and to create conditions conducive to their own well-being. Patients must become collaborative participants in the process if such treatments are to have any chance of success. A detailed discussion of strategies for establishing collaborative relationships with patients is available elsewhere.[4]

ALTERING PAIN SENSATIONS

Some interventions are designed to reduce physical discomfort. Relaxation training and transcutaneous electrical stimulation are the major treatments in this category.

Relaxation Training

Relaxation training appears to be effective in reducing a number of types of clinical pain.[5–7] The mechanism(s) of action is unclear. There are at least three possibilities, which are not mutually exclusive:

1. Muscle tension may cause or exacerbate pain; if so, relaxation of involved muscles should reduce pain. However, no consistent relationship has been found between the amount of muscular relaxation achieved during training and the degree of subjective relief.[6,7]
2. Relaxation may result in a sense of control that increases the patient's sense of well being.[8]
3. Relaxation training apparently induces changes in the sympathetic nervous system;[9] it is conceivable that unspecified alterations in the nervous system underlie the subjective sense of improvement.

Two methods of relaxation training. EMG biofeedback and progressive relaxation training, are used widely.

EMG BIOFEEDBACK

Attempts have been made to train people to relax muscles by providing them with ongoing information about EMG levels of target muscles.[5–8] Commercial equipment that transforms EMG readings into auditory or visual signals is available. The patient may, for instance, hear a clicking signal that increases in rate as EMG level rises and decreases as EMG level falls. The patient's task is to learn to relax with the assistance of this feedback.

This treatment has not been evaluated adequately with back problems. The limited available data suggest that while some back patients benefit considerably from this treatment, a substantial proportion do not; results vary across studies.[5] Refinement in patient selection and treatment procedures could conceivably lead to more predictable results. However, at present the credibility of the approach is open to question since no consistent relationship has been found between EMG changes and subjective improvement.[6–8] Also, progressive relaxation training may be a more cost-efficient alternative to EMG feedback.[6,7]

PROGRESSIVE RELAXATION TRAINING

Jacobson[10] introduced progressive, or deep muscle, relaxation training. A number of procedural variations have been developed.[11] All involve having the patient learn to relax major muscle groups throughout the body. Relaxation instructions[12] may be delivered by the therapist or by tape recording.

Progressive relaxation training appears to be used widely to treat patients with back pain. However, surprisingly little information exists about its effectiveness with this population.

One report describes results of treatment with 111 chronic low back patients.[13] The progressive relaxation training was supplemented with EMG biofeedback. The biofeedback was used "to help patients become more aware of excessive muscular activity in specific muscle groups, to concentrate on relaxing these muscle groups, and to increase motivation to practice general relaxation procedures." Patients learned to relax not only while reclining but also while sitting, standing, and walking. The average number of treatment sessions was 10.6. Biofeedback was faded gradually from the program, so that patients were relaxing without the equipment by the end of treatment.

Steps were taken to promote the use of relaxation skills in environments other than the immediate treatment situation. For instance, patients were asked to practice at least twice a day on their own using taped relaxation instructions. Also, they were given adhesive-backed dots to place in conspicuous places in their natural environment: These dots were to cue them to engage in a "mini-practice" technique, which involved relaxing while carrying on normal activities. Patients were encouraged to learn to relax first in situations where relaxation was relatively easy (e.g., while lying down), then to progress to relaxing under conditions that tended to increase pain (e.g., walking relatively long distances).

By the end of treatment, average pain ratings dropped 29%, 49.2% of patients decreased medication use, and 63.2% reported increased activity. EMG levels dropped with treatment, but patients with good outcomes did not have greater EMG reductions than those who responded poorly.

Comparison of good and poor responders revealed that the good responders had (1) fewer years of continuous pain, though they did not differ from poor responders in number of years since onset; (2) a lower incidence of multiple surgery; and (3) a lower incidence of disability payments. Good and poor responders did not differ in MMPI scores, incidence of psychiatric diagnoses, or anatomical plausibility of pain descriptions.[13]

Our clinical experience suggests that several things can be done to enhance patients' involvement in relaxation training. First, if the original relaxation induction can be conducted under conditions that produce a marked result, this seems to increase the credibility of the procedure, thereby motivating the patient to both learn and use the skill. For instance, we have sometimes seen patients who reported that because of their pain they had had little sleep for several days, despite taking soporific medications; when a leisurely relaxation induction put them into a sound sleep, they were subsequently very impressed by and enthusiastic about the procedure. Second, asking patients to rate and record levels of subjective distress and serenity before and after relaxation may help to maintain a sense of progress even if residual discomfort remains. Third, patients wary of psychological formulations of their problems may be reassured by the introduction of supplementary EMG feedback: The equipment tangibly communicates the physical focus of the treatment.

Transcutaneous Electrical Stimulation

As the name suggests, transcutaneous electrical stimulation (TES) involves the application of electrical current using surface electrodes. Melzack[14] found that among a group of patients with longstanding, intractable back pain, TES yielded an average pain decrease of 60%, although outcomes were variable and unpredictable. Relief was sometimes short-lived, sometimes more enduring. Approximately 50% of patients seemed to experience continuing benefit 6 to 18 months after treatment ended. TES seems to produce more pain relief than placebo.[14,15]

Clinical guidelines for TES therapy emphasize the need to explore different electrode placements with each patient. Melzack[14] placed electrodes (1) over trigger zones (areas that trigger pain, identified through palpation) in the painful region; (2) over distant trigger zones (a map of trigger zones was used to search for these if no local zones were found); (3) over major peripheral nerves associated with the painful area; or (4) over acupuncture points. Melzack noted that there was considerable correspondence between trigger zones and acupuncture points designated for the same pain patterns and that these regions tended to lie over major sensory nerves. With the electrodes in place, voltage was increased gradually until the patient found it painful, then lowered slightly to a level that the patient thought would be tolerable for 20 minutes. Each treatment session lasted 20 minutes, with voltage adjusted up or down as necessary to maintain intense but tolerable stimulation. Most patients had one to three treatments per week; some had two sessions a day over 4 consecutive days. Some apparently had few treatments; others were treated over a period of weeks or months. Those who responded were allowed to borrow a stimulator for home use, with instructions to use it once daily for 20 minutes.

TES appears to be quite safe.[16] However, it has been recommended that the technique not be used with patients who have demand cardiac pacemakers or who are in the first trimester of pregnancy; also, electrodes should not be placed over the carotid sinus.[16]

REDUCING PAIN BEHAVIOR

An important treatment goal, in addition to pain relief, is to help the patient reestablish or maintain a lifestyle that is as normal and satisfying as possible. Two general treatment strategies, not mutually exclusive, may be used to this end. The first, operant treatment, emphasizes the importance of creating an environment where "pain behaviors" are disregarded and "well behaviors" are actively encouraged. The second, adaptive response training, concentrates more on the patient than on the environment: It involves training the patient how to deal more effectively with personal difficulties.

Operant Treatment

Wilbert Fordyce and his colleagues[1,17] developed a treatment program based on the principles of operant conditioning. The basic premise of the program is that behaviors leading to positive consequences tend to persist or to increase in frequency, whereas behaviors that are followed by neutral consequences tend to decrease in frequency or even to disappear altogether. For instance, in a familiar application of these basic principles, it is often noted that if a child's temper tantrums pay off, they become more frequent; if ignored, they tend to become less frequent and usually stop entirely.

Formal operant treatment of pain patients is conducted on an inpatient basis over a period of weeks. Staff members are trained to ignore pain behaviors (e.g., complaints, wincing, groaning, limping); "well behaviors" (e.g., socializing, physical activity) are expected and systematically encouraged. Detailed records of ongoing progress are maintained for the benefit of patients and staff alike; Fordyce[1] has published a detailed description of his program and procedures.

The operant approach to detoxification is noteworthy. Medication is not provided on demand. This arrangement makes pain relief (a positive experience) contingent on pain complaints and may therefore serve to maintain or increase complaints. Instead, drugs are provided at fixed intervals. Medications are mixed with a flavored syrup in a "pain cocktail" that makes it possible to reduce active medication gradually without the patient's awareness (although the patient should know in advance what is planned and agree to the tapering).

Operant programs seem to result in improvement in difficult patients. For instance, Fordyce et al[17] described results obtained with 36 patients who had had two to seven major operations for pain and who had had pain for 92.7 months on average. With treatment, average weekly "up-time" (i.e., time not reclining) increased from 59.2 hours to 88.9 hours; average daily walking distance doubled to more than a mile; use of analgestic medication dropped to approximately one sixth of pretreatment levels. Patient follow-ups after discharge were encouraging, though incomplete. Results that are generally similar have been obtained in response to similar programs in other settings.

Although the cumulative results seem impressive, it is difficult to interpret the data with confidence. For instance, most reports are based most on uncontrolled outcome studies. Also, since operant programs have been used with other treatments (physiotherapy, vocational therapy, etc.), the absence of control groups makes it impossible to know how much of the apparent treatment effect is the result of the operant program itself.[18,19]

There are drawbacks and limitations to operant treatment. It is costly, time consuming, and complex (despite its conceptual simplicity, all staff members in contact with the patient need to be cooperatively involved in the program). Although treatment seems to reduce pain behavior, many patients still report considerable discomfort.[17] Finally, treatment gains may be reversed quickly if people interacting with the patient discontinue the systematic encouragement of normal behaviors. Fordyce[1] attempts to forestall such relapse by training members of the patient's family to respond selectively to normal behaviors.

Even though it is not feasible to offer a formal operant program in many settings, it should be noted that the basic principles can be implemented in the context of other common treatments (Fordyce's book contains specific, practical suggestions). The general practice of systematically monitoring and encouraging gains in normal behavior, while carefully avoiding inadvertent encouragement of pain behaviors, appears prudent.

Adaptive Response Training

Patients sometimes appear to be engaging in self-defeating patterns of behavior that exacerbate their general malaise or deprive them of rewarding experiences. In such cases, treatment may focus on establishing more adaptive behavior patterns. In recent years, psychologists have become interested in the therapeutic value of training in basic adaptive skills (e.g., effective communication strategies, general problem-solving skills).[20] The potential role of adaptive response training can be illustrated in relation to two problems commonly experienced by back patients, namely, social inhibition and insomnia.

SOCIAL INHIBITION

People who feel shy, insecure, sexually inadequate, etc. may discover that their pain enables them to avoid stressful situations in a socially acceptable way. If such patients can acquire the skill and confidence required to deal directly with stressful situations, they may benefit considerably. For example, a woman reported that she had difficulty refusing unreasonable requests. In the past, she had found herself yielding to pressures to take on commitments that she resented and worried about. She also had trouble resisting demands from her family, especially her aging parents who lived nearby. After she developed pain, however, she discovered that she was asked to do less and others were willing to help more. Her pain seemed to serve to fend off others and enlist their cooperation without her appearing to be "offensive" or "selfish." The treatment program included training in how to be directly assertive in ways that would be satisfactory both to her and to those with whom she interacted. The value of training pain patients to respond more effectively in social relationships has not been systematically evaluated. However, a follow-up of 81 patients treated in a rehabilitation program revealed that those who improved were more likely to have received assertive skill training than those who had not improved.[21]

INSOMNIA

Adaptive responding may also be used in the treatment of insomnia, a common complaint among patients with back pain. People who experience insomnia may exacerbate their sleep difficulties in a variety of ways. For instance, they may compensate for lost sleep by napping through the day or by oversleeping in the morning, so that they are not tired at bedtime. Sleep difficulties have been treated with some success by training poor sleepers how to establish routines, skills, and conditions conducive to a normal sleep pattern. The following guidelines, for instance, have been recommended:[22]

1. Lie down to sleep only when sleepy.
2. Do not do anything (aside from sexual activity) in bed except sleep.
3. If you are not asleep within 15 minutes after getting into bed, get up and leave the bedroom.
4. If still unable to sleep, repeat step 3 as often as necessary.

5. Set the alarm for the same time evey morning and get up then, regardless of how much sleep time was achieved.
6. Avoid daytime naps.

It may also be prudent to avoid caffeine and alcohol before retiring.

Adaptive response training may serve to enhance the general quality of the person's life even if there is no clear evidence that the pain or associated problems are being aggravated by maladaptive behavior patterns. For instance, we have sometimes worked with patients who were interested in improving relationships or in personal productivity. Although no demonstrable decrease in pain or pain behavior occurred, some of these people reported that it was satisfying to have a positive focus and to see evidence of constructive change in their lives. They hurt as much as ever and had to continue restricting activities, but somehow, in the overall context of their lives, these things seemed to bother them less.

THE PATIENTS THOUGHTS AS A FOCUS FOR TREATMENT

The way the patient thinks about problems may influence the way he or she feels and behaves. Our main objectives are to promote realistic thinking and a sense of personal control.

Encouraging Realistic Expections and Attitudes

Patients' expectations and attitudes may affect treatment response, whether the treatment is physical or psychological.

Those who have unrealistically optimistic expectations about treatment may be disappointed with what would normally be regarded as a good outcome if there are lingering problems that they had not anticipated. Similarly, those who have serious reservations about treatment (e.g., those who are unusually apprehensive about surgery because they have known people whose operations seemed to worsen their problems) may overreact to residual difficulties if these are misinterpreted as evidence that the treatment really was ill-conceived. Patients with misgivings about proposed treatments may be reluctant to express them unless they are actively encouraged to discuss questions or concerns.

Realistic expectations can be promoted through careful pretreatment discussion of the probable outcome of successful treatment, with emphasis on any residual difficulties or limitations that are likely. Patients who are very apprehensive may gain confidence if they are encouraged to get a second opinion or given an opportunity to talk to patients successfully treated with the procedure.

Misinterpretations that lead patients to overestimate the severity of their problems also cause difficulties occasionally. A rather dramatic case illustrates this point. A man was admitted to a surgical ward for nonsurgical treatment. He was a source of concern because he was subdued, withdrawn, and appeared to be surprisingly incapacitated. During the course of a long interview he eventually said that he was distressed because he was receiving what he erroneously perceived to be mere palliative treatment rather than "corrective surgery." He had misconstrued all this as meaning that he was beyond surgical help ("I guess they can't operate or they'll paralyze me or something") and on a degenerative course. Unearthing and correcting such misunderstandings may have therapeutic value.

Patients who make sinister misinterpretations of their symptoms may sometimes benefit from structured opportunities to engage in experiences that invalidate their fears. For instance, an athletic middle-aged woman who had surgery discovered that her back subsequently bothered her when she was active. She saw this as evidence that she had a permanent disability that would make it impossible to engage in vigorous activity, so she gave up sports. She became reclusive and depressed, since much of the personal recognition and social contact she received came through participation in athletic competition. We encouraged her to attribute her activity-related discomfort provisionally to being out of shape and urged her to see if it could be relieved by systematically working back into good condition. She resumed athletic activities gradually, under supervision, and was soon fully active with minimal discomfort. The improvement had been maintained at a 2-year follow-up. Graduated resumption of normal activities with reassuring supervision appears to be a useful strategy for managing patients who are overly cautious and self-restricting.[23]

Fostering a Sense of Control

Patients whose pain and disability cannot be eliminated may feel overwhelmed, helpless, and desperate. There is evidence that a sense of helplessness in the face of adversity may have wide-ranging debilitating effects.[24,25] People who believe that they can do nothing about their difficulties tend to give up. The less they do to help themselves, the worse the problems become, and the more overwhelmed and hopeless they feel. This can become a vicious cycle.

A major challenge of rehabilitation is to reverse or forestall this cycle, to promote a sense that patients can, indeed, take effective action on their own behalf. Much psychological research is currently being devoted to clarifying the processes involved in the development of self-efficacy.[26] Although a detailed discussion of this work is not possible here, it would appear that at a gross level of analysis two conditions must be met before patients can be expected to help themselves.

First, they must recognize that there is something constructive they can do. Pain and disability tend to be seen as medical problems requiring professional treatment. It may not be evident to patients that they themselves often have it within their power to reduce their own discomfort and to counteract secondary psychological or interpersonal difficulties. Any psychological (e.g. relaxation training) or other rehabilitative treatment (e.g., physiotherapy exercises) that explicitly equips them to help themselves has the potential to enhance their morale and sense of control. Making such treatments available, and presenting them with enthusiasm, may boost the patient's morale and lay the goundwork for self-help behavior.

Second, given that patients have the capacity to respond effectively and recognize this, they must put this capacity to use by actually engaging in efforts to help themselves. Clear evidence of progress may be the best spur to continued effort and confidence.[26] A sense of progress may be engendered by setting realistic, attainable goals (e.g., walking progressively longer distances beginning with a distance well below potential and increasing slowly and steadily). Modest, specific, short-term goals (e.g., to walk a half mile this morning) are more likely to be useful in this process than more ambitious, vague, long-term goals (e.g., to be back to normal by the end of June). Once initiated, continued progress may be encouraged by keeping records of daily accomplishments: Patients who continue to experience diminished walking endurance, for instance, are less likely to become discouraged if they have authentic evidence that walking endurance has been increasing steadily. It may be advantageous to monitor positive (how much the patient was able to accomplish) rather than negative (level of discomfort or amount of continuing restriction) indexes of progress, since the latter may contribute to preoccupation with pain.

Stress inoculation training[4,27] refers to a treatment strategy specifically designed to establish and promote self-help capabilities and a sense of control. Patients go through an educational or conceptualization phase, during which they carefully examine their own experiences with pain. The data of their own experiences are then used to educate them, in a collaborative way, about the complex nature of pain. This is followed by a skills acquisition and rehearsal phase, which involves having patients learn and practice strategies for coping with the various aspects of the pain experience. Finally, there is an application phase during which the patient gains experience testing out the skills in pain-engendering situations under clinical supervision. More detailed descriptions of this approach are available elsewhere.[4]

MANAGING EMOTIONAL FACTORS

Chronic pain is often associated with anxiety, depression, anger, and fears. This is not surprising, considering the multiplicity of problems often faced by the pain-sufferer: financial uncertainty, family role changes, adversarial relationships with compensation agencies, iatrogenic symptoms from excessive quantities of pharmaceuticals, not to mention the exhausting effect of the chronic pain itself.

Depression

It is often noted that there are many clinical similarities between chronic pain and chronic depression. Lesse[28] took the position that some cases of chronic pain could be seen as "masked depression." Blumer and Heilbronn[29] and Blumer et al.[30] discovered in "pain-prone" individuals, many characteristics that would identify them with affective disorder, includ-

ing many clinical features of depression, a family history of depressive spectrum disorders, and positive response to antidepressants. In an epidemiological survey, Crook and Tunks[31] found that chronic pain patients referred to a specialty pain clinic were likely to suffer disturbed emotional states more than persistent pain sufferers in the community who were not being referred. There are many reports of successful use of antidepressants in relieving the symptoms of patients with chronic pain.[32–34] Clearly, some chronic pain patients are markedly depressed and show striking improvement in their mood and distress as a result of antidepressant therapy. With chronic back pain, the best results are in those whose depression is obvious, with insomnia, loss of energy, ruminations, agitation, and with evidence that the depression is not a lifelong or personality problem. As a diagnostic point, it should be noted that the agitation, which often accompanies depression, frequently resembles severe anxiety or anxiety attacks but is similarly responsive to antidepressant therapy.

Beyond the element of depression, pain itself may also improve in some circumstances with antidepressant therapy. After the initial report by Paoli et al.[34] of tricyclic antidepressants for cancer pain, numerous reports have confirmed their usefulness in a variety of conditions, particularly neuralgia, chronic headache, diffuse fibromyalgia (called "fibrositis" or "nonarticular rheumatism"), and in pain associated with cancer.[35–37] Unfortunately, improvements are less often produced in back pain sufferers, and Pilowsky et al.[38] found that amitryptyline was no better than placebo for a group of chronic pain patients in a double-blind trial.

The antidepressants most preferred have been amitryptyline, doxepin, and clomipramine. Butler[37] speculated that the serotinergic effects of these drugs gives them analgesic properties. However, other antidepressants, including the monoamine oxidase inhibitors or lithium, are not infrequently beneficial in specific cases.

Amitryptyline and the related tricyclic antidepressants have a host of potential side effects, and therefore prescriptions are best introduced gradually with 10 to 25 mg given at night. This offers some welcome sedation and alleviates some of the insomnia. The dose then may be increased at weekly or biweekly intervals. For pain alone (as in neuralgia), benefits may be seen at a daily dose of 25 to 75 mg, whereas for depression higher doses of from 50 to 150 mg are usually required.

Several indicators suggest that antidepressant therapy should be instituted: (1) severe depression, possibly suicidal, with reduced energy, or with marked agitation, insomnia and other vegetative signs, or with inability to cooperate with treatment due to affective distress; (2) previous history of a depressive episode or of a good response to antidepressant, or (3) a clear family history of affective disorder. They may also be prescribed as analgesics for the specific conditions previously mentioned. To ensure the patient's compliance, when offering the prescription it is important to explain the possible major side effects, the method of slowly increasing the dose, and the fact that the therapeutic effect may take 2 weeks or more to be obvious. After therapeutic response has been obtained, the medication usually has to be maintained for several months to avoid relapse in depression. However, in most individuals, antidepressants should not be perpetuated indefinitely.

Anxiety and Fear

As in the case of many chronically debilitating illnesses, chronic back pain sufferers may show anxiety, regression, and dependency, with a sense of helplessness. The cognitive component of this is beliefs concerning loss of control over illness and pain and reduction in the sense of self-efficacy. This cognitive aspect of anxiety is best dealt with by cognitive therapy.[4]

Patients with chronic back pain commonly display evidence of somatic preoccupation, fearful to attempt activity lest they may further injure themselves and anxious or hypochondriacal about bodily perceptions. This is linked to the illness behavior problems that occasion much of their functional disability and that mark them as "psychologically disturbed" in the view of consultants. Specific back education programs, and pain programs that use behavior modification techniques, are the most appropriate and effective in managing this aspect of anxiety.[39–42]

As mentioned in the discussion of depression, more severe manifestations of anxiety occasionally represent the agitation component of a severe depression, in which case one obtains good results by prescription of antidepressants. However, there is also always a cognitive and illness behavior component to the anxiety and depression: While medications are being offered, attention must still be directed to dealing with the cognitive and behavioral elements of the problem, as previously described. It is wise, at the time of writing the prescription, to emphasize the fact that the drug is offered to alleviate some of the unpleasant symptoms so that the patient's energy may be directed to the work of rehabilitation.

The problem of back pain often overshadows phobic symptoms, particularly if the pain originated in a road or work accident. Unless the examiner asks, it may not be appreciated that many patients harbor phobias regarding the situation in which they were injured; for example, many are afraid of being in a workplace, in an automobile, or in a noisy or busy environment. These fears inhibit the process of reintegrating the patient into a normal way of life. Phobias of this sort usually respond well to specific desensitization procedures, which can be linked to the relaxation techniques commonly taught to patients with chronic pain. In brief, the patient is asked to participate in the phobic situation, while carrying out the relaxation procedure. The degree of exposure to the phobic situation is regularly increased as the patient gradually masters the sense of anxiety experienced in each situation.

Anxiolytic drugs, primarily those of the benzodiazepine series, may seem to be a logical choice for patients who suffer chronic back pain with its attendant anxiety and insomnia. It may also be assumed that since patients with low back pain seem to have pain in their muscles, sedatives and muscle relaxants ought to relieve the pain. However, in the case of low back pain, in the long term this sort of medication is neither analgesic nor helpful, and may be harmful, by adding the iatrogenic effects of anergy, depression, memory problems, and sometimes drug habituation. Furthermore, the prescription may be perpetuated indefinitely because the pain is not alleviated, becoming then a daily reminder or symbol to the patient of the disabled or incurable status. Discontinuing analgesics and sedatives is usually a major step in helping these individuals reassert a sense of control and self-efficacy, with the additional benefit of improvement in mental status that comes from detoxification.

In dealing with the symptoms of anxiety or fear, inquiry must be directed to (1) whether there are symptoms of a serious depression, (2) the possible presence of a phobic element that merits specific management, (3) the cognitive components of the problem that may respond to back education or to cognitive therapy, and (4) illness behavior, which likely will require a program of physical activation or behavior modification in some form.

Clinical Approach

In management of the problems of anxiety and depression that frequently accompany chronic back pain, the vast majority of patients improve with education and psychological techniques. In the majority of cases, medication is not necessary, and indeed most patients do much better after all of their analgesic and psychotropic medication is withdrawn. A minority of patients will be found to suffer major affective disorders, which can usually be diagnosed clinically from their presentation, previous history, and family history. These patients do well with antidepressant therapy for both the depressive and anxiety components of the disorder. If medications are given, it is still necessary to combine such therapy with psychological treatment, making it clear to the patient that the goal is rehabilitation of function and quality of life, in which effort the patient must be actively involved.

A PERSPECTIVE ON PSYCHOLOGICAL TREATMENT

Preliminary evidence suggests that psychological and psychiatric treatments may be useful for managing patients with back pain. Although a scientific literature is developing, current clinical practice often goes beyond well-established findings. It is to be hoped that, whenever possible, rehabilitative programs will be structured so that they permit reasonable evaluation of the treatments offered. A self-critical approach appears prudent if we are to be self-correcting (i.e., to ensure that management programs are revised on an ongoing basis to enhance their efficacy and economy).

ACKNOWLEDGMENT

We are grateful to C. Barr Taylor and Kenneth Prkachin for their valuable comments on an earlier draft of this material.

REFERENCES

1. Fordyce WE: Behavioral Methods for Chronic Pain and Illness. CV Mosby, St. Louis, 1976
2. Holzman AD, Turk DC, (eds): Pain Management: A Handbook of Psychological Treatment Approaches. Pergamon Press, New York, 1986
3. Sternbach RA: Pain Patients: Traits and Treatment. Academic Press, Orlando, FL 1974
4. Turk D, Meichenbaum D, Genest M: Pain and Behavioral Medicine. Guilford Press, New York, 1983
5. Linton SJ: Behavioral remediation of chronic pain: a status report. Pain 24: 125, 1986
6. Jessup BA, Neufeld WJ, Mersky H: Biofeedback therapy for headache and other pain: an evaluative review. Pain 7: 225, 1979
7. Turk DC, Meichenbaum DH, Berman WH: Application of biofeedback for the regulation of pain: a critical review. Psychol Bull 86: 1322, 1979
8. Holroyd KA, Penzien DB, Hursey KG, et al: Change mechanisms in EMG biofeedback training: cognitive changes underlying improvements in tension headache. J Consult Clin Psychol 52: 1039, 1984
9. Hoffman JW, Benson H, Arns PA, et al: Reduced sympathetic nervous system responsivity associated with the relaxation response. Science 215: 190, 1982
10. Jacobson E: Progressive Relaxation. University of Chicago Press, Chicago, 1938
11. Borkovec TD, Sides J: Critical procedural variables related to the physiological effects of progressive relaxation: a review. Behav Res Ther 17: 119, 1979
12. Ferguson JM, Marquis JN, Taylor CB: A script for deep muscle relaxation. Diseases of the Nervous System 38: 703, 1977
13. Keefe FJ, Block AR, Williams RB, Surwit RS: Behavioral treatment of chronic low back pain: clinical outcome and individual differences in pain relief. Pain 11: 221, 1981
14. Melzack R: Prolonged relief of pain by brief, intense transcutaneous somatic stimulation. Pain 1: 357, 1975
15. Thorsteinnson G, Stonnington HH, Stillwell GK, Elveback LR: The placebo effect of transcutaneous electrical stimulation. Pain 5: 31, 1978
16. Rosenberg M, Curtis L, Bourke DL: Transcutaneous electrical nerve stimulation for the relief of postoperative pain. Pain 5: 129, 1978
17. Fordyce W, Fowler R, Lehmann J, et al: Operant conditioning in the treatment of chronic clinical pain. Arch Phys Med Rehabil 54: 399, 1973
18. Fordyce WE, Roberts AH, Sternbach RA: The behavioral management of chronic pain: a response to critics. Pain 22: 113, 1985
19. Keefe FJ, Gil KM, Rose SC: Behavioral approaches

in the multidisciplinary management of chronic pain: programs and issues. Clin Psychol Rev 6: 87, 1986

20. Goldfried M: Psychotherapy as coping skills training. In Mahoney MJ (ed): Psychotherapy Process. Plenum, New York, 1980

21. Morgan CD, Kremer E, Gaylor M: The behavioral medicine unit: a new facility. Compr Psychiatry 20: 79, 1979

22. Bootzin RR, Nicassio PM: Behavioral treatments for insomnia. In Hersen M, Eisler RM, Miller PM (eds): Progress in Behavior Modification. Vol. 6. Academic Press, Orlando, 1978

23. Dolce JJ, Crocker MF, Moletteire C, Doleys DM: Exercise quotas, anticipatory concern and self-efficacy expectancies in chronic pain: a preliminary report. Pain 24: 365, 1986

24. Lefcourt HM: Locus of Control: Current Trends in Theory and Research. Lawrence Erlbaum, New Jersey, 1976

25. Seligman MEP: Helplessness. WH Freeman, San Francisco, 1975

26. Bandura A: Social Foundations of Thought and Action: A Social Cognitive Theory. Prentice-Hall, Englewood Cliffs, 1986

27. Meichenbaum D, Cameron R: Stress-inoculation training: toward a general paradigm for training coping skills. In Meichenbaum D, Jaremko M (eds): Stress Prevention and Management. Plenum, New York, 1983

28. Lesse S: The multivariant masks of depression. Am J. Psychiatr. Suppl., 124: 35, 1968

29. Blumer D, Heilbronn M: Chronic pain as a variant of depressive disease: the pain-prone disorder. J Nerv Ment Dis 170: 381, 1982

30. Blumer D, Zorick F, Heilbronn M, Roth T: Biological markers for depression in chronic pain. J Nerv Ment Dis 170: 425, 1982

31. Crook J, Tunks E: Defining the "chronic pain syndrome": an epidemiological method. In Fields HL, Dubner R, Cervero (eds): Advances in Pain Research and Therapy. Vol. 9. Raven Press, New York, 1985

32. Lascelles RG: Atypical facial pain and depression. Brit J Psychiatry 112: 651, 1966

33. Ward NG, Bloom VL, Friedel RO: The effectiveness of tricyclic antidepressants in the treatment of coexisting pain and depression. Pain 7: 331, 1979

34. Paoli F, Darcourt G, Cossa P: Preliminary note on the action of imipramine in painful states. Rev Neurol (Paris) 102: 503, 1960

35. Merskey H, Hester RA: The treatment of chronic pain with psychotropic drugs. Postgrad Med 48: 594, 1972

36. Watson CP, Evans RJ, Reed K, et al: Amitriptyline versus placebo in postherpetic neuralgia. Neurology (NY) 32: 671, 1982

37. Butler S: Present status of tricyclic antidepressants in chronic pain therapy. In Benedetti C, Chapman CR, Moricca G (eds): Advances in Pain Research and Therapy. Vol. 7. Raven Press, New York, 1984

38. Pilowsky I, Hallett EC, Bassett DL, et al: A controlled study of amitriptyline in the treatment of chronic pain. Pain 14: 169, 1982

39. Doleys DM, Crocker M, Patton D: Response of patients with chronic pain to exercise quotas. Phys Ther 62: 1111, 1982

40. Flor H, Turk DC: Etiological theories and treatments for chronic back pain. I. Somatic models and interventions. Pain 19: 105, 1984

41. Turk DC, Flor H: Etiological theories and treatments for chronic back pain. II. Psychological models and interventions. Pain 19: 209, 1984

42. Fordyce WE, McMahon R, Rainwater G, et al: Pain complaint-exercise performance relationship in chronic pain. Pain 10: 311, 1981

23

The Pain Clinic in the Management of Low Back Pain

Gordon M. Wyant

Chronic back pain is by far the most common nonmalignant condition encountered in a pain management clinic. It is the example *par excellence* of a chronic pain condition that embodies, like no other, all the elements which call for an interdisciplinary team approach of management. Many of these patients are young, and there is an overwhelming necessity to reintegrate them into the economic mainstream of life by a process of rehabilitation involving orthopaedic surgeons, pain clinicians, physiotherapists, and chiropractors. The ravages of inability to work, with its demoralizing and economic consequences, play havoc with the family unit and frequently require the services of a social worker skilled in dealing with problems of this kind. Moreover, psychologists or psychiatrists must assess resentment against employers, on whose premises or in whose service many of these injuries have occurred, as well as the patient's perceived entitlement to compensation, depression, and pain perception dysfunctions. All these various experts must be brought together as a team to treat the patient in a rational, logical and integrated fashion.

Many of the characteristics of chronic pain have been described in earlier chapters of this book, but it is appropriate here to consider them once more, this time from the perspective of the pain clinician. In particular, is it imperative to differentiate between acute and chronic pain to understand why time-honored pain remedies usually fail so miserably when applied to chronic pain situations.

DEFINITIONS AND PRINCIPLES OF PAIN

Acute Pain

Acute pain is a self-limiting, purposeful condition that warns of an anatomical derangement or other pathological situation and thus precipitates protective action. It responds readily to analgesics with or without immobilization and subsides as healing progresses. Everyone has acute pain at one time or another, and physicians are quite capable of dealing with it in one of several traditional ways.

Chronic Pain

Chronic pain, on the other hand, has no purpose, does not necessarily point to an organic change, and tends to perpetuate itself through a vicious cycle in-

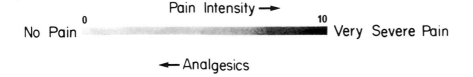

ACUTE PAIN

Pain Intensity ⟶

0   10

No Pain   Very Severe Pain

⟵ Analgesics

CHRONIC PAIN

Fig. 23-1 Graphic comparison of acute and chronic pain.

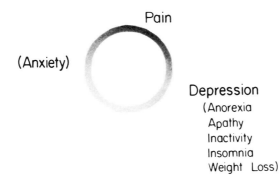

Pain

(Anxiety)

Depression
(Anorexia
Apathy
Inactivity
Insomnia
Weight Loss)

volving depression with all its signs and symptoms, which in turn increases the perception of pain while at the same time decreasing the individual's ability to deal with it. This further increases the depression and despondency. (Fig. 23-1).

From a clinical perspective as well, there is a fundamental difference between acute and chronic pain. Acute pain presents as catecholamine release, the result of the "fight and flight" response of the body to threatening or actual danger and is characterized by an elevation in blood pressure and pulse rate, sweating, mydriasis, restlessness, and apprehension. Treatment ranges from mild analgesics such as acetylsalicylic acid (ASA) up to one of the opioids; anxiolytics, such as diazepam (Valium), and other benzodiazepines are also of value. As mentioned before, chronic pain in its purest form is accompanied by depression, not by signs of anxiety. Hence anxiolytics can actually increase pain perception dysfunction by deepening the existing depression. On the other hand, antidepressants, such as amitriptyline (Elavil), doxepin (Sinequan), trimipramine (Surmontil) or any others in a large array of tricyclics or a few quadricyclics, are the agents of primary choice. This is a fact of fundamental importance, still all too often disre-

garded. This does not mean, of course, that anxiolytics are never indicated, as episodes of acute anxiety might occur concomitantly from time to time with chronic pain; however, their use must be strictly limited.

ASSOCIATED FEATURES OF PAIN

Injury anywhere, but particularly to the musculoskeletal system, tends to cause muscle spasm, originally a protective mechanism designed to splint the injured part and thus promote healing. However, if the contraction is abnormally prolonged, the resultant metabolic events initiate a self-perpetuating myospastic cycle in which the accumulation of pain-producing (algesic) substances, such as KC1, serotonin, bradykinin, and prostaglandin E, plays a significant role (Fig. 23-2). Eventually, the prolonged muscle contraction results in replacement of contractile elements by fibrous tissue and consequent irreversibility of the process. At the same rate, certain socioeconomic developments occur that exercise a significant influence on the progress of the pain syndrome and that might,

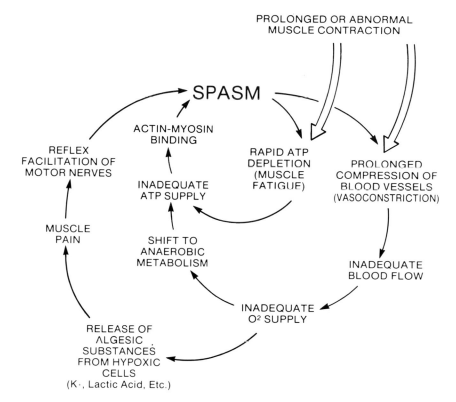

Fig. 23-2 The myospastic cycle. (Hendler NH, Long DM, Wise TN (eds): Diagnosis and Treatment of Chronic Pain. John Wright PSG Inc, Littleton, Massachusetts, 1982.)

in some instances, become the predominant factor preventing successful treatment or at least rendering it immeasurably more difficult. If not recognized and treated energetically by a competent social worker and psychologist, it will lead to deepening depression, total withdrawal from society, deeply ingrained pain behavior, and reinforcement of the irreversibility.

ORGANIZATION OF PAIN CLINICS

Most pain management services take patients only by referral. Patients might be referred either by their family physician; by another medical consultant; or by a health worker, such as a physiotherapist, chiropractor, or the like. The majority of low back pain patients will have been seen by an orthopedic surgeon at one time or another, and appropriate reports supported by x-rays, CT scan where applicable, and other workup should be made available. Many clinics have the patient complete a pain questionnaire, either before the appointment or at the time of the first visit. Although these questionnaires vary from clinic

to clinic, they all should solicit information about the individual's work status, compensation and litigation data, date and circumstances of the onset of pain, severity rating, aggravating and ameliorating factors, previous similar complaints, treatments to date and results, and a pain drawing. Much other useful information can be elicited by means of such a questionnaire which, if submitted before the first appointment, can serve as a screening mechanism and even as a deterrent to frivolous "doctor shopping."

AIMS OF TREATMENT

The aims of treatment are identical to those of most kinds of chronic pain, depending on the underlying condition. The following goals are presented in their order of importance:

1. Restoration of function and return to a normal productive life.
2. Prevention of pain. To achieve this goal, treatment should precede the onset of the next episode of pain. Many treatment modalities can be applied in this fashion, such as the administration of drugs,

TENS, exercises, acupressure, self-hypnosis, and others that do not call for large nonportable or difficult to operate equipment or for intervention by another person.

3. Ease of administration. Drugs must be active by mouth, sublingually, or by suppository; and equipment must be portable and affordable.

4. Trust and confidence. Referral to a pain clinic is often only the latest step in a series of hitherto unsuccessful attempts at treatment. The patient therefore is skeptical, possibly even hostile, and has lost all confidence in the physician. Restoration of confidence in the physician and optimism is absolutely essential for success.

5. Erasure of the memory of the pain. If subsequent recurrences of pain are prevented or at least ameliorated in intensity, the recollection of the pain will gradually fade, and the individual will relax, confident that whatever permissible activities are planned will not hurt and that the pernicious process of pain–spasm–pain has been broken.

6. Avoidance of habituation and addiction. Although the temptation often is great under pressure from patients or relatives to take the path of least resistence and prescribe opioid analgesics, the course must be strenuously resisted. The majority of these individuals are young and have a normal life expectancy. It would be quite unforgivable to expose them to the need for ever-increasing doses of opioids for a number of decades when other less harmful alternatives are now readily available.

7. Lesser considerations. It is important that any treatment chosen should have a prolonged effect, so that it does not need to be repeated so often that patients become unwilling to comply. It also goes without saying that treatments must be free from undesirable side-effects or they must at least be so mild as to be outweighed by the benefits of treatment. Moreover, normal affect and alertness should not be impaired by treatment.

CLINICAL CONSIDERATIONS

Causes of Low Back Pain

The causes of low back pain are as diverse as the structures that contribute to the maintenance of the erect posture. Aside from the nonorganic factors, backache can arise from the bone and joint components of the spine, from the muscle elements, and from neighboring structures, such as the urinary and genital tracts. It is not always appreciated that the severity of symptoms does not necessarily bear much relation to radiologically demonstrable abnormalities; and thus, quite considerable degenerative changes might be incidental findings in an individual with relatively few symptoms, whereas the opposite is frequently also the case. Thus, the physician is faced with formidable difficulties in diagnosis. The temptation is great to ascribe a patient's complaints to malingering, secondary gain, and similar nonorganic causes, when in fact there are unrecognized organic reasons for the pain aggravated by greater or lesser pain perception dysfunction, anxiety or depression. These, in turn, are fuelled by the long duration of the pain and the apparent inability or unwillingness of others to recognize the reality of the individual's suffering. Hence, it becomes a matter of paramount importance to identify the presence and intensity of the organic component. To that end, a number of techniques have been devised, among them the induction of an epidural or subarachnoid differential block. However, I have found examination under light thiopentone (Pentothal) anesthesia the most informative of these procedures. General anesthesia is induced just until the lid reflex is lost, a state in which actual antanalgesia or hypersensitivity to pain exists. If repetition of stimuli that had been painful in the awake state now fail to evoke a response from the patient, it can be safely assumed that the organic component of the complaint is negligible or entirely absent.

Patient History

Bearing in mind the multitude of factors that contribute to the genesis and maintenance of low back pain, the physician must begin by obtaining a thorough patient history. This history should include not only the origin and progression of the present symptoms with localization, character, and radiation of the pain but also previous complaints and injuries, other musculoskeletal relieving and aggravating factors, sleeping patterns, occupational and domestic stresses, the degree of activity or inactivity, metabolic diseases, family history, and the relation of onset of the backache to concomitant symptoms in other organ systems. A thorough physical examination is then done, including the thoracic and abdominal organs;

central nervous and musculoskeletal systems, with special emphasis on the spine and associated structures, and other organs as might be suggested by the presenting signs and symptoms. The findings so recorded should be corroborated by appropriate laboratory and imaging investigations that have not yet been done.

Plan of Action

Having assembled all available information, the pain clinician will now formulate a plan of action. Such plan will involve other members of the pain management team—in particular the orthopedic surgeon, anesthetist, physiotherapist, chiropractor, psychologist, and in some instances the social worker, occupational therapist, and nursing consultant. A sound relationship with insuring agencies, such as workers' compensation board and others, recognizing and respecting their different goals and responsibilities, can be of great help. These not infrequently involve members of the legal profession who again have quite distinct aims and often bring novel perspectives to a particular case. Whereas the physician recognizes that the expectation of financial gain and a feeling of injustice suffered might engender a delay in improvement and thus desires a speedy resolution of any litigation, the lawyer is loathe to accept a final disposition of the case until he is assured of the severity and duration of any sequela, information that cannot be supplied reliably until a considerable period of time has passed.

TREATMENT

A great variety of drugs, belonging to many different pharmacological groups, is available and can be useful adjuncts to the treatment of patients with low back pain. Many kinds of analgesics, both the more common over-the-counter ones and those requiring a physician's prescription, should be considered. Despite the insistence of some patients for more and more potent drugs, the temptation of prescribing opioids and their derivatives must be strenuously resisted, except in the very elderly with a short life expectancy and even then only if other treatments have failed.

Since the pain in many instances is musculoskeletal, it is obvious that the nonsteroidal anti-inflammatories (NSAIDs) can often be of significant benefit in low back pain, as they are able to break the myospastic cycle. This might be the only residual organic abnormality left in those cases in which the original lesion has subsided. So-called muscle relaxants are often also prescribed, although their specific relaxant action is doubted by many pharmacologists. Diazepam (Valium) does relax muscles because of its central sedative effects, but it is not recommended, not only because of habituation but also because it increases any coexisting depression if used for any length of time. If anxiolytic agents are indicated, hydroxyzine (Atarax) is as good as any, whereas in more severe cases fluphenazine (Moditen) or thioridazine (Mellaril) have been found useful.

Depression, as has been pointed out earlier, frequently occurs concomitantly with chronic pain and hence antidepressant drugs are often indicated. Their secondary sedating properties enhance sleep, which is so often disturbed in these patients.

It cannot be stressed too emphatically, however, that pharmacological treatment is only one of many tools available; several others are often used simultaneously. Many of the treatment modalities available clearly fall within the sphere of competence of the orthopedist, but others are more appropriately supplied by members of the pain team or by professionals co-opted specifically in a particular case. Some orthopedic surgeons will prefer to use the services of the anesthetist for such procedures as steroid lumbar or caudal epidural injections; injection of trigger points of deep muscles, such as the piriformis or quadratus lumborum; and injection of facet joints. Others prefer to attend to these procedures themselves. The details of these divisions of labor will depend on the team's structure and expertise of its members.

There is no uniform agreement regarding the precise indications for steroid epidural injections and even less agreement regarding the efficacy of employing the lumbar or caudal route. However, a case could be made that frank disc prolapse with nerve root involvement calls for surgical intervention, unless the patient's general condition contraindicates that approach, but that injections for cases without root involvement, of disc bulging, or of minor stenoses are indicated and not infrequently successful in alleviating the presenting symptoms, especially when combined with physical therapy. We have found that such injections can have prophylactic value in patients prone to develop root fibrosis as demonstrated at reoperation. Caudal steroid injections, administered at the first signs of pain recurrence often will prevent progression of fibrous tissue formation and maturation.

One of the major new tools in pain management is neuroaugmentation. Spinal epidural implants have proven to be particularly effective in long-term, severe root fibrosis presenting with neuralgic pain in one or both lower extremities, especially since all other treatment modalities are usually unable to control these symptoms. If a trial with transcutaneous nerve stimulation (TENS) has proven effective, the chances are excellent that implantation of such a device will achieve pain relief in at least 80% of patients. Root fibrosis is one of the prime indications for this method. In those patients who fail to benefit from TENS it is suggested that a double-blind, morphine-naloxone test be given, since a positive test might be an indication for a deep brain implant. Recent improvements in the available hardware and the refinement of the indications for these procedures have made these recommendations possible after early disappointing beginnings. In long-neglected cases, the patient may enter a state of chronic pain behavior. This diagnosis should be suspected when, despite previous treatment, symptoms fail to improve or even progress even though physical findings are absent or minimal. These situations are by no means rare and clearly call for the services of the psychologist supported by the social worker and the physiothera-pist. Frequently, treatment cannot proceed on an outpatient basis. While some patients can be helped by patient and prolonged intervention, the overall prognosis for this group of individuals is not good.

SUMMARY

This chapter has attempted to sketch the role of a pain management team organized in a pain clinic in the comprehensive treatment of patients with chronic low back pain. Unfortunately this multidisciplinary approach is often sought only after months and even years of a piecemeal therapy, which not infrequently fails to recognize the complicated nature of the problem until chronic pain behavior has become well established, the will or ability to work has been lost, and irretrievable harm has come to patient and family, not to mention the loss of productivity to society as a whole.

SUGGESTED READINGS

Hendler NH, Long DM, Wise TN: Diagnosis and Treatment of Chronic Pain. John Wright, Boston, 1982

Stanton-Hicks M, Boas RA: Chronic Low Back Pain. Raven Press, New York, 1982

Swerdlow M: Relief of Intractable Pain. Elsevier Science Publishing, North Holland, 1983

Wall PD, Melzack R: Textbook of Pain. Churchill Livingstone, Edinburgh, 1984

24

Neuroaugmentive Surgery

Charles V. Burton

Pain is nature's way of informing the brain that something is amiss in a body part. Acute injury produces high intensity sharp pain that is well localized and elicits reflex withdrawal from the insult. A study of the brain's representation of body parts (the "homunculus") reveals that the cortical area for the low back is miniscule when compared with that for mouth, fingers, toes and special senses. This should not be surprising when we consider that during early life the storage banks of our brain "computer" are being programmed by a high volume of sensory information from the latter but not from the former. It is only in later decades of life that sensory information in the guise of pain is likely to be directed to the brain. Thus it is not difficult to understand that this input is deciphered as diffuse and nonspecific in light of the very small area of representation.

Following acute injury a phase occurs in which sharp, localizing pain is replaced by dull, aching discomfort (agony), which is nature's way of reminding us not to use or further injure the afflicted body part. We now appreciate that pain can be potentiated by many means, and the end perception represents an interplay of organic and functional entities. Pain is basically a protective system, but when constant and severe, it is a liability and can be destructive and incapacitating.

Pain-relieving analgesics and narcotics serve effectively to manage acute pain. They are, however, because of their endorphin-suppressing effect, a disaster for the chronic pain patient in whom they potentiate (rather than alleviate) the pain problem.

In the search for means of relieving incapacitating pain the medical profession turned to electrical stimulation over 2,000 years ago, as documented by the Roman writer Scribonius Largus.[1] Painful extremities (usually from gouty arthritis) were placed in buckets of water along with an electric eel (torpedo fish). The inevitable electrical "jolt" produced a state of immediate pain relief. It also often produced pain relief lasting for many hours. We know now that this phenomenon resulted from the release of endogenous opiates from the brain in response to the electrical stimulation.

In recent centuries scientists and physicians, Benjamin Franklin among them, have tried mightily to harness electricity for pain relief. Figures 24–1 and 24–2 show a battery-operated transcutaneous electrical nerve stimulator (TENS) manufactured in Paris by Gaiffe and described by Beard and Rockwell in 1871.[2] It is basically similar to modern TENS devices with the exception that its maximum output was only about 3 mA (modern devices output over 90 mA with similar resistive loads). The "electreat," which has been manufactured in the United States since 1918 represents the first of recent TENS units

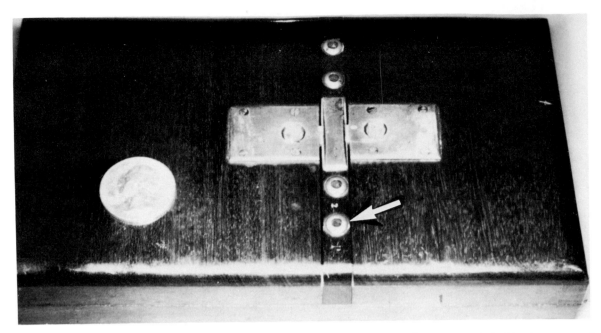

Fig. 24-1 A battery-operated TENS device manufactured in Paris by Gaiffe prior to 1871. Size is compared with a U.S. quarter. The arrow points to one of the lead wire "plug-ins."

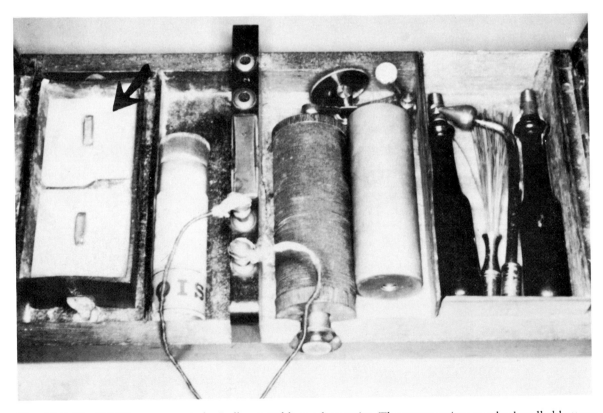

Fig. 24-2 The TENS components basically resemble modern units. The arrow points to a lead-walled battery containing mercury sulfate. The battery is removable and the contact points in the case are similar to those in modern flashlights. At the right is a vial of mercury sulfate and next to it a cylindrical inductorium. The last compartment contains contact probes and a wire brush with wooden handles. With a higher electrical output this TENS unit would have been clinically effective.

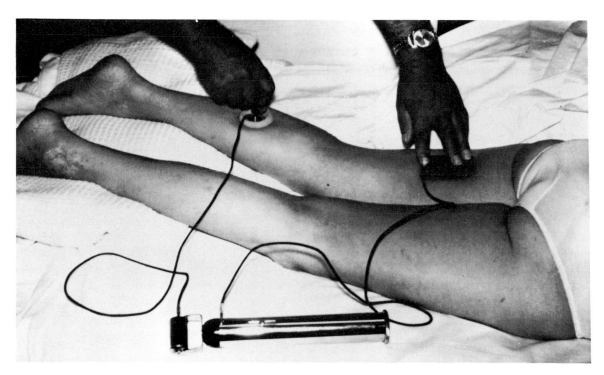

Fig. 24-3 The "electreat" TENS unit is shown in use. The electrodes are moistened sponges. Note the roller at the end of the unit used for electrical "massage." It is estimated that over 300,000 of these devices have been sold since 1918. Although crude, they are capable of producing pain relief where TENS is of value.

(Fig. 24-3). The advent of solid state electronics after World War II and the development of the cardiac pacemaker allowed a modern refocusing of medical interest on electrical stimulation as a means of potentiating (augmenting) function of the intact nervous system. Present TENS units are solid state and designed to be used with a high level of safety.

Following the publication, in 1965 of the "Gate Theory of Pain" by Melzak and Wall,[3] it was thought by many that the neuromechanism of electronic pain relief was evident. The discovery of endogenous opiate systems passing between brain and spinal cord has served both to enlighten and to confuse understanding of this complex subject.[4]

Modern TENS devices continue to have application as a reasonable means of producing pain relief when the pain is mild and is well localized to a single area. Although efficacy for acute use (60% to 80%) is higher than for chronic use (35% to 60%) the device has the advantage of enhancing (rather than depressing) endogenous opiates and is inherently safe. Basic efficacy, precautions, and practical limitations of TENS

have been reviewed by Burton[5] who notes that the most common complication has been skin reaction to electrodes.[6]

In addition to pain relief TENS systems are now being used to potentiate bone healing[7] and for the electronic stimulation of muscle groups.[8] Muscle stimulation by this means has been used during surgery to avoid thrombophlebitis and to reduce risk of postsurgical pulmonary embolus.

IMPLANTED NEUROAUGMENTIVE DEVICES

In 1967 neurosurgeon C. Norman Shealy developed the first implanted electronic device intended to relieve pain.[9] Initial tests of his dorsal cord neurostimulator (DCN) were successful in relieving pain from metastatic carcinoma, and when these DCN units entered the commercial market in 1970[10] there was a high level of initial enthusiasm. Unfortunately, the lack of knowledge regarding patient selection and techniques of surgery combined with initially high device malfunction rates led to a subsequent period of disenchantment during which time device design, surgical techniques, and indications for use were improved.

A major problem from the beginning was the difficulty in determining which patient with chronic pain was a potential candidate for a neuroaugmentive implant.[11] Although neural tissue-destructive procedures were still being used to treat some acute pain problems in the early 1970s (e.g., rhizotomy, cordotomy, tractotomy, thalamotomy), it became evident that these procedures had very little role in managing chronic pain because they produced deafferentation pain states. These problems, of which anesthesia dolorosa is an example, were often more disabling than the original chronic pain problem. It also became evident that the DCN was not capable of relieving *all* pain. Patients using these devices were able to appreciate sharp and localized pain (neo-spinal—thalamic) normally with the device activated, but were relieved of the dull and aching pain (paleo—spinal-thalamic). It was also found that patients on narcotic medications often felt the electrical parasthesias but obtained no pain relief and that pain relief could sometimes be enhanced by using nutritional supplements and tricyclic anti-depressant medications that potentiated endorphin release and action. A significant disadvantage was the inability to determine by testing prior to implantation of the DCN if a patient would benefit from its use. TENS devices were tried for such screening but proved unreliable.

In 1973, Hoppenstein[12] first reported on the use of percutaneously inserted epidural neurostimulating electrodes (PENS) that could be implanted on a temporary basis under local anesthesia to allow the patient to determine the degree of pain relief. Through rapid development and improvement, PENS systems have become the most extensively used neuroaugmentive devices for pain relief. Although the usual period of testing for an ambulatory patient is 2 to 5 days, in debilitated patients it is possible to maintain the epidural electrodes with their percutaneous extensions for many months. Normally, after the testing period the epidural electrodes are internalized and can serve as a definitive electronic pain relief device. Today many PENS systems have been functional for more than 5 years. If after internalization a malfunction

occurs (approximately 30% of cases) the clinical efficacy information is utilized to place a directly implanted dorsal cord neurostimulator system optimally with the electrode placed either epidurally or within a dural pocket (endodural). DCN systems are the most stable, effective, and long-lasting when used in conjunction with PENS systems for screening. DCN development has been well documented in a number of publications.[13]

Although spinal neurostimulators are the most frequently used neuroaugmentive devices to relieve low back and/or leg pain, there are occasional patients whose pain is so severe and widespread throughout the body that deep brain neurostimulators (DBS) are necessary. In these cases the stimulating electrode is usually located in the periventricular gray matter (limbic system) or in a thalamic sensory nucleus. DBS systems are the most effective in relieving pain but also carry the highest risk.[14] They are, however, potentially capable of relieving some elements of sharp, well localized pain. The DBS appears to function more by endogenous opiate release than be "gating" which seems to be more characteristic of spinal stimulators.

Peripheral nerve stimulation (PNS) devices have been used for pain relief in some patients over the past decade but have been significantly limited in use because of the common complication of muscle spasm accompanying pain relief. A very important advantage of spinal stimulation over PNS has been the consistent observation that the former is capable of not only relieving pain but also increasing peripheral blood flow into impaired extremities.[15,16] This phenomenon is particularly noticeable in patients with causalgia of an extremity because of both the neurological and vascular bundle injuries. Existing tissue anoxia and chronic ulceration usually disappear within 1 to 2 weeks following initiation of stimulation. The author has seen a number of cases where patients with peripheral arteriosclerotic vascular disease have been referred for treatment of a postamputation pain syndrome (usually due to neuroma). Following the initiation of spinal cord stimulation for pain relief, blood flow in the impaired contralateral extremity has dramatically improved. The improvement in blood flow appears to reflect a direct modification of autonomic function at the spinal level and promises to be an important area for future investigation.

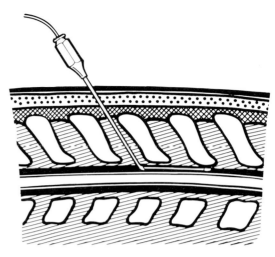

Fig. 24-4 Under local anesthesia an epidural guide needle is passed to the epidural space. The flexible PENS electrode is passed to the appropriate level, usually in the midline. Skew of position to either side usually produces an appreciation of stimulation only on that side. (Courtesy of Cordis Corporation.)

Fig. 24-5 A solid-state battery operated pulse generator is used for initial testing. Amplitude, frequency, and pulse width of waveform are usually varied as part of multiparameter testing at different spinal levels and locations (Insert A). In Insert B a flexible PENS electrode (arrow) has been passed through the guide needle. In this case, monopolar testing is in progress using the guide needle as "ground." (TENS skin electrodes may also be used for this purpose). If initial testing is successful, the guide needle is removed leaving the epidural electrode(s) in place. Extension leads are connected to the end of the electrode and placed under the skin so that the ends of the extension pass through the skin and can be connected to a pulse generator for ambulatory testing. (Courtesy of Cordis Corporation.)

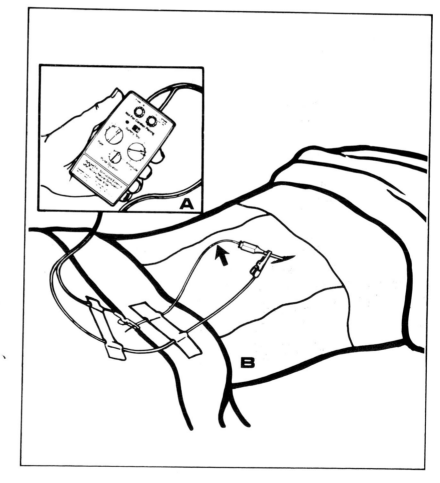

PATIENT SELECTION

As previously noted, patients with constant dull and aching pain (often referred to as "agony") tend to obtain the best results from neuroaugmentive devices. This type of pain is typical of a number of clinical entities involving nerve injury. Causalgia is an example of this. The term was coined by neurologist Weir Mitchell during the U.S. Civil War. He observed and described the "burning and searing" agony produced by incomplete lesions of peripheral mixed nerves. The author believes that causalgia is caused by atypically patterned sensory information (resulting from partial injury to the conducting system) reaching the brain and being interpreted in an adverse manner. This entity is often dramatically alleviated by electrical nerve stimulation that modifies the pattern of information being sent to the brain.

One of the most difficult therapeutic problems known, and unfortunately a problem affecting approximately 25% of patients who have undergone lumbar spine surgery is the "failed back surgery syndrome" (FBSS). This is a complex entity reflecting organic and functional disease as well as learned pain behavior and socioeconomic incentives that tend to enhance incapacitation. From the work of Burton et al.[17] many of the primary organic causes of FBSS have been identified in large populations of patients who were referred for rehabilitation. Although the majority of patients (57% to 58%) were found to have lateral spinal stenosis (potentially treatable by surgical decompression), 6% to 16% had adhesive arachnoiditis and 6% to 8% epidural fibrosis as the primary pathological process* responsible for chronic pain. The last two are pathological entities that are usually not improved by surgical treatment and the associated pain reflects the chronic nerve impairment resulting from swelling and irritation. These particular problems are the most difficult therapeutic challenges. Following alleviation of functional and chemical dependency and abuse problems by special programs, these patients are primary candidates for implanted neuroaugmentive pain relief devices. The lateral spinal stenosis patients may also have permanent nerve injury and may require neuroaugmentive

devices as a secondary procedure. Statistics at our institute indicate that over the past 5 years approximately 11% of FBSS patients being referred for rehabilitation have had a neuroaugmentive device implanted as part of the comprehensive rehabilitative process.

TECHNIQUE

As previously noted, PENS systems have the advantage of being relatively easy to implant and test. Their disadvantage is their instability in the spinal

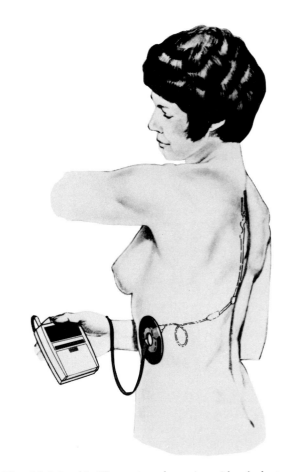

Fig. 24-6 In this illustration the twin epidural electrodes (bipolar) have been connected to a subcutaneous radio-frequency receiver. The battery-operated pulse generator is external and patient controlled. The silicone antenna is placed over the skin and the signal is pulsed through the skin received, demodulated, and passed to the epidural electrodes. In actual use the tips of the electrodes are separated by at least one vertebral level. (Courtesy of Medtronic, Inc.)

---

*It was not possible to document intraneural fibrosis clinically.

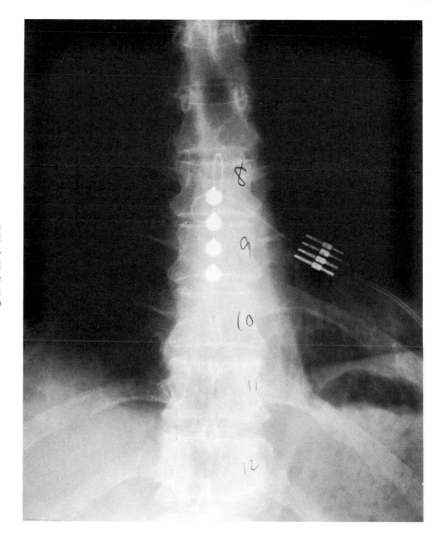

Fig. 24-7 Intractable left leg pain adequately relieved by a dorsal cord neurostimulator over a 10-year period. Failure of the device required revision and this Medtronic Resume spinal neurostimulator was placed in the epidural space at the T8–9 level skewed to the left of midline.

canal. Approximately 30% need to be replaced by a surgically placed DCN because of malfunction.

In Figure 24-4 a monopolar electrode has been passed under local anesthesia through a guide needle into the epidural space. This should be carried out under bi-plane fluoroscopic control. For back and leg pain control one or more electrodes are passed to approximately the T8 level and multiparameter (multiple locations and variable) testing is performed. Most optimal results are obtained at the T9–10 levels. Figure 24-5 shows a single electrode (monopolar) being tested with the guide needle serving as "ground." A solid-state pulse generator provides the electrical stimulation. Should initial testing provide pain relief the epidural electrodes can be connected

to extension leads that run under the skin and exit laterally where they can be connected to a pulse generator operated by the patient. At our institute, twin leads (bipolar) are usually preferred to a single lead (monopolar). Successful ambulatory testing indicates that the system can be internalized (Fig. 24-6). Since publication of the first edition of this text, percutaneous epidural electrodes have been used less frequently at our institution. A directly placed epidural 4-contact electrode array carried out under local anesthesia with supplementation through a small incision, is increasing in popularity. The latter system is easier to use, more stable and consistent, fraught with less complications, more versatile, and can provide higher intensity of local stimulation than PENS (Fig. 24-7).

From the standpoint of simplicity of use and reliability RF-coupled systems have consistently remained the most popular. Following the introduction of totally implanted pulse generators (Figs. 24–8 and 24–9) they have become more "user friendly," allowing the patient the opportunity of turning the device on and off with an external magnet and allowing the physician to change stimulation parameters and patterns with an external control unit. At the present time, the disadvantages of the totally implanted systems are their complexity, greater expense, and requirement for additional surgery to replace batteries. With continued improvements, these factors will probably become less significant.

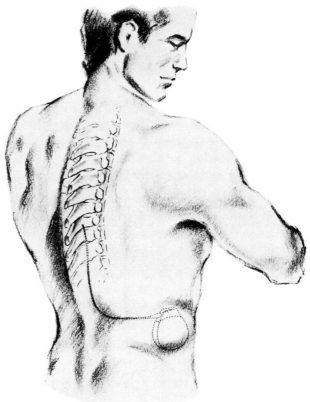

Fig. 24-9 A monopolar system is represented here. The pulse generator itself serves as the opposite pole of the circuit. This basic system is a forerunner of the future "smart" implant systems. (Courtesy of Cordis Corporation.)

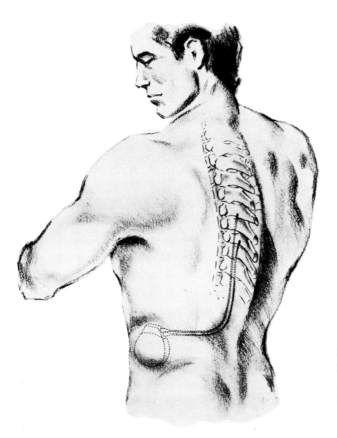

Fig. 24-8 A more recent option is a totally implanted system that can be programmed from an external device and turned on and off by an external magnet. With small size and high output the total implant is becoming increasing popular. In this case the system is bipolar. After 5 years the chest incision must be opened and the batteries replaced. (Courtesy of Cordis Corporation.)

SAFETY AND EFFICACY

Following their introduction by C. Norman Shealy in 1967, implanted spinal neurostimulators in general neurosurgical use were fraught with a myriad of complication including spinal cord compression, spinal fluid leak, implant injury or failure, infection, etc. It has also been recognized that an important requirement for success is the complete cessation of narcotic use by the patient. After almost two decades of clinical use, however, these implanted neurostimulators have become reliably commonplace in centers dealing with failed back surgery patients and causalgia, reflecting improvements in technique, instrumentation, and patient selection.

Table 24–1 Neuromodulation: Use and Estimated Improvement

Pain Control Device	Estimated Number Worldwide	Estimated Significant Improvement	
		Short-Term %	Long-Term %
Transcutaneous electrical nerve stimulator (TENS)	100,000	80	35
Percutaneous epidural neurostimulator (PENS), acute and chronic	1,200	80	†
Dorsal cord neurostimulator (DCN)	7,500	80	35
Peripheral nerve neurostimulator (PNS)	500	80	50
Depth brain neurostimulator (DBS)	100	90	70

* Significant improvement = 50% or more (moderate to marked) improvement in pretreatment pain. Criteria are variable and depend on patient population, clinical pain problem, selection criteria, device used, and method of use. Long-term improvement averages over 2 years in patients who continue to use the device.
† Thought to be about 50% to 60%.

In 1977 my associate Charles Ray published a general review of the efficacy of neurostimulation devices.[18] (Table 24-1). General estimates such as these are always difficult to interpret because they are so sensitive to proper patient selection and, therefore, can easily be skewed negatively. These reports, however, do tend to reflect the results of the most experienced surgeons. In 1981 Ray et al.[19] reviewed the efficacy of neurostimulation with PENS and DBS at our institute. From 1976 to 1981 after an average follow-up of 19.4 months, 58% of patients were still using PENS, with a 49% good-to-excellent result. After a 2 year follow-up,, the DBS group had a 75% good-to-excellent response. The author's 15-year experience with spinal cord stimulation in a patient population essentially limited to adhesive arachnoiditis and causalgia has demonstrated a long-term good-to-excellent result rate of about 50% to 55%. At the 1986 American Academy of Neurological Surgeons meeting Donlin Long indicated that the present over-all initial success rate for dorsal cord neurostimulation was about 50%, with long-term success decreasing to 30%. Initial depth brain stimulation was reported in 57% of patients and decreasing to 32% after long-term follow-up.

Although these results may not seem impressive at first glance, the reader must appreciate that neurostimulation devices replace destructive procedures such as rhizotomy, cordotomy thalamotomy, topec-

tomy and labotomy with a relatively benign procedure designed to enhance the body's own natural pain relief mechanisms. One must also appreciate that the low level of efficacy represents a dramatic improvement over what was previously possible in a group of patients who clearly represent the single most difficult management problem confronting the medical profession.

SUMMARY

External and implanted neuroaugmentive devices in the treatment of pain continue to be increasingly effective in pain relief. The implanted systems are more reliable today and long-term use has now been observed in many patients. Key elements to success remain careful patient selection and well-trained surgeons, familiar with electronic systems and and well versed in potential pitfalls. Further potentiation of good results requires the use of ancillary comprehensive facilities and programs with adequate medical and technical support.

ACKNOWLEDGMENTS

The author would like to take this opportunity especially to express to Dr. Charles D. Ray, friend and colleague over many years, Director of the Neuroaugmentive Surgery section of the Institute for Low Back Care, our appreciation for the many contributions made to the field of neurostimulation. Dr. Ray has been an innovative pioneer in this area and much of the present state of the art reflects his contributions.

Appreciation for support and consideration is also directed to Drs. Alex Lifson and Harvey Aaron, Mr. Kevin Gracie, and the staff of the Institute for Low Back Care and to Medtronic, Inc. and the Cordis Corporation for use of illustrations and quality products for our patients.

REFERENCES

1. Scribonius L: De compositione medicamentorum liber. Translated in Kellaway P: The part played by electric fish in early history of bioelectricity and electrotherapy. Bull Hist Med 20: 112, 1946

2. Beard GM, Rockwell AD: A Practical Treatise on the Medical and Surgical Uses of Electricity. William Wood, New York, 1871

3. Melzak R, Wall PD: Pain mechanisms: a new theory. Science 150: 971, 1965

4. Burton CV, Ray DC: Neurostimulation. In DeVita V, Hellman S, Rosenberg SA (eds): Cancer: Principles and Practice of Oncology. JB Lippincott, Philadelphia, 1982

5. Burton CV: Transcutaneous electrical nerve stimulation to relieve pain. Postgrad Med 59: 105, 1976

6. Burton CV, Maurer DD: Pain suppression by transcutaneous electronic stimulation. JEEE Trans Biomed Engin BME 21: 81, 1974

7. Bassett CAL, Pawluk RJ, Pilla AA: Acceleration of fracture repair by electromagnetic fields: a surgically non-invasive method. Ann NY Acad Sci 238:242, 1974

8. Burton CV, Maurer DD: Solvent-activated current passing tape electrode for transcutaneous electrical stimulation of the peripheral nervous system. JEEE Trans Biomed Eng BME 33: 346, 1976

9. Shealy CN, Mortimer JT, Reswick JB: Electrical inhibition of pain by stimulation of the dorsal columns: preliminary clinical report. Anesth Analg 46:489, 1967

10. Shealy CN, Mortimer JT, Hagfors NR: Dorsal column electroanaglesia. J Neurosurg 32: 560, 1970

11. Ray, CD (ed): Electrical stimulation of the human nervous system for the control of pain. Minneapolis Pain Seminar. Surg Neurol 4:61, 1973

12. Hoppenstein R: Percutaneous implantation of chronic spinal cord electrodes for control of intractable pain. Preliminary report. Surg Neurol 4: 171, 1973

13. Burton CV, Ray CD, Nashold BS: Symposium on the safety and clinical efficacy of implanted neuroaugmentive devices. Neurosurgery 1: 185, 1977

14. Ray CD, Burton CV: Deep brain stimulation for severe, chronic pain. Acta Neurochir, suppl., 30:289, 1980

15. Cook A, Oygar A, Baggenstros P, et al: Vascular disease of extremities: electric stimulation of spinal cord and posterior roots. NY State J Med 76: 366, 1976

16. Dooley DD, Kasprak M: Modification of blood flow to extremities by electrical stimulation of the nervous system. South Med J 69: 1309, 1976

17. Burton CV, Kirkaldy-Willis WH, Yong-Hing K, Heithoff KB: Causes of failure of surgery on the lumbar spine. Clin Orthop 157: 191 1981

18. Ray CD: New electrical stimulation methods for therapy and rehabilitation. Orthop Rev 6: 29, 1977

19. Ray CD, Burton CV, Lifson A: Neurostimulation as used in a large clinical practice. Appl Neurophysiol 45: 160, 1982

25

Functional Restoration: New Concepts in Spinal Rehabilitation

Holly Mayer
Tom G. Mayer

Until recently, rehabilitation for spinal disorders has not been standardized and is of questionable effectiveness. In contrast to other areas of musculoskeletal medicine in which rehabilitation generally implies restoring physical functional capacity to the highest level possible, care in the low back patient has taken an aberrant turn. The fine work of early investigators into the psychosocial concomitants of long-term disability led to recognition of relationships between illness behavior to operant conditioning and stress to muscular tension.[1-3] This has led to a large community of 2,000 American treatment facilities known as pain clinics, which have increased in popularity in the past 25 years. Possible drawbacks of this approach are (1) the high cost of some of these clinics and (2) their unsubstantiated benefits.

Important barriers to restoring function may be inherent in the disability system. A generation of employers have grown up convinced that the high incidence of recurrent back problems in the previously back-injured population and the frequently ambiguous circumstances of back injury, make these patients of dubious reemployment value. This thinking is abetted by insurance companies, attorneys, and state workers' compensation boards who, in ardently disagreeing over financial compensation to be granted to back patients (the highest cost benign condition in industrialized countries), create a hostile, adversarial atmosphere.

Additionally, the lack of visual feedback to the joints and muscles of the back and the lack of a contralateral side for comparison in the spine makes spinal disorders, unaccompanied by deformity or measureable neurological deficit, a "hidden disability." Opinions about the seriousness of this "hidden disability" have polarized views of health professionals into two opposing camps. This polarization has caused a hardening of the attitudes, so that some believe most back-injured patients are "fakers," whereas others believe that the vast majority are "totally and permanently disabled." The absence of clinical visual feedback makes this distinction more often legal than medical.

Meanwhile, from the human cost standpoint, the patient is clearly the victim. In any given year, 3% to 4% of the working population has a disabling injury. Though more than 90% of patients resolve their problem spontaneously within 3 to 4 months, the remaining small group (about 10%) accounts for approximately 80% of the money spent on back injuries and half of the group (about 5%) remain disabled for 1 to 2 years.[4,5] Patients of this small group then go on to develop the attendant psychosocioeconomic changes of prolonged disability with which we have become so familiar: depression, anxiety neurosis, divorce, drugs, litigation, multiple surgery, and, all too frequently, suicide.

DIAGNOSIS AND TREATMENT

It is into this strained atmosphere that a new approach to spinal rehabilitation, termed "functional restoration," has been introduced. The treatment basically consists of an amalgam of a sports medicine approach to restoring physical capacity and a cognitive crisis intervention technique for dealing with psychosocial issues in patients suffering from chronic spinal disability.

Quantification of Physical and Psychological Function

The key diagnostic element is quantification of physical and psychological function. The derivation of this concept results, quite simply, from the recognition of the hidden nature of spinal impairments. Unlike the extremities, spinal anatomy does not lend itself to simple visual inspection or palpation. We, as clinicians, have been seduced by progressively more sophisticated imaging techniques into believing that (1) a correctable structural lesion usually exists, and (2) that an anatomical lesion is the most common basis for ongoing complaints. We have inadvertently lent credence to the grossly erroneous conclusion that "if surgery can't fix it, the lesion must be in the head." An error equally damaging to the doctor/patient relationship is the belief that "if the imaging tests are normal, there is probably nothing wrong."

Of course, unsubstantial beliefs fly in the face of all evidence. Surgery is useful in only a small percentage of patients with degenerative spinal disorders. Furthermore, we know that rehabilitation can dramatically improve musculoskeletal function in the extremities by altering joint motion, muscle strength, endurance, and neuromuscular coordination through

training. Such treatment is also possible for spinal disorders; however, the precondition for such treatment is objective and reliable recognition requiring measurement technology that is currently available and slowly emerging in clinical settings.

It is beyond the scope of this chapter to discuss in detail the loss of physical functional capacity, termed the deconditioning syndrome, which is responsible for maintaining the organic component of disability in most chronic spine patients. However, extensive information concerning these issues is now available in the literature, specifically regarding measurement of range-of-motion,[1,6-8] trunk strength in sagittal and axial planes,[9-13] aerobic capacity,[14] and functional task performance such as lifting and bending.[6,15,16]

Measurement of physical capacity in the lumbar spine imposes test demands not usually encountered in the extremities. First of all, nonbilaterality implies that use of intra-individual controls, long used in the extremities, must be replaced by reliance on a large interindividual normative database in the spine. It also has become empirically evident that such databases must be made specific for gender and age. Furthermore, tests of muscular performance (i.e., trunk strength or lifting capacity) can have reduced population variability if normalized to body weight, and, in some instances, to the Davenport index. Ultimately, databases may become large enough to relate anticipated physical capacities to the ergonomic demands of a specific job. A clinical example of a quantitative impairment evaluation using physical measurement technology is shown in Table 25-1

A second test demand is that, because there are no intra-individual controls, an effort factor must be identified for each test. Terminology may be confusing, though, and the reader must understand that limitations of effort are only infrequently the result of conscious attempts to defraud the examiner. They usually result, at least on initial testing, from pain, fear of injury, and patient perception. Patients usually have been conditioned by personal experience, as well as advice from friends and physicians, that "if it hurts, don't do it." This results in a vicious cycle of overprotectiveness, leading to additional disuse, and resultant susceptibility to recurrent injury with minimal additional trauma, until a steady state is reached at low functional tolerance. The effort factor, together with a variety of psychological tests and patient self-report measures, identifies the cognitive and psychosocial barriers to function. The clinician's recognition of low effort helps direct subsequent interventions to a greater emphasis on education and counseling. It also identifies the degree to which the testing has been invalidated and shows the clinician that a higher degree of physical performance than was demonstrated may be expected from this individual on subsequent testing.

The range of motion effort factor is clearly delineated in other publications.[6,17] Endurance tests can usually be calibrated for effort by use of a target heart rate (with notable exceptions, such as intercurrent cardiovascular disease or use of rate-limiting medications). Reaching the target heart rate in bicycle ergometry, upper body ergometry, or psychophysical lifting tests indicates that the patient has high motivation in achieving this work performance level. From this point on, the patient is usually able to continue reaching the target heart rate as reconditioning leads to achievement of progressively higher work rates.

Dynamic strength testing (sagittal and axial trunk strength and isokinetic lifting) permits identification of another effort factor. This factor is related to the empirical observation that only a maximum voluntary contraction (MVC) is truly reproducible through multiple trials. Although isometric testing may provide for comparison of peak forces, a dynamic test gives a curve of force versus distance, which allows for improved characterization of function through comparison of curve shape and work integral (or area beneath the curve). In time, it should be possible to provide a normal database of acceptable variability between trials with regard to peak forces, curve shape, or work performance, leading to a fully quantified strength effort factor.

Finally, a variety of quantified psychosocial tests and self-report measures are combined[18] to give a comprehensive view of other potential barriers to functional recovery. Armed with this information, plus repeated self-report testing of patient pain/disability/depression perception at scheduled intervals, the psychological counselor can become a potent force in advising the physical treatment team and in supporting the patient through the functional restoration program.

Functional Restoration Treatment Programs

The functional restoration treatment program for the chronic back patient involves a multidisciplinary team approach using physical and occupational therapy, psychology, and nursing and is guided by a supervising physician who is not necessarily a surgeon. The physician must have an understanding of neurological and musculoskeletal disorders and must clearly recognize the difference between previous passive interventions and the patient's active participation in functional restoration. The nurse generally functions as a physician–extender, providing counseling on medical matters, patient education, medication control, communication with outside agencies, and examinations for minor intercurrent illnesses.

The physical therapists are concerned with mobilizing and strengthening the injured part of the body. Their focus on the "weak link of the lifting chain" causing the problem involves them in guiding a sequential reconditioning program and deals with the minor overuse problems of rebuilding a severely deconditioned anatomical area.

By contrast, occupational therapists have two main roles. First, they provide training in task performance—that is, synchronizing the injured part with the whole body in tasks such as lifting, bending, twisting, squatting, and climbing. A variety of physical tasks is employed, and improving positional tolerance for sitting and standing are also major training goals. Second, occupational therapists become involved in the socioeconomic consequences of disability and the various societal outcomes that must be dealt with to promote the patient's recovery, such as employment and litigation.

Psychologists involved in this type of program also are involved in a dual role. First, they have a general crisis intervention role in which they must coordinate with the occupational therapist to help the patients deal with the termination of disability, as well as the economic, vocational and family goals associated with this change. Second, they must help other team members recognize the barriers to functional recovery in an individual patient and help the patient to deal with these barriers. We have found that a cognitive-behavioral treatment orientation is appropriate and effective for a functional restoration approach. This orientation emphasizes the importance of simultaneously dealing with thoughts and feelings, as well as overt behavior in correcting maladaptive behaviors and dysfunctions. Under medical supervision, the psychologist may also provide valuable assistance in dealing with habituating drugs, as well as with appropriate medication for withdrawal, depression, or anxiety neurosis. Counseling for specific individual problems identified through psychological testing is a critical part of the program. Long-term psychother-

apy, however, is inappropriate in such a program because of its tendency to produce dependency.

Initially, the patient is evaluated by a physician who must determine whether surgery has been ruled out and the type of rehabilitation to be performed. The evaluation includes a QIE (Table 25-1), psychology consult, and appropriate structural diagnostics. A preprogram period designed to remobilize and assess patient attitudes is followed by a 2 to 3 week

Table 25-1 Example of a Thoracolumbar Quantitative Functional Evaluation

Patient Name: Carol
SS#: 336–46–
Test Date: 1–31–86

This patient underwent a Quantitative Impairment Evaluation which is a battery of tests of spinal physical functional capacity. This information may be used to determine medical impairment of function. % Normal ratings are based on a limited clinical sample: a large standardized normative database is being assembled and constantly updated.

I. Self-report scores
  1. Beck Depression Inventory — 15
  2. Pain drawing
    a. Intensity score — 5/10
    b. Trunk — 2/72
    c. Extremities — 0/136
  3. Dallas Analog Scale — 70/150

II. Physical capacity
  1. Physical status — Right/Left
    a. Neurological deficit — Negative/Negative
    b. FABER — Positive/Negative
    c. Spasm — Negative/Negative
  2. Deformities/posture — Negative

  3. Range of motion — Degrees — % Normal
    a. Sagittal
      1. Gross motion F/E — 115(Ad)/25(MoD) — 92/56
      2. True lumbar (T12–S1 only) F/E — 45(MoD)/20(MoD) — 68/67
      3. Hip motion F/E — 70 (NL)/5(SeD) — 117/33
      4. Straight leg raise R/L — 90 (NL)/95(NL) — 106/112
      5. True spine/hip flex ratio — 64% Abnormal: True spine flexion deficit
    b. Coronal
      1. True lumbar R/L — 30 (NL)/30 (NL) — 100/100
      2. Hip motion R/L — 10 (NL)/10 (NL) — 100/100
    c. Effort factor — Good
  4. Trunk strength (CYBEX)
    a. Isokinetic (sagittal (ft-lb/lb) — Torque/Body weight — % Normal
      1. 60°/second F/E — 77(MiD)/36(SeD) — 84/33
      2. 120°/second F/E — 31(SeD)/23(SeD) — 35/22
      3. 150°/second F/E — 41(SeD)/35(SeD) — 49/36
      4. F/E ratios (60°/120°/150°) — 214%/135%/117% — (Abn)/(Abn)/(Abn)
      5. High speed drop off (120°/60°) — 40/64 — (Abn)/(Abn)

(Table continues.)

Table 25-1 (*Continued*).

		Bicycle Ergometry	Upper Body Ergometry
5. Cardiovasular endurance			
a. Target heart rate(BPM)		158	158
b. Work rate (KGM)		700	500
c. Endurance time		7	4
d. Heart rate achieved		160	160
e. Effort factor		Excellent	Excellent

III. Occupational capacity

1. Occupational status

a. Working		Yes	
b. Job demand category—Previous		1	
c. Job demand category—Present/anticipated		1	
d. Job lifting requirements		Floor-Waist	Waist-Overhead
1. Frequent (lbs)		—	—
2. Occasional (lbs)		0–10	0–10

2. Positional tolerance

		Job requires	Patient capacity
a. Timed observation			
1. Sitting		N/A	N/A
2. Standing		N/A	N/A
3. Leg use		N/A	N/A
4. Upper body use		N/A	N/A
b. Timed obstacle course		N/A	

3. Lifting Capacity (Psychophysical Protocol)

		Floor-Waist	Waist-Overhead
a. Frequent lifting capacity			
1. Weight lifted(lbs)		21	21
2. Force/body weight		17(SeD)	17(MoD)
3. Endurance time		90	90
4. Heart rate achieved		112	112

	Max. force(lbs)	Force/BW(%)	% Normal
b. Isometric lifting			
1. Leg lift capacity	31	25%(SeD)	27
2. Torso lift capacity	39	32%(SeD)	35
c. Dynamic isokinetic lift (Cybex)			
1. Lumbar (0–4 ft)	Max. force(lbs)	Force/BW(%)	% Normal
a. 18″/second	60	49%(MoD)	55
b. 30″/second	52	43%(MoD)	50
c. 36″/second	54	44%(MoD)	55
d. Effort factor	Fair		

4. Global effort rating

a. Physical therapy		Good
b. Occupation therapy		Fair

SUMMARY

This patient with moderate disability and mild pain/depression self-report has significant spine flexion impairment with reversed spine/hip ratio, severe trunk strength deficit and associated lifting capacity deficits with mild barriers to functional recovery requiring significant efforts at functional restoration.

Test Interpretation By:
Tom G. Mayer, M.D.

TGM:prt

A lumbar quantitative impairment evaluation (QIE) report from the Productive Rehabilitation Institute of Dallas for Ergonomics (PRIDE) demonstrating patient results in quantified self-report, range of motion, trunk strength, aerobic and lifting capacities. Normal databases are utilized to calculate a ''% normal'' based on the mean scores of the specific test group. Symbols (e.g., NL = Normal; SeD = Severely Deficient) categorize the degree of physical deficit into simplified groupings.

comprehensive 10-hour/day treatment program. Follow-up lasting up to 6 weeks balances physical capacity with anticipated job demands.

Evidence also suggests that a large number of postoperative patients, even those with relatively minimal symptoms, continue with physical capacity deficits that make them susceptible to recurrent injury.[19] In general, it appears that the longer the time of disability and the more extensive the surgery, the greater the postoperative physical capacity deficits to be rectified. Since pain perception is an individual phenomenon with wide population variance, self-report is an extremely unreliable method for judging who may or may not be at risk.[20] For these postoperative individuals, relatively simple outpatient reconditioning or work hardening programs may be instituted with subsequent use of home equipment or a fitness center to maintain higher levels of physical capacity. Routine reemployment physicals and education programs that stress the importance of maintaining high levels of physical capacity in industry to prevent recurrence may well be established in the future.

SOCIETAL OUTCOMES

Low back disability is not just a disease but a manifestation of a complex system. The process also involves employers, attorneys, physicians, unions, insurance companies, and governmental agencies, all of whom may have fixed perceptions and deeply-rooted resistance to change. These groups must be made aware not only of the problems of disability but also of multiple accompanying problems that range from the loss of productivity to the financial drain on society. Once aware of the problems, these groups will in time be able to accept that functional restoration plays a crucial role in the ultimate solution.

All industrialized societies have a variety of social systems set aside to compensate individuals for injury, illness, or lost wages. From the relatively low reporting rates of back disability in emerging third world countries that have limited compensation systems, we can deduce that compensation for lost time may also be a factor in a worker's decision to miss work after an injury. However, the literature is ambiguous regarding its role in maintaining disability. From the previous discussion of the deconditioning syndrome,

it should now be clear to the reader that once the disability process has begun, a new set of mediators may take over to maintain it.

Some treatment facilities only attempt to alter the patient's pain report. Functional restoration is similar to most musculoskeletal rehabilitation, whose primary goal is to return patients to their highest level of physical capacity and productivity. Extensive evaluation at the PRIDE clinic now documents the ability of such a program to influence significantly important societal issues such as return to work, settlement of litigation, additional medical cost, recurrent injury, functional capacity, and pain reduction.[21-23]

It is worth pointing out a few salient observations from articles concerning functional restoration treatment outcome results. With regard to return to work, more than 85% of PRIDE patients who completed the functional restoration treatment program were able to return to productive employment. Furthermore, these patients returned to work at an average of 10 weeks after the program and have remained at work with a low rate of recurrence at 2-year follow-up, similar to back injury rates of the general population. Unlike prior rehabilitation efforts in which patients were often placed on permanent "light duty" jobs for which they were unsuited (security guard, computer operator), patients who are functionally restored and who have achieved high levels of physical capacity generally are able to return to heavy employment in positions similar to those they previously occupied. A return-to-work rate of more than 80% was noted in functional restoration treatment graduates, whereas the majority of the nontreatment comparison group chronic patients (averaging more than 1 year of disability) have been found to remain unemployed. The costs of compensation for nonproductivity are, of course, ultimately borne by the employer, consumer, and taxpayer.

The analysis of chronic patients also confirms that, under certain circumstances, the "green-back poultice" is effective in settling litigation a particular case. This leads some observers to believe that rehabilitation should only be offered selectively on the basis of unspecified predictors of outcome success. However, the high rate of a subsequent work-related injury, for which another employer is liable, in unrehabilitated patients whose cases were settled and the loss of productivity from patients denied the opportunity to do heavy work makes the denial of the rehabilitation opportunity both undemocratic and ultimately unprofitable. Furthermore, the questionable efficacy of other forms of treatment must be borne in mind, as no controlled trial has demonstrated effectiveness of pain clinic treatment or of multiple surgery for chronic back disability. The former may be no better than placebo,[23] and the latter may produce more disability than it resolves.

Functional restoration is not a cure for pain. It has been noted empirically that patients whose functional capacity has improved generally show an inversely proportional decrease in pain/disability self-report scores.[22] However, these patients, many of whom have somatization disorders, often continue to endorse higher pain/disability scores at their best functional levels than other population groups do at their worst.[20] This evidence of the variability in individual pain perception further reinforces our impression that pain report used by itself is *not* a valid outcome measure for low back disability. It should thus be used with extreme caution as the sole parameter for surgical decision-making in chronic low back pain patients. The physician must always keep in mind that functional restoration primarily emphasizes the return of productivity and functional capacity while accepting as a secondary benefit the lessening of pain and disability self-report.

REFERENCES

1. Fordyce W, Roberts A, Sternbach, R: The behavioral management of chronic pain: a response to critics. Pain, 22: 112, 1985
2. Sternbach R: Pain Patients: Traits and Treatment. Academic Press, Orlando, 1983
3. Turk D, Meichenbaum D, Genest M: Pain and Behavioral Medicine: A Cognitive-Behavioral Perspective. Guilford Press, New York, 1983
4. Bigos S, Spengler D, Martin N, et al: Back injuries in industry: a retrospective study. II. Injury factors. Spine 11: 246, 1986
5. Bigos S, Spengler D, Martin N, et al: Back injuries in industry: a retrospective study. III. Employee-related factors. Spine 11: 252, 1986
6. Mayer T, Kishino N, Keeley J, et al: Using physical measurements to assess low back pain. J Musculoskel Med 2: 44, 1985
7. Mayer T, Tencer A, Kristoferson S, Mooney V: Use of noninvasive techniques for quantification of spinal range-of-motion in normal subjects and chronic low-back dysfunction patients. Spine 9: 588, 1984
8. Pearcy M: Measurement of back and spinal mobility. Clin Biomech 1: 44, 1986
9. Davies G, Gould J: Trunk testing using a prototype Cybex II isokinetic stabilization system. J Orthop Sports Phys Ther 3: 164, 1982
10. Mayer T, Smith S, Keeley J, Mooney V: Quantification of lumbar function. II. Sagittal plane trunk strength in chronic low back pain patients. Spine 10: 765, 1985
11. Mayer T, Smith S, Kondraske G, et al: Quantification of function. III. Preliminary data on isokinetic torso rotation testing with myoelectric spectral analysis in normal and low back pain subjects. Spine 10: 912, 1985
12. Smith S, Mayer T, Gatchel R, Becker T: Quantification of lumbar function. I. Isometric and multispeed isokinetic trunk strength measures in sagittal and axial planes in normal subject patients. Spine 10: 757, 1985
13. Thompson N, Gould J, Davies G, et al: Descriptive Measures of Isokinetic Trunk Testing. J Orthop Sports Phys Ther 7: 43, 1985
14. Mayer T: Assessment of lumbar function. p. 101. In Mooney V (ed) Assessment of Musculoskeletal Function. Vol. 221. JB Lippincott, Philadelphia, 1987
15. Chaffin D, Herrin G. Keyserling W: Pre-employment strength testing: an updated position. J Occup Med 20: 403, 1979
16. Kishino N, Mayer T, Gatchel R, et al: Quantification of lumbar 4: isometric and isokinetic lifting simulation in normal subjects and low back dysfunction patients. Spine 10: 921, 1985
17. Keeley J, Mayer T, Cox R. et al: Quantification of function 5: reliability range of motion measures in the sagittal plane and in vivo torso rotation measurement technique. Spine 11: 31, 1986
18. Capra P, Mayer T, Gatchel R: Adding psychological scales to your back pain assessment. J Musculoskel Med 2: 41, 1985
19. Mayer T: Quantifying postoperative functional capacity deficits utilizing novel technology. Proceedings of the International Society For The Study Of The Lumbar Spine, Dallas, Texas, May 1986.
20. Gatchel R, Smith D, Barnes D, Mayer T: Relationships among common self-report measures of pain and disability in chronic back pain patients. Proceedings of the International Society For The Study Of The Lumbar Spine, Dallas, Texas, May 1986
21. Mayer T: A two-year follow-up study of functional restoration in industrial back pain patients utilizing physical capacity quantification technology. Proceedings of the International Society For The Study Of The Lumbar Spine, Dallas, Texas, May, 1986.

22. Mayer T, Gatchel R, Kishino N, et al: Objective assessment of spine function following industrial injury: a prospective study with comparison group and one-year follow-up; Volvo award in clinical sciences, 1985. Spine 10: 482, 1985

23. Mayer T, Gatchel R, Kishino N, et al: A prospective short-term study of chronic low back pain patients utilizing novel objective functional measurement. Pain 25: 53, 1986

26

Back Pain and Work

William H. Kirkaldy-Willis

The physical, mental, emotional, and spiritual aspects of personality combine to form an individual's unique response to pain (Fig. 26-1). As described in Chapter 7, these individual qualities are acted upon by environmental conditions. The four main components of an individual's environment—home, workplace, hobbies, and contacts with others—are diagrammed in Figure 26-2.

The psychological factors that affect people with low back pain have been considered at some length in Chapter 8. Sociological factors are also very important both within and outside the work environment. The role of the patient in the home and the help and support he or she gets from the family affect very considerably his or her attitude to the present disability, the speed of recovery, and the necessary adjustment to any residual disability. An unhappy home environment can and often does delay the patient's recovery. Similarly, the personality characteristics of the patient and the way in which he or she interacts or fails to interact with friends, neighbors, other people in community activities such as clubs and associations for games, and with members of a church community play a very important role. Part of the task of the physician and the psychologist is to give the patient advice about these matters and to encourage an active role in all these situations. All of these factors can interact significantly with the efforts of the employer and of compensation boards to get the patient back to work.

SOCIOLOGICAL FACTORS

Our Environment

Our environment is the atmosphere in which we live and work and play. In this modern age we live in an environment that is full of stress and noise and bustle. To be bigger is equated with being better. Fortunately, some among us are rebels and seek a life that is not full of stress, that is quiet, and that proceeds at a slower tempo regardless of financial gain. Nevertheless many men and women work for a firm, a business, or an industry in which profit is the main concern of management. For many the workplace represents an environment where they are not consulted, they do not enjoy their work, and subconsciously they are ready for any excuse not to work. North American industry could well take a look at the new approach now common in Japan, in which management considers the well-being of their employees, tries to make work interesting for them, consults them, and plans to make them feel that their place of work is one to which they belong.

The Work Atmosphere

For many the environment at work sets the stage for the first attack of low back pain. In a sense, the man or woman caught up in such an environment

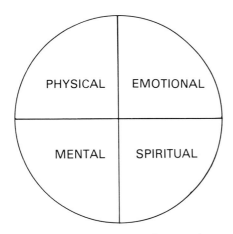

Fig. 26-1 Four aspects of personality.

almost hopes to be afflicted by something like low back pain as a means of escape.

The work environment operates in another way. The patient laid up by a first attack of low back pain often has little incentive to recover and return to the impersonal, boring grind. Pain, fear, lack of understanding, and uncertainty make matters worse. The author recently stood in the wings and observed a young man with a moderately severe episode of posterior joint dysfunction. Before the attack he worked as a plasterer for a company that demanded a full day's work or nothing. Simple measures of treatment dealt with the pain but not with the sense of despondency he felt. After some weeks it suddenly occurred to him that he could work for himself and start by doing half a day of work each day. Almost immediately he ceased to have any problem with his back and the worry and anxiety left him. What appeared to be a very difficult matter for the physician suddenly ceased to be a problem at all for physician or patient.

Delay in Obtaining Adequate Treatment

Fortunately most patients with an episode of low back pain (dysfunction) recover quickly on rest, aspirin, and reassurance. One figure given is 17 to 21 days, depending on the measures employed. A small percentage of patients do not respond to simple measures in what is considered a reasonable period of time. These plague both the physician and their employers. Symptoms and signs are often minimal and the radiograph is considered normal. It is in fact very difficult to say what adequate treatment is for such patients. Some years ago the author himself had a minor episode of low back pain. After a week of rest at home, he was able to return to work as a physician. Certain activities—getting in and out of the car, sitting in a boat, attempts at gardening— were painful for many weeks. He was aware that he would not have been able to work as a carpenter, plasterer or laborer for 3 months.

One result of an apparently unavoidable delay in seeking expert help in such cases is a back that is stiff and painful in a patient who is fearful and apprehensive.

In some patients the pain becomes "fixed" and a point is reached at which no form of treatment is effective in returning the patient to work.

The Return to Work

Returning to work depends on the attitudes of both the patient and the employer. The patient must want to go back to work. This is much less of a problem for people who are self-employed and who thus can gradually increase the amount of work done in a day until they are back to normal. The incentive is greatest in someone like a farmer: It is often impossi-

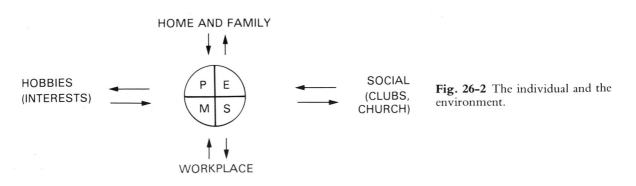

Fig. 26-2 The individual and the environment.

ble to prevent him from engaging in activities that are not wise at the stage reached in his recovery, but it is better to let him run some risk—riding his tractor or lifting bales of hay—than to have him chomping at the bit. Work has a therapeutic value. During all work, and especially that involving physical exertion, muscles contract, joints move, and the mechanoreceptors are stimulated and tend to close the gate to pain impulses (see Chapter 5).

The attitude of the employer is also vitally important. Fortunate the patient who has an employer considerate of his well-being. A phone call from the doctor helps. The employer should be asked if he can arrange things so that the patient does a half day's work for 2 or 3 weeks and so gradually reconditions himself for the job. Activities that produce pain should be avoided. The principles learned during the spine education program in regard to standing, sitting, lifting, and resting to relax after a few hours of work should be practiced. Under these conditions return to work is much more rapid. Recently, the author saw two patients in one afternoon. Both were recovering from minor episodes of posterior joint dysfunction. Both were apprehensive about their return to work. They were told that at this stage in their recovery return to work was an important part of treatment. The writer then phoned both employers, explained the situation, and arranged for a gradual return to work under the employer's supervision.

Many employers and supervisors say that they are unable or unwilling to make special concessions that would enable the employee to return to work until he or she is completely fit for the job. Inevitably this means that time off work is prolonged for weeks or months. Days spent at home without employment are bad for the patient mentally and physically, compound the problem, and sometimes result in the patient never returning to work.

Some large business concerns, such as the Vauxhall Company in the United Kingdom and the Volvo Company in Sweden, encourage consultation between the physician and the steward on the shop floor. A program of work is planned that is within the patient's capability and is gradually increased until the patient is back to a full day of normal work. This is ideal. We need a quiet but persistent publicity campaign to make this enlightened approach common practice in industry. A Saskatchewan firm, recently stimulated by one of its employees who had under-

gone treatment for a disc herniation, asked for help in setting up a day's program of instruction in spine education for supervisors and workers in the factory.

Insurance Companies and Compensation Boards

These should be, and often are, concerned not only with financial assistance while the patient is unable to work but also with making it as easy as possible for him to return to work. Often there is a lack of understanding and a lack of liaison between the physician and the officer of the company or board. Both can be at fault. Part of the difficulty is that each looks at the problem from a different point of view. The result can be many additional weeks away from work.

Compensation board officers do try to help the patient back to work. In talking to employers they often encounter the difficulties referred to previously. Perhaps more thought and more effort should be directed to this aspect of their work.

In some patients the spinal disorder, though not grave, makes it impossible for a laborer or heavy worker ever to return to the job he did before his injury. Here it is of vital importance to find lighter work for the patient or to retrain him for other work that is within his capacity. In the writer's opinion, companies and boards are sometimes slow to make such essential arrangements. On other occasions their officials encounter the very real problem of decreasing opportunities for employment in a shrinking economy.

There is a value in making a final decision regarding the degree of permanent disability as quickly as possible. It may not be possible for the physician to produce the necessary information for some weeks or months. At this stage further official delay often takes place. It can be tough but is often effective to make a definite decision, compensate the patient, and leave him on his own to sink or swim. The chances are greater that the patient will swim.

PREVENTION OF LOW BACK PAIN

It is well to remind ourselves of the vision granted to Nicolas Andry, a great French surgeon and one of the pioneers of orthopedics, in the middle of the

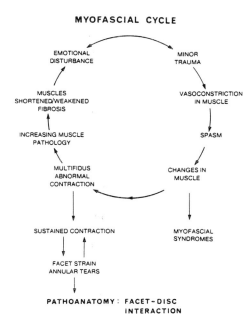

Fig. 26-3 Overview of pathophysiology.

18th century. In his book "L'Orthopédie ou l'art de prévenir et de corriger dans les enfans les difformitées du corps." (Orthopaedics or the art of preventing and correcting in children the deformities of the body), published in 1741, he put preventive orthopedics on an equal footing with the curative art. In trying to follow Andry's example, it is useful to look again at the Overview of Pathophysiology and Myofascial Cycle first presented in Chapter 4. (Fig. 26-3).

Two factors have to be considered: (1) communicating the necessary knowledge of the causes and management of this condition to individuals, the community, and those responsible for industrial plants and factories; and (2) practicing basic spine mechanics by individuals in the community and in industrial environments.

The Spine Education Program

This program has been described in some detail as it applies to the management of low back pain in Chapter 16. It is designed not only to relieve an existing episode of pain but also in practice to prevent future attacks of pain. The knowledge gained of the normal back and the way it functions, of the abnormal back and the ways in which pain results, of exercises that maintain the back in a healthy condition, and

of basic spine mechanics that reduce the risk to the back during daily activities is the most effective way of preventing back pain for the individuals who have attended the sessions of such a program. There is of course room and need for many more such programs in every country.

Publications on Back Care for the Lay Public

A number of books are now available. The individual who reads and carefully studies one of these should understand the problem much better and be able to put what he has read into practice. Undoubtedly to attend a well planned spine education program is of greater value than reading the best of books, but the program is so far only available for a limited percentage of any population.

Spine Education Program for School Children and the Lay Public

Programs for children in school, adapted from that described above, would certainly be most useful. Some such programs are already run for adults in institutions such as the Y. M. C. A. We need to develop and increase the number of such programs.

At the present stage quality (a well-run program) is probably more important than quantity (starting a large number of poorly run programs).

Television Programs

Television authorities are beginning to appreciate the value of educational broadcasts for both school children and adults. The writer knows of two such programs now being planned in Canada. A great deal of thought and hard work is being put into these. Any such program needs to be as short and as simple as possible, based on the spine education program previously described.

Spine Education in Industry

The Spine Education Center in Dallas, Texas has already started to arrange educational sessions in factories in that area. This is an example that many of us should follow. As already mentioned, the Vauxhall and Volvo factories have been doing this for a number of years. Management, i.e., shop stewards and employers, need to know as individuals the things that are taught in the spine education program, and the knowledge that is available needs to be put into practice in the factory. Each task should be planned so that it can be done with minimum risk to the back. Poorly designed plants that place the worker's back at risk should be replaced. To do this requires much tact on the part of advisors from outside. Clearly management must want to make changes. In the long run the company will benefit not only from a decrease in absenteeism due to back pain but also from a happier, more contented group of workers. Industrial psychologists have been working as advisors in factories for at least 50 years, but the problem of low back pain has not yet received adequate attention. It should be no more difficult to persuade management that our present problem needs attention than it has been in the past to convince them of the importance of temperature, light, space, and noise in affecting the health and the output of their employees.

A Combined Approach for the Future

The author approaches this section with some initial hesitancy. All too often the "combined approach" results in a great deal of energy and time expended by many experts with little final achievement. It has been stated frequently, and with good reason, that, when a group of specialists, let us say in a hospital, wishes to make no change, the best way to be certain of maintaining the status quo is to appoint a committee. This should not and must not apply as we study together what now needs to be done for the further prevention of low back pain. We need to be aware of the dangers.

It seems likely that the teams should consist of communications experts; sociologists; psychologists, including industrial psychologists; and physicians, surgeons, and allied therapists concerned with and interested in this field.

The immediate need is for further research into every aspect of the problem of prevention. A great deal of research has been done over past years into the basic science and clinical aspects of low back pain. Much time and energy—some say too much—has been expended on devising new and more effective surgical procedures. Research into prevention demands a new slant and a new approach. We do not yet know what form this will assume.

Research in this field will lead to practical applications. Indeed it will intermingle with the latter. Much of this research will have to be undertaken in the environment in which individual persons or the group of people live, work, and play.

CONCLUSION

In this book a number of different aspects of the management of low back pain have been considered and a large number of facts have been described. They all lead to this conclusion—what are we going to do from now on to prevent the lesions that we have tried to understand and to treat?

INDEX

Page numbers followed by *f* denote figures; those followed by *t* denote tables.